Amyotrophic Lateral Sclerosis

Concepts in Pathogenesis and Etiology

Amyotrophic lateral sclerosis, known as ALS and sometimes as Lou Gehrig's disease, is an invariably fatal disease of the nervous system. A remarkable feature of ALS is its extremely high incidence in regions of the Western Pacific. Such endemic occurrences of any disease carry a particularly ominous aspect.

A symposium in Vancouver examined some of the concepts on pathogenesis arising out of studies on Western Pacific ALS; it also dealt with new concepts on the 'classical' disease that is seen the world over. From that symposium come the papers collected in this volume. They address the complex problems of mechanisms and cause of ALS.

Contributors include Carleton Gajdusek, Nobel prize winner; S.A. Hirano, neuropathologist, and Peter Spencer, toxicologist, both of New York; and Jack Antel, neurologist-in-chief of the Montreal Neurological Institute, as well as a number of other Canadian and American experts.

ARTHUR J. HUDSON, MD, is Professor of Neurology and Medicine, University of Western Ontario. He founded the Amyotrophic Lateral Sclerosis Society of Canada in 1976.

Amyotrophic Lateral Sclerosis:
Concepts in Pathogenesis and Etiology

Edited by ARTHUR J. HUDSON

UNIVERSITY OF TORONTO PRESS

Toronto Buffalo London

© University of Toronto Press 1990
Toronto Buffalo London
Printed in Canada

ISBN 0-8020-3446-2

Printed on acid-free paper

Canadian Cataloguing in Publication Data

Main entry under title:
Amyotrophic lateral sclerosis

Based on a symposium held in Vancouver, B.C., on June 26, 1987 as part of
the 22nd Canadian Congress of Neurological Sciences.
ISBN 0-8020-3446-2

1. Amyotrophic lateral sclerosis.   2. Amyotrophic lateral sclerosis –
Guam.   I. Hudson, Arthur J. (Arthur James), 1924–   .   II. Canadian Congress
of Neurological Sciences (2nd : 1987 : Vancouver, B.C.)

RC406.A24A59 1990   616.8′3   C89-095148-9

Contents

Preface

This book is the outcome of a symposium on amyotrophic lateral sclerosis (ALS) that was held in Vancouver, British Columbia, on 26 June 1987 as part of the 22nd Canadian Congress of Neurological Sciences. The symposium dealt with classical ALS and with ALS as it occurs on the island of Guam in the Western Pacific, and with other important related areas of interest such as neuronal culture and virus infection of neurons, but some contributions to the book are based on lectures delivered in a series at the University Hospital, London, Ontario, a few months before.

ALS is a fatal and much-feared paralytic disease causing death within a few years of clinical onset. In Europe and North America ALS afflicts about 1 in 20,000 persons though the ratio increases to 1 per 1000 *adults* by later life. In some other areas of the world, such as West Irian in the Western Pacific, the prevalence is a thousandfold greater. It is an inexorably progressive wasting disease of voluntary muscles from an as yet unexplained and widespread degeneration of the motor neurons in the brain and spinal cord that sustain these muscles. The muscles affected include those of speaking, swallowing, and breathing in addition to those of the limbs and trunk. For reasons that remain unclear the extraocular muscles (with rare exceptions) and the sphincters of the bowel and bladder are spared. Sometimes intellect is impaired but as a rule it is retained throughout the illness and the patient has, therefore, full awareness of the outcome. Because the extraocular muscles tend to be spared the ability to blink and shift gaze is retained, permitting communication with the eyes in those patients who are severely paralysed. Complete paralysis of all voluntary muscles is infrequent because at almost any stage of the illness paralysis of the respiratory muscles and pulmonary failure intervene to cause death. When placed on a respirator the patient's life can be extended indefinitely but there is then absolute dependence on others and a life-supporting machine.

ALS is an age-related disease, its incidence increasing with longevity and, like Alzheimer's and Parkinson's diseases, it is of increasing concern because of its greater prevalence among the elderly, a population that, at least in the economically developed world, now has improved life expectancy. But this is not the entire story because on the Western Pacific island of Guam ALS and parkinsonism-dementia (PD) have diminished incidence in recent years. This decline has accompanied Western acculturation and, therefore, many investigators believe that the environment plays an important role in the cause of these diseases. If environment is an important factor, then the effects undoubtedly begin decades before clinical onset. This problem is addressed in this volume, but two groups of authors have markedly different views on the possible cause of the disease on Guam. The disease has been ascribed by one group to calcium deficiency leading to toxic mineral deposition in neurons, but the affected indigenous population, the Chamorros, until recently also consumed the cycad seed (*Cycas circinalis* L.) containing an intensely cytotoxic amino acid, which is the focus of the second group. Thus, the debate is partly concerned with the possible contribution of these factors to the disease.

There may be (and it seems there always are) many factors that influence susceptibility, age of onset, and severity of disease. In about 5% of ALS cases the disease is dominantly inherited, suggesting genetic predisposition in all ALS cases. The expanding and important area of molecular genetics is addressed by one author in terms of viral/genetic studies on motor neuron disease of mice. There is a broad spectrum of motor neuron diseases and there are some, such as occur in the gangliosidoses, post-polio syndrome, and motor neuropathies of various kinds, that may be confused with ALS. These are discussed because they offer particular insights into the specific pathophysiology of motor neurons found in ALS. Special techniques such as neuronal culture and positron emission tomography are included to demonstrate their value to the study of the pathophysiology of motor neurons.

Knowledge of cell metabolism is not, of course, essential to finding treatment for disease. Gastric intrinsic factor and insulin were discovered when little basic knowledge was available on the disorders they treat. The mere undertaking of research has, of itself, inestimable value in stimulating enquiry and heightening awareness of the processes of disease and, thereby, the possibilities of treatment. Hence, this book has as one of its intentions the facilitation of further ideas on the possible cause and treatment of this disease. Essential to this, however, has been the opportunity to assemble those who are distinguished in the field of ALS study and who could offer not only the excitement of their discoveries but many other 'state of the art' advantages.

The editor is grateful to the following colleagues for assistance in the review of manuscripts: Dr Charles Bolton, Dr William F. Brown, Dr George Cherian, Dr Bruce Gordon, Dr Alan Hrycyshyn, Dr John Kaufmann, Dr Donald Lee, Dr Peter Merrifield, Dr John Noseworthy, Dr James Redshaw, Dr George Rice, and Dr Brian Weinshenker. Gratitude is also extended to the following whose contributions made publication possible: the ALS Society of Canada chapters of Alberta, Hamilton, London, Manitoba, New Brunswick, Nova Scotia, Windsor; ALS Foundation of Saskatchewan; Mr Gunther Baatz; Baatz Tire Rebuilders Ltd.; Mrs Doris Galant; Mr and Mrs William Hayman; Mrs Mabel Sproule; and many private donors. Special gratitude is extended to the University Hospital Foundation, London, Ontario, who made possible the symposium of the Canadian Congress of Neurological Sciences on ALS and this work through financial contributions and raising of funds. It is effort such as theirs that brings recognition to those whose lives depend on the discovery of a cure for ALS.

Arthur J. Hudson, MD
London, Ontario

Contributing Authors

Jack P. Antel, MD, Professor and Chairman, Department of Neurology, McGill University, and Neurologist-in-Chief, Montreal Neurological Institute and Hospital, Montreal, Quebec

Carmel Armon, MD, Departments of Neurology and Health Sciences Research, Mayo Clinic and Mayo Clinic Foundation, Rochester, Minnesota

Catherine Bergeron, MD, Assistant Professor, Department of Pathology, University of Toronto, and Staff Neurologist, Toronto General Hospital, Toronto, Ontario

Donald B. Calne, MD, Professor and Head, Division of Neurology, Department of Medicine, Health Sciences Centre Hospital, University of British Columbia, Vancouver, British Columbia

Raman Chirakal, MSc, Department of Nuclear Medicine, Chedoke-McMaster Hospital, Hamilton, Ontario

Marinos C. Dalakas, MD, Head, Unit on Neuromuscular Diseases, National Institute of Neurological and Communicative Disorders and Stroke, Bethesda, Maryland

Glyn Dawson, PhD, Professor, Departments of Biochemistry, Molecular Biology, and Pediatrics, University of Chicago, and Joseph P. Kennedy, Jr., Mental Retardation Research Center, University of Chicago, Chicago, Illinois

Herbert M. Dembitzer, PhD, Associate Professor, Department of Pathology, Albert Einstein College of Medicine, Montefiore Medical Center, Bronx, New York

Marjorie G. Driver, MA, Director of Spanish Documents, Micronesian Area Research Center, University of Guam, Guam

Andrew A. Eisen, MD, Professor, Department of Medicine, Division of Neurology, University of British Columbia, and Head, Neuromuscular Diseases Unit, Vancouver General Hospital, Vancouver, British Columbia

Gunter Firnau, PhD, Department of Nuclear Medicine, Chedoke-McMaster Hospital, Hamilton, Ontario

D. Carleton Gajdusek, MD, Chief, Laboratory of Central Nervous System Studies, National Institute of Neurological and Communicative Disorders and Stroke, National Institutes of Health, Bethesda, Maryland

E. Stephen Garnett, MD, Professor of Radiology, McMaster University, and Director, Department of Nuclear Medicine, Chedoke-McMaster Hospital, Hamilton, Ontario

Etienne A. Grima, BSc, Department of Physiology, University of Toronto, Toronto, Ontario

Mark Gurney, PhD, Assistant Professor, Departments of Neurology and Pharmacological and Physiological Sciences, University of Chicago, Chicago, Illinois

Tomasa Q. Guzman, Research Associate, National Institute of Neurological and Communicative Disorders and Stroke, National Institutes of Health, and Veterans Administration Medical Clinic, Naval Hospital, Guam

Larry W. Hancock, PhD, Research Associate and Assistant Professor, Departments of Biochemistry, Molecular Biology, and Pediatrics, University of Chicago, and Joseph P. Kennedy, Jr., Mental Retardation Research Center, Chicago, Illinois

Lanny J. Haverkamp, PhD, Instructor, Department of Neurology, Baylor College of Medicine, Houston, Texas

Leroy F. Heitz, PhD, PE, Director, Water and Energy Research Institute, University of Guam, Guam

Asao Hirano, MD, Professor, Department of Pathology, Albert Einstein College of Medicine, and the Bluestone Laboratory of the Division of Neuropathology, Montefiore Medical Center, Bronx, New York

Michio Hirano, MD, Department of Neurology, Neurological Institute, Columbia Presbyterian Hospital, New York, New York

Arthur J. Hudson, MD, Professor, Departments of Medicine and Clinical Neurological Sciences, University of Western Ontario, and Director of Research, University Hospital, London, Ontario

Paul Jolicoeur, MD, PhD, Professor, Department of Microbiology and Immunology, University of Montreal, and Director, Laboratory of Molecular Biology, Clinical Research Institute of Montreal, Montreal, Quebec

Frank H. Kilmer, PhD, Professor Emeritus, Geology, Humboldt State University, California, and College of Arts and Sciences (Geology), University of Guam, Guam

Seung U. Kim, MD, PhD, Professor, Department of Medicine, Division of Neurology, University of British Columbia, Vancouver, British Columbia

Glen Kisby, PhD, Assistant Staff Scientist, Center for Occupational Disease Research, Oregon Health Sciences University, Portland, Oregon

Leonard T. Kurland, MD, DrPH, Senior Consultant and Professor of Epidemiology, Department of Health Sciences Research, Section of Clinical Epidemiology, Mayo Clinic and Mayo Clinic Foundation, Rochester, Minnesota

Norah R. McCabe, PhD, Research Associate, Departments of Biochemistry, Molecular Biology, and Pediatrics, University of Chicago, and Joseph P. Kennedy, Jr., Mental Retardation Research Center, Chicago, Illinois

Donald R. Crapper McLachlan, MD, Professor of Physiology and Medicine, Departments of Physiology and Medicine, Centre for

Research in Neurodegenerative Diseases, University of Toronto, Toronto, Ontario

Claude Nahmias, PhD, Department of Nuclear Medicine, Chedoke-McMaster Hospital, McMaster University, Hamilton, Ontario

Ronald W. Oppenheim, PhD, Professor, Department of Anatomy, Bowman Gray School of Medicine, Wake Forest University, Winston-Salem, North Carolina

Carolyn M. Parker, MS, Department of Food Science and Human Nutrition, University of Hawaii, Hawaii

Ann M. Pobutsky, MA, Research Associate, National Institute of Neurological and Communicative Diseases and Stroke, Veterans Administration Medical Clinic, Naval Hospital, Guam

Stephen M. Ross, PhD, Associate Staff Scientist, Center for Occupational Disease Research, Oregon Health Sciences University, Portland, Oregon

Dwijendra N. Roy, DSc, PhD, Associate Staff Scientist, Center for Occupational Disease Research, Oregon Health Sciences University, Portland, Oregon

Peter S. Spencer, PhD, MRCPath, Director, Center for Occupational Disease Research, Oregon Health Sciences University, Portland, Oregon

Bluebell R. Standal, PhD, Professor of Food Sciences and Human Nutrition, Department of Food Science and Human Nutrition, University of Hawaii, Hawaii

John C. Steele, MD, Professor of Medicine, University of Hawaii, and Veterans Affairs Medical Clinic, Naval Hospital, Guam

Kari Stefansson, MD, Associate Professor, Departments of Neurology and Pathology, University of Chicago, Chicago, Illinois

William Zolan, MSc, Laboratory Manager, Water and Energy Research Institute, University of Guam, Guam

AMYOTROPHIC LATERAL SCLEROSIS:

CONCEPTS IN PATHOGENESIS AND ETIOLOGY

Human Spinal Cord Neurons in Culture

SEUNG U. KIM

In amyotrophic lateral sclerosis (ALS), spinal and cortical motor neurons die. At present, there are no satisfactory explanations for pathogenesis of ALS. Viral infections, environmental toxins, lack of a specific neurotrophic factor, and circulating endogenous toxin(s), all have been proposed as causative mechanisms [1, 2]. Until recently, the study of human spinal motor neurons in disease has been delayed and hampered by the lack of suitable material or models.

Most ideal experimental models for the study of human spinal motor neurons and ALS can be found in spinal cord cultures. Neural tissue grown and maintained in culture provides an excellent opportunity to study properties of neurons under a simple and well-controlled environment. Since the first report of neural tissue culture by Harrison almost 80 years ago [3], numerous studies have described the structural and functional properties of neuronal and glial cells, as well as their interactions [see reviews 4 and 5]. However, the majority of these studies have been concerned with neural tissues from avian or non-human mammalian sources. Several tissue culture studies using human central nervous system (CNS) tissues have been carried out [6–12], but the information available about the structure and function of human spinal cord neurons in culture is scant and spotty at best.

In this chapter, morphological, immunocytochemical, and neurophysiological properties of human spinal cord neurons in culture will be presented.

Explant and Monolayer Cultures

Tissues were obtained from 8–11 weeks' gestational human fetal materials 3–4 hours after therapeutic abortion (legal abortions were performed in an authorized clinic and a certificate of approval was obtained from the Ethics Committee of the author's university). Spinal cord was removed following dorsal laminectomy, and sliced manually into 1.0-mm-thick sections in Hanks' balanced salt solution (HBSS) with a care to position the ventral side of sections so as to face towards the investigator. The sections were used for explant and dissociated cell cultures. For explant cultures, spinal cord fragments were placed on collagen-coated 12-mm round Aclar plastic coverslips (Allied Corporation, Morristown, NJ) The coverslips were placed in 24-well plastic multiwell plates, and the explants were covered with 0.1 ml feeding medium and incubated at 36°C under a water-saturated atmosphere of 5% CO_2/95% air. Twenty-four hours later, 0.4 ml of feeding medium was added to each well.

Dissociated cell monolayer cultures were prepared by trypsin treatment of spinal cord fragments following the procedures developed for the monolayer culture of chick spinal cord neurons [13]. In brief, spinal cord fragments were incubated in 0.25% trypsin and 20 μg/ml DNAse in calcium- and magnesium-free HBSS for 30 minutes at 36°C, and dissociated into single cells by repeated pipetting. After a low-speed centrifugation (1000 rpm for 5 minutes), cells were resuspended in feeding medium at the final cell density of 1–2 × 10^5 cells/ml, and plated on collagen-coated or polylysine-coated 12-mm round Aclar coverslips. Twenty-four hours later, 2.5 ml of feeding medium was added to each 60-mm petri dish, which housed nine coverslips.

Feeding medium consisted of Eagle's minimum essential medium supplemented with 20% human placental cord serum or fetal bovine serum, 5 mg/ml glucose, and 20 μg/ml gentamicin. The medium was renewed twice weekly. Collagen-coated coverslips prepared by exposure to ammonia vapour [14] were air-dried under a laminar flowhood. Approximately 1 hour before culture, collagen coverslips were conditioned with 0.1 ml of feeding medium.

When transected explants of fetal spinal cord were placed on collagen-coated coverslips, the ventral portion of the explant was directed toward the investigator and a mark was made on the plastic coverslip. Within 2–3 days, all of the explants were found to adhere to the collagen substrate (Fig. 1). The earliest features in the development of the spinal cord explants were occurrences of fine nerve fibres and clusters of fibroblasts and astrocytes appearing along the margin. These early outgrowths were found during the first week *in vitro*; the outgrowth zone, consisting of fibroblasts, astrocytes, and nerve fibres, then increased in size eventually to cover the entire margin of an explant. At this stage of the outgrowth, a large number of nerve fibres were found radiating out of the explants,

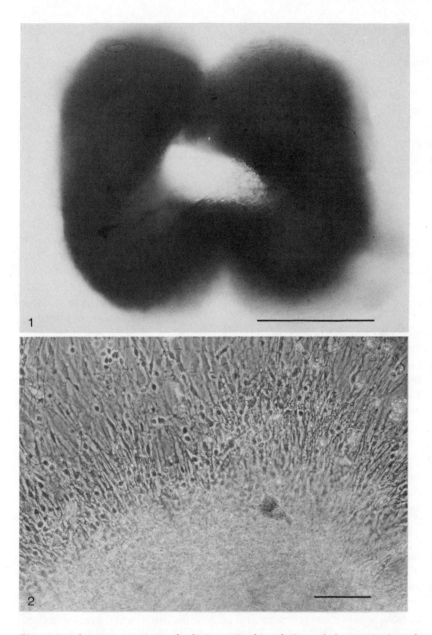

Figure 1. A low-power view of a living spinal cord (8 weeks' gestation) explant grown for 2 days *in vitro*. Bar indicates 1 mm.

Figure 2. A living spinal cord (8 weeks' gestation) explant culture grown for 2 weeks *in vitro*. Extensive outgrowths of nerve fibres, flat astrocytes, and bipolar cells (young neurons) are observed in the outgrowth zone. Bar indicates 100 μm.

often reaching beyond the outgrowth zone and occurring either singularly or in fascicular bundles. From 2 weeks onward, numerous small round or oval bipolar cells (8–10 μm diameter) migrated from the explants (Fig. 2). They had dark nuclei and scanty cytoplasm and long, thin processes. They were identified as young neurons upon immunostaining with neurofilament and A2B5 monoclonal antibodies (Fig. 4). They migrated singly or in groups and usually were found on top of large, flat cells, identified as fibroblasts or astrocytes by their reaction to fibronectin or glial fibrillary acidic protein (GFAP) immunostaining. For the ensuing weeks, and up to 6 months *in vitro*, the areas occupied by the outgrowths of astrocytes and fibroblasts increased, and young neurons, usually in groups of 6–12 cells, were found to be very distant from the explant proper. These neurons had cell bodies of 8–12 μm diameter, became multipolar in shape, and were interconnected by long, thin axons which formed rather intricate networks. The size and shape of neurons in the outgrowth did not change significantly for periods as long as 6 months in culture. The majority of the neurons did not exhibit the sizes (20–40 μm diameter) or characteristic morphology (multipolar and finely branched) reported for embryonic avian and non-human mammalian spinal cord neurons grown in culture [12, 13, 15–17].

One day after plating, dissociated cells were found to adhere firmly to the coverslip surface. Most of these cells were flat cells identified as fibroblasts or astrocytes, by their reaction to fibronectin or GFAP immunostaining. Small spherical cells (8–12 μm diameter) were also found among the more numerous flat cells. Within a week, these small cells began to acquire thin, long processes and to aggregate into small clumps. These small cells could be identified as neurons, by their positive immunostaining by neurofilament and A2B5 antibodies (Fig. 5). As shown in the explant cultures, the size and morphology of these neurons in monolayer did not increase appreciatively during their growth in culture, even after 4 months in culture, the longest period some of these monolayer cultures were maintained.

Neuron-Specific Markers

Identification of spinal neurons and differentiating them unambiguously from other neural cell types are prerequisite to the understanding of their property and function. Several cell-type specific markers are available which make it possible to identify neurons, oligodendrocytes, astrocytes, and fibroblasts in culture derived from human spinal cord tissues. The neurofilament protein is the most specific marker for neurons [18, 19], while GFAP for protoplasmic and fibrous astrocytes [20–22] and galactocerebroside and myelin basic protein for oligodendrocytes [17, 21, 23] have been considered as selective and specific cell-type markers. A2B5 monoclonal antibody which is specific for G_Q polysialic ganglioside [24] has been shown to label all of fetal human CNS neurons in addition to a small number of astrocytes [25]. We have utilized the neurofilament protein (neurons), glial fibrillary acidic protein (GFAP; astrocytes), and galactocerebroside (oligodendroctyes) as cell-type specific markers for the various neural cell types found in spinal cord cultures. In addition, fibronectin was used as a specific fibroblast antigen marker [22].

Cultures were washed briefly in HBSS and then incubated for 30 minutes at room temperature with A2B5 mouse monoclonal antibody (specific for G_Q ganglioside) [24] or rabbit anti-galactocerebroside serum diluted in HBSS containing 2% horse serum and 10 mM HEPES (HBSS-HS). The cultures then were washed in HBSS-HS and incubated for 30 minutes at room temperature with rhodamine-conjugated goat anti-mouse or goat anti-rabbit immunoglobulin (Cappel Laboratories) diluted in HBSS-HS. After being washed three times in HBSS-HS, the cultures were fixed in acid alcohol (5 ml glacial acetic acid in 95 ml ethanol) for 15 minutes at $-20°C$, washed in phosphate-buffered saline (PBS), and incubated for 60 minutes in monoclonal rat anti-150kd neurofilament protein (NF) antibody [19] or monoclonal rat anti-glial fibrillary acidic protein (anti-GFAP) diluted in PBS. The cultures were incubated in fluorescein-conjugated goat anti-rat immunoglobulin (Cappel Laboratories, rat-specific and not cross-reacting with mouse) diluted in PBS for another 60 minutes, washed in PBS, and mounted on slides with glycerol-PBS. Similarly, double-labelling experiments were performed using rabbit anti-galactocerebroside serum and A2B5 monoclonal antibody concurrently. These antibodies were mixed and applied to cultures. All incubation and washing processes were performed at room temperature. Immunostained cultures were examined under a Zeiss Universal microscope equipped with fluorescence and phase contrast optics.

Astrocytes with GFAP-positive immunoreaction were the most conspicuous and numerous in the spinal cord cultures (Fig. 3). These had the appearance of an 'astrocytic carpet.' In contrast to the large number of GFAP-positive astrocytes, galactocerebroside-positive oligodendrocytes were far fewer in spinal cord cultures. They were small, round cells (8–10 μm) with several short processes.

Neurons at the top of the 'astrocytic carpet' were identified by their immunoreactivity with neurofilament protein (NF) antibody (Figs. 4 and 5). NF-positive cells were reactive also to A2B5 antibody (Figs. 4 and 5), thus indicating that A2B5 antigen (G_Q ganglioside) may be used as cell-type specific marker of neurons in human neural cell cultures. A2B5

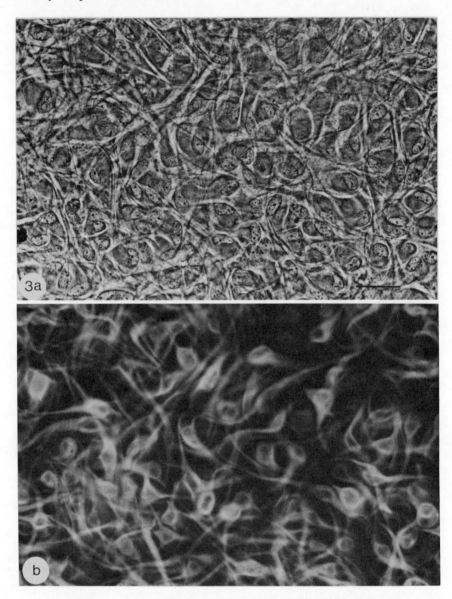

Figure 3. GFAP-positive astrocytes found in the outgrowth of a spinal cord explant culture grown for 4 weeks. These astrocytes form an extensive carpet-like layer. a: phase contrast microscopy; b: GFAP immunostaining. Bar indicates 50 μm.

immunostaining was detected only in the population of neurofilament-containing neurons and not in GFAP-positive astrocytes of galactocerebroside-positive oligodendrocyte populations.

Using a panel of cell-type specific markers that include NF for neurons, GFAP for astrocytes, as well as galactocerebroside for oligodendrocytes, we demonstrated that GFAP-positive astrocytes were the most conspicuous and numerous among the cells found in spinal cord cultures. Relatively small numbers of galactocerebroside-positive oligodendrocytes and more numerous NF- and A2B5-double positive neurons were found in our cultures. In the past, several criteria have been utilized by previous authors in order to identify neurons in culture and distinguish them from other cell types; these involve morphological examination with light and electron microscopy, silver and Nissl staining, cytochemical demonstration of neurotransmitter-associated enzymes, and autoradiographic demonstration of transmitter uptake [10, 26].

In the present study, the majority of neurons found in the spinal cord cultures were unambiguously identified by the immunofluorescence technique by NF and A2B5 immunoreaction. It should be noted that NF antibody is the most specific cell-type marker for cultured neurons [18, 19, 25], whereas A2B5 antibody can be used as a neuronal marker with some caution because of its reactivity with a subclass of astrocytes [25, 27].

In addition to NF and A2B5 immunostaining, we have recently applied immunocytochemical techniques of neuron-specific enolase (NSE), an isoenzyme of the glycolytic enzyme enolase localized exclusively in neurons and neuroendocrine cells [28]. Specific localization in cultured mouse spinal cord neurons was also reported [29]. A strong positive immunostaining by rabbit anti-NSE serum (DAKO), in groups of small neurons, was demonstrated in spinal cord cultures (data not shown). Similarly, acetycholinesterase immunoreactivity-positive neurons were demonstrated in human fetal spinal cord cultures using a monoclonal antibody directed against human acetylcholinesterase protein [30].

Electron Microscopy

Spinal cord cultures were prepared for electron microscopy in order to examine the structural changes in spinal cord neurons during their development and maturation in culture. Coverslips carrying spinal cord cultures were fixed in 3% glutaraldehyde in 0.12 M phosphate buffer (pH 7.4) for 30 minutes after a brief rinse in PBS, followed by fixation in 2% osmium textroxide in the same buffer for 30 minutes, and after dehydration in ethanol, were embedded in Epon 812 [10]. Semi-thin and

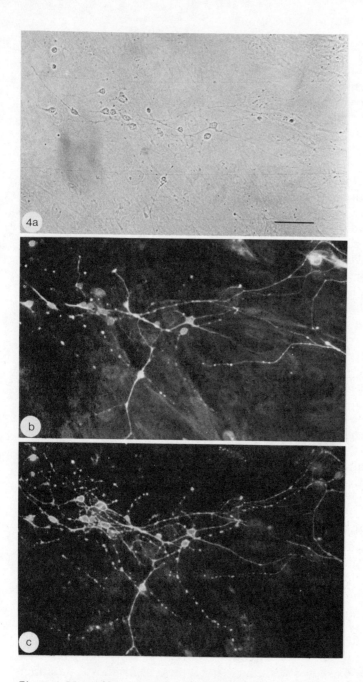

Figure 4. Neurofilament and A2B5 double immunostaining of spinal cord neurons found in the outgrowth of a 4-week-old culture. a: phase contrast microscopy; b: neurofilament-FITC; c: A2B5-rhodamine fluorescence. Bar indicates 20 μm.

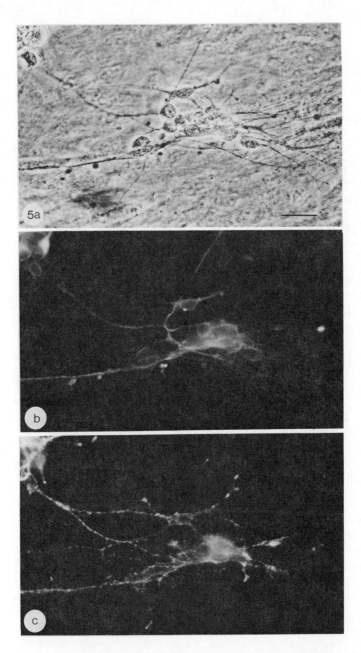

Figure 5. Neurofilament and A2B5 double immunolabelling of spinal cord neurons in a 5-week-old monolayer culture. Note the double labelling of small neurons by both NF and A2B5 antibodies. a: phase contrast microscopy; b: neurofilament-FITC fluorescence; c: A2B5-rhodamine fluorescence. Bar indicates 20 μm.

ultra-thin sections were prepared from selected areas of the blocks, stained with lead citrate and uranyl acetate, and examined under a Philips 300 electron microscope.

The following account concerns mostly spinal cord neurons found in explant cultures because structural integrity and preservation were better in the explants than in monolayer cultures.

In early cultures (2–3 weeks) large numbers of small cells (8–10 μm) containing chromatin-rich round or ovoid nuclei which were surrounded by a thin rim of cytoplasm were found in the outgrowth and in the midst of explants. Cytoplasm in these cells contained a few, rather small mitochondria, short elements of rough endoplasmic reticulum, and occasionally a small Golgi apparatus and moderate numbers of ribosome clusters (Fig. 6).

It is interesting to note that large neurons with cell bodies exceeding 20 μm in diameter were frequently demonstrated in cultures grown for 2–3 months under electron microscopic examination. These neurons were usually found in the midst of the explants, in contrast to the smaller neurons of approximately 12 μm diameter which were found in the outgrowth of the explants or in dissociated cell cultures. In addition to the marked increase in the size of the cell body (20–30 μm) an increased number of mitochondria and Golgi apparatus and further development of rough endoplasmic reticulum and Golgi apparatus were observed in the cytoplasm of such cells (Fig. 7). The cells often were observed to possess long, slender processes; these contained numerous microtubules, which ran parallel to the long axis of the process. These cells were identified unambiguously as neurons by the presence of axo-somatic synapses on their perikarya (Fig. 7).

Although only a smaller number of axo-somatic synapses were found in cultures examined, axo-dendritic synapses were seen more frequently. The most immature and incipient synaptic profiles occurred in 3-week-old cultures; these structures, which contained just perceptible membrane thickenings, a few synaptic vesicles, and no mitochondria, were exclusively axo-dendritic (Fig. 8). Similarly, the earliest axo-somatic synapse was observed to contain a small number of synaptic vesicles and to terminate on structurally immature neurons with few cytoplasmic organelles (Fig. 6). There were indications that a large number of synapses in culture underwent structural development with increased age. This synaptic development is characterized by the appearance of mitochondria, a greater number of synaptic vesicles, and denser, conspicuous membrane thickenings in synaptic terminals (Figs. 9–11). The synaptic vesicles which were found in these terminals were mostly clear and spherical and measured 30–60 nm in diameter. Dense-cored vesicles of

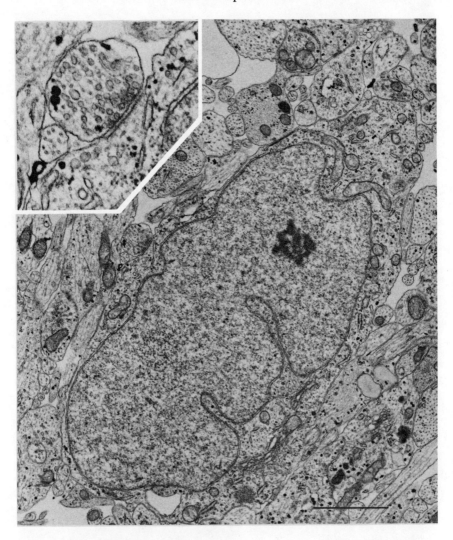

Figure 6. This electron micrograph shows a small cell (N) with ultrastructures indicative of young neurons which include scanty cytoplasm with a few mitochondria ribosome clusters, and Golgi apparatuses. A synapse terminating on the cell body is shown in the inset at higher magnification. Bar indicates 1 μm.

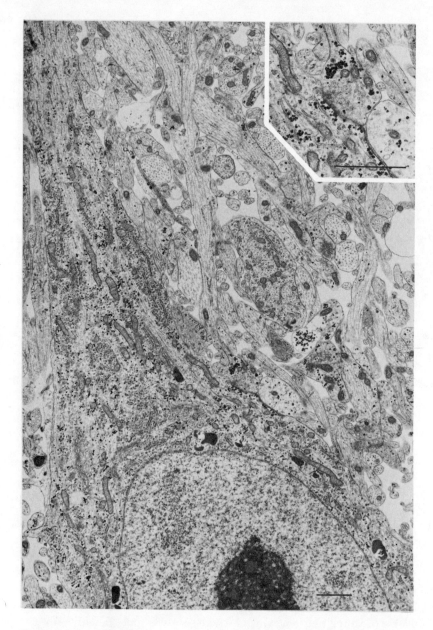

Figure 7. This electron micrograph shows a well-developed neuron of 9-week-gestation spinal cord cultured for 3 months. Several components of Golgi apparatus, numerous mitochondria and rough endoplasmic reticulum, and microtubules are found in the cytoplasm. An axo-somatic synapse terminating on this neuron is shown in the inset at higher magnification. A rich array of microtubules is found in the proximal portion of the dendrite. Bar indicates 1 μm.

60–90 nm were also found within the synaptic terminals. Large synaptic terminals which made contacts to several dendritic spines were demonstrated (Fig. 11).

The formation of synaptic terminals in culture has been described previously for embryonic chick [13, 15, 31], fetal mouse [4, 16, 17], fetal rat spinal cord [32], and fetal human cerebellum cultures [10]. The distinguishing difference noted in the present study from others was the demonstration of axo-somatic synapses. The eliminating of extraspinal and extrasegmental afferent fibres during the slicing of spinal cord for the culturing was considered by Guillery et al [16] to be the reason for the paucity of axo-somatic synapses in their cultures. It is reasonable to infer that the extraspinal and extrasegmental afferent fibres contribute to a large number of synaptic connections in spinal cord *in situ*. However, in the human spinal cord cultures described here, in which all the afferent fibres were severed, a considerable number of synapses could be demonstrated. This indicates that the fibres of surviving spinal neurons can generate a well-organized, neuronal circuitry in culture.

The earliest recognizable synapses in our spinal cord cultures were demonstrable after 2 weeks in culture, and fully matured synapses were seen after 2 months in culture. The starting material for our cultures was fetal spinal cord of 8–11 weeks' gestation at which time only young neurons had begun to assume their final position at the anterior and posterior horns following active migration from the ventricular layer. It is evident from these results that fetal human spinal neurons grown in culture continue to differentiate, to interact with other neurons, and to form synaptic connections. The electron microscopic demonstration of synapse formation in this study and the generation of action potentials observed in fetal human spinal neuron cultures as reported previously [33] suggest the operation of a well-developed neuronal network in human spinal cord cultures described herein.

Electrophysiology

The electron microscopic evidence of a high degree of synapse formation in fetal human spinal cord cultures is also reflected in the electrophysiological intracellular recordings from the cultured neurons. These recordings were obtained in collaboration with Drs E. Puil and I. Spigelman.

Coverslips carrying spinal cord explants were attached with petroleum jelly to the glass bottom of the recording chamber, which was mounted on the stage of a Leitz microscope. The cultures were bathed in HBSS buffered with 25 mM HEPES with pH adjusted to 7.4. The temperature

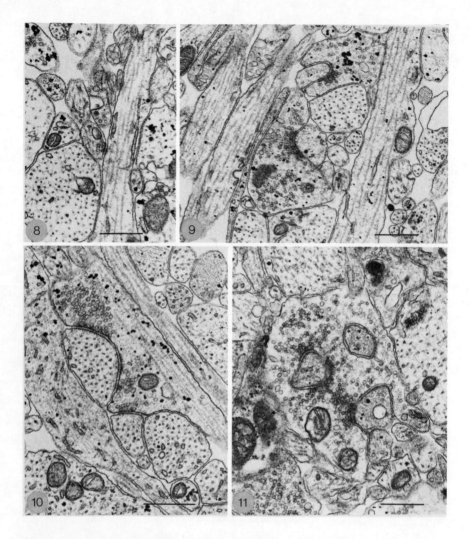

Figure 8. A small axo-dendritic (arrow) synapse found in a 3-week-old culture of 9-week-gestation spinal cord explant. Note the small number of synaptic vesicles and insignificant junction area indicating this as an early synapatic terminal. Bar indicates 1 μm.

Figure 9. Two axo-dendritic synapses with numerous synaptic vesicles as well as glycogen particles are shown here. A 2-month-old culture of 8-week-gestation spinal cord. Bar indicates 0.5 μm.

Figure 10. An axo-dendritic synapse terminating on two dendritic processes is shown here. A 2-month-old culture of 10-week-gestation spinal cord. Bar indicates 0.5 μm.

Figure 11. Multiple synaptic contacts formed by an axon terminal and 2 dendritic spines are shown here. A 2-month-old culture of 8-week-gestation spinal cord. Bar indicates 0.5 μm.

of the bathing solution was controlled at 36°C throughout the electrical recording period (2–8 hours). Intracellular recordings were made using glass micropipettes filled with 3 M potassium chloride pulled from 1 mm glass blanks such that the tip resistances ranged from 35 to 75 MΩ. The microprobe system (M-701, WP Instruments) which was used to measure potentials allowed intracellular injections of current-pulses via an active bridge circuit for conventional measurement of membrane resistance [33]. Resting membrane potential of the cell was continuously monitored on a chart recorder and the zero level was determined upon withdrawal of the electrode from a cell. Cell input resistances were calculated from the linear-slope portions of the established voltage/current relationships.

Intracellular recordings were obtained from 50 cells in 14 spinal cord explant cultures. Most of these cells were small bipolar or multipolar cells located in the outgrowths as shown in Figure 4. Twenty-six of the cells were identified as neurons by their non-linear, local (5–20 mV) responses or spikes elicited by intracellular injections of depolarizing current pulses. These neurons had stable resting membrane potentials between −20 and −80 mV (mean −52 ± 2.3 mV SEM, n = 24) and exhibited voltage/current relationships which were linear over a 30−mV range of membrane potentials. The average input resistance was 31 ± 3.4 SEM (n = 26) and the membrane time constant was 5.7 ± 0.8 ms SEM (n = 12). An example of an action potential elicited from a neuron is shown in Figure 12. Other neurons displayed smaller-amplitude 'local' responses to depolarizing stimuli.

There have been few electrophysiological studies of human spinal cord in culture in the past. Crain and Peterson reported on an occurrence of synaptically mediated bioelectric activity in spinal cord explant cultures [6]. Investigations by Hosli et al have described electrophysiological properties of glial cells as well as resting membrane potentials recorded from neurons [8]. Kato et al have also described the recordings of resting membrane potentials and action potentials in their cultured human fetal neurons [9]. However, despite a very similar membrane time constant (<10 ms), the mean input resistance value for the 8 neurons in their investigations is more than 20 times that of the 26 neurons reported here. The neurons studied by Kato et al were at a much earlier stage of development (19 days) than those in this study (60–120 days). This suggests that an increase in resting ionic conductances may occur during development.

Conclusions

There are at present few satisfactory clues as to the cause of ALS. Viral infections, lack of a neurotrophic factor, environmental toxins, and cir-

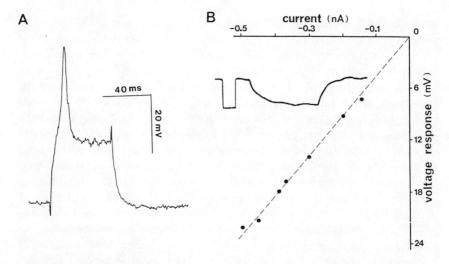

Figure 12. Responses of a human spinal cord neuron to intracellular injections of step currents. A: action potential evoked by 0.6 nA depolarizing current pulse. B: voltage/current plot showing linear relationship in response to hyper-polarizing current pulses. Example of hyperpolarizing response of membrane potential is shown as an inset. Calibration pulses (20 mV, 10 ms) precede neuronal response in B. From a 9-week-old culture of a 10-week-gestation spinal cord explant.

culating endogenous cytotic factors have all had proponents at one time or another. The truth may lie in a multifactoral interplay of many of the above mechanisms.

Recently, persistent virus infection as the cause of ALS has received attention from many investigators. Three different viruses have been implicated. They are Creutzfeldt-Jakob disease virus, human immuno-deficiency virus, and human T-cell leukemia virus type I (HTLV-I) [2]. To understand the pathogenesis of viral pathology, it is important to demonstrate that these viruses are capable of infecting human neurons and glial cells. In this connection, we are currently studying infectivity of HTLV-I in primary mixed glial cell (oligodendrocytes and astrocytes) cultures obtained from autopsied adult human brains [21] and in human fetal spinal cord cultures. In adult human glial cell cultures, approxi-mately 3% of GFAP-positive astrocytes and 1% of galactocerebroside-positive oligodendrocytes were found to contain virus antigen (Fig. 13). We are continuing our effort to investigate whether HTLV-I is capable of infecting human spinal cord neurons in culture.

Previous studies have demonstrated in culture that addition of skeletal

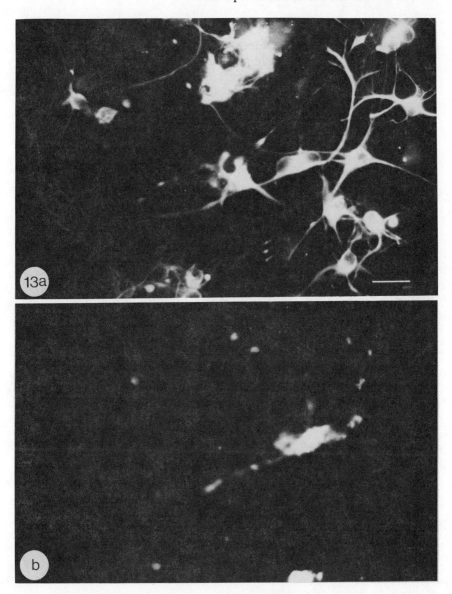

Figure 13. Double immunofluorescence microscopy of adult human astrocyte culture infected by HTLV-I. Cells were isolated from the brain of a 49-year-old male 5 hours post-mortem and grown for 14 days. a: GFAP-FITC staining; b: HTLV-I *gag* p19 protein-rhodamine staining. Bar indicates 20 μm.

muscle to spinal cord enhances long-term survival of neurons and promotes axonal growth and increased choline acetyltransferase activity [34]. In addition, media conditioned on muscle cells or muscle extracts can reproduce some of these neurotrophic effects [34–37]. Recently, we have obtained a 60,000-molecular-weight protein from conditioned media of human fetal skeletal muscle cultures. Preliminary work indicates that this protein promotes neurite growth extensively when tested in quail and mouse spinal cord neuron cultures. We are currently examining neurotrophic activity of this protein in human fetal spinal cord neuron cultures (unpublished data).

Previously, Wolfgram and Myers reported that sera from ALS patients contained a cytotoxic activity directed against motor neurons in newborn mouse spinal cord cultures [38]. Roisen et al have also confirmed these results [39]. However, other investigators were unable to demonstrate the cytotoxic activity in sera of ALS patients [40, 41]. We have examined the possible cytotoxic activity of ALS sera using human fetal spinal cord neuron cultures. Cultures were incubated in medium containing sera from ALS patients and controls (at 20% final concentration) for a week, and then viewed under a phase contrast microscope. At light microscopic level, we did not detect any toxic effects of ALS sera (6 samples tested) over normal controls (4 samples). It is too early to discredit and abandon the circulating cytotoxic factor theory; further study is necessary.

It is obvious from our studies that the use of cultured human fetal spinal cord neurons currently represents the most promising model system with which to explore the cause of ALS.

Acknowledgments

This work was supported by grants from the Medical Research Council of Canada (MT 7700), the Amyotrophic Lateral Sclerosis Society of Canada, and the Jacob W. Cohen Fund for Research into Multiple Sclerosis. The author wishes to thank A. Eisen, M. Kim, D. Osborne, E. Puil, D. Shin, and I. Spigelman for their help in this study.

References

1 Rowland L. Human Motor Neron Diseases. New York, Raven Press, 1982
2 Rowland L. Motor neuron disease and amyotrophic lateral sclerosis. Trends Neurosci 1987;10:393–397
3 Harrison RG. Observations on the living, developing nerve fiber. Proc Soc Exp Biol 1907;4:140–143
4 Crain S. Neurophysiologic Studies in Tissue Culture, New York, Raven Press, 1976

5 Nelson P. Nerve and muscle cells in culture. Physiol Rev 1975;55:1–61

6 Crain S, Peterson ER. Complex bioelectric activity in organized tissue cultures of spinal cord (human, rat and chick. J Cell Comp Physiol 1964;1–14

7 Hogue MJ. Human fetal brain cells in tissue cultures: Their identification and motility. J Exp Zool 1947;106:85–108

8 Hösli L, Andres P, Hösli E. Ionic mechanisms associated with the depolarization by glutamate and aspartate on human and rat spinal neurons in tissue culture. Pflugers Arch Physiol 1976;363:43–48

9 Kato A, Tourzeau G, Bertrand D, Bacler CR. Human spinal cord neurons in dissociated monolayer cultures: Morphological, biochemical and electrophysiological properties. J Neurosci 1985;5:2750–2761

10 Kim SU. Tissue culture of human fetal cerebellum: A light and electron microscopic study. Exp Neurol 1976;50:226–239

11 Lapham LW, Markesbery W. Human fetal cerebellar cortex: Organization and maturation of cells in vitro. Science 1971;173:829–832

12 Peterson E, Crain S, Murray MR. Differentiation and prolonged maintenance of bioelectrically active spinal cord cultures (rat, chick and human). Z Zellforsh 1965;66:130–154

13 Kim SU, Wenger E. De novo formation of synapse in cultures of chick neural tube. Nature 1972;236:152–153

14 Bornstein MB. Reconstituted rat-tail collagen used as substance for tissue culture on coverslips. Lab Invest 1958;134–137

15 Grainger F, James DW, Tresman RL. An electron microscope study of the early outgrowth from chick spinal cord in vitro. Z Zellforsch 1968;90:53–67

16 Guillery RW, Sobkowicz HM, Scott G. Relationship between glial and neuronal elements in the development of long-term cultures of the spinal cord of the fetal mouse. J Comp Neurol 1970;140:2–34

17 Ramson B, Neale E, Henkart M, et al. Mouse spinal cord in cell culture. I. Morphology and intrinsic neuronal electrophysiologic properties. J Neurophys 1977;40:1132–1150

18 Bennett GS, Tapscott SJ, Dilullo C, et al. Differential binding of antibodies against the neurofilament triplet proteins in different avian neurons. Brain 1984;304:291–302

19 Lee V, Wu L, Schlaepfer WW. Monoclonal antibodies recognize individual neurofilament triplet proteins. Proc Natl Acad Sci 1982;79:6089–6092

20 Bignami A, Eng L, Dahl D, Uyeda C. Localization of the glial acidic protein in astrocytes by immunofluorescence. Brian Res 1972;43:429–435

21 Kim SU. Antigen expression by glial cells grown in culture. J Neuroimmunol 1985;8:255–282

22 Raff M, Fields K, Hakomori S, et al. Cell type-specific markers for distinguishing and studying neurons and glial cells in culture. Brain Res 1979;174:283–308

23 Raff M, Mirsky R, Fields K, et al. Galactocerebroside is a specific cell-surface antigenic marker for oligodendrocytes in culture. Nature 1978;274:813–816

24 Eisenbarth GS, Walsh F, Nirenberg M. Monoclonal antibody to a plasma membrane antigen of neurons. Proc Natl Acad Sci 1979;76:4913–4917

25 Kim SU, Moretto G, Lee V, Yu RK. Neuroimmunology of gangliosides in human neurons and glial cells in culture. J Neurosci Res 1986;15:303–321

26 Weiner H, Hauser S. Neuroimmunology: Antigenic specificity of the nervous system. Ann Neurol 1982;12:499–509

27 Raff M, Miller R, Noble M. A glia progenitor cell that develops in vitro an astocyte of oligodendrocyte depending on the culture medium. Nature 1983;303:390–396

28 Marangos PJ, Zis A, Clark R, Goodwin F. Neronal, non-neuronal and hybrid forms of enolase in brain: Structural, immunological and functional comparisons. Brain Res 1978;150:117–133

29 Schmechel DE, Brightman MW, Barker JL. Localization of neuron-specific enolase in mouse spinal cord neurons grown in culture. Brain Res 1980;181:391–400

30 Fabrough DM, Engel A, Rosenberry T. Acetycholinesterase of human erythrocytes and neuromuscular junctions: Homologies revealed by monoclonal antibodies. Proc Natl Acad Sci 1982;79:1078–1082

31 Lyser KM. Early differentiation of the chick embryo spinal cord in organ culture: Light and electron microscopy. Anat Rec 1971;169:45–64

32 Bunge R, Bunge M, Peterson E. An electron microscope study of cultured rat spinal cord. J Cell Biol 1965;163–191

33 Puil E, Spigelman I, Eisen A, Kim SU. Electrophysiological responses of human spinal neurons in culture. Neurosci 1986;71:77–82

34 Giller EL, Neale JH, Bullock PN, et al. Choline acetyltransferase activity of spinal cord cell cultures increased by co-culture with msucle and by muscle conditioned medium. J Cell Biol 1977;74:16–29

35 Calof A, Reichardt LF. Motoneurons purified by cell sorting respond to two distinct activities in myotube conditioned medium. Dev Biol 1984;106:194–210

36 Henderson C, Hucht M, Changeux JP. Neurite outgrowth from embryonic chicken spinal neurons is prompted by media conditioned by muscle cells.. Proc Natl Acad Sci 1981;78:2625–2629

37 Tanaka H, Sakai M, Obata K. Effects of serum, tissue extract, conditioned medium, and culture substrate on neurite appearance from spinal cord explants of chick embryo. Brain Res 1982;4:303–312

38 Wolfgram F, Myers L. Amyotrophic lateral sclerosis: Effect of serum on anterior horn cells in culture. Science 1973;179:579–580

39 Roisen FJ, Bartfeld H, Donnenfeld H, Baxter J. Neuron-specific in vitro cytotoxicity of sera from patients with amyotrophic lateral sclerosis. Muscle & Nerve 1982;5:48–53

40 Horwich MS, Engel WK, Chauvin PB. ALS sera applied to cultured motor neurons. Arch Neurol 1974;30:332–333
41 Liveson J, Fry H, Bornstein MB. The effect of serum from ALS patients on organotypic nerve and muscle tissue cultures. Acta Neuropathol 1975; 32:127–131

Death of Motoneurons by Accident and Design: Neurotrophic Interactions of Anterior Horn Cells with Their Targets

LANNY J. HAVERKAMP AND
RONALD W. OPPENHEIM

When mature motoneurons are disconnected from their target muscles by cutting or crushing their projecting axons, a well-described series of events takes place collectively referred to as chromatolysis. There are changes in the appearance and a redistribution of the cell nucleus and organelles, RNA and protein synthetic patterns undergo wholesale alterations, afferent synapses to the cell are withdrawn, and dendrites may be partially reabsorbed [1–4]. With the onset of chromatolysis, regeneration of the damaged axon commences, the neuron is eventually reconnected to its target muscle, and normal neuronal properties are restored.

Neuronal Death and Loss of Target Contact

In contrast to the reversible effects of axotomy on mature motoneurons, damage to the nerves of neonatal or very young animals is devastating. While various factors influence the result of such trauma, most notably the precocity of the species' neuromuscular system at the time of birth, section of the sciatic nerve of newborn rats, for example, results in the death of virtually all motoneurons which project through this nerve. As the animal matures, so does the motoneuron response to nerve damage [5, 6]. While the lethal effect of nerve damage is dependent upon the type of injury inflicted as well as the type of muscle to which the nerve projects [6, 7], maturation of response to axotomy can be quite sudden and dramatic. When the rat's sciatic nerve is crushed (rather than sectioned) within 1 day of birth, 60–70% of the neurons innervating the leg muscles die. If the crush is delayed until day 5–6 post-natal, however, there is only negligible motoneuron loss [8, 9].*

What maturational change in the motoneurons might account for this altered response to axotomy? In 1967, Prestige reported a developmental study of the effects of limb amputation on toad motoneurons [10]. When the leg was removed very early, at the time of onset of reflex movements, motoneuron degeneration occurred with 3–4 days. Removing the leg at a slightly later stage resulted in loss of motoneurons which did not conclude until 3 weeks following amputation. Duration of motoneuron survival was directly proportional to limb maturation: amputation of the hindlimbs of juvenile toads did not result in motoneuron death until 5–7 months after the trauma. Prestige concluded from these data that the motoneuron loss could not be a direct effect of axotomy itself, but must be a result of a loss of peripheral influence on the motoneurons – a loss which the cells were able to endure for longer times as they matured, but one to which they all ultimately did succumb [11].

If we hypothesize that the developmental change in mammalian motoneuron reaction to axotomy is based upon a progressive ability to endure temporary withdrawal of a target factor, as in the amphibian, then the large-scale cell death seen after nerve crush at birth, and that is absent after nerve crush at 5–6 days post-natal, may be ascribed to the inability of neonatal motoneurons to endure the absence of target factor for even that time necessary to regrow and re-establish contact with the muscle. Kashihara et al [12] provided direct evidence for this possibility when they sectioned the nerve to the rat medial gastrocnemius muscle on day 4 post-natal. The cut nerve reinnervated the muscle in about 14 days, with only a 20% loss of neurons. If the sectioned nerve was prevented from regrowth into the muscle, however, the motoneurons were able to survive for about 2 weeks, after which more than 80% were lost.

These data indicate, therefore, that one developmental change which motoneurons undergo with maturation is the time over which they can survive in the absence of connection with their target. For immature motoneurons, this period is very short – a matter of days. Mature mo-

---

*It has been generally assumed that an inability to label neurons by injection of a retrogradely transported marker (such as horseradish peroxidase) into either the muscle or the nerve to which those neurons normally project is indicative of the death and degeneration of those neurons. With the advent of a new generation of retrograde labels such as fluoro-gold and rhodamine beads, which may remain unmetabolized within cells for weeks without diffusion, this assumption is being challenged [76–78]. While we refer throughout this chapter to death of neurons as a result of axotomy, the possibility that motoneurons assumed to die as a result of injury may rather simply atrophy and withdraw peripheral projections should be kept in mind.

toneurons, however, in the absence of reconnection with their target muscles, may survive for months or years. Even mature neurons may have limits of endurance without target to innervate, however. Limb amputations of both adult rats and humans result in eventual loss of significant numbers of motoneurons [13, 14].

In the chick, a precocial species, motoneurons are relatively mature at hatching and predictably show little acute degeneration in response to axotomy. Hindlimb removal between embryonic days 8 and 10 (E8–E10), however, produces a rapid and large-scale motoneuron degeneration [15]. Furthermore, when the hindlimb bud is removed from the chick embryo at E2, a stage prior to outgrowth of axons into the tissue, 8 days later nearly all of the motoneurons which would have innervated that limb have died [16–18]. That is, while the neurons' processes are not themselves directly injured, the absence of target musculature results in their death. Target ablation does not affect the neurons' proliferation or migration, for at 4-1/2 days of incubation embryos from which a limb bud was removed on E2 possess lateral motor columns which are indistinguishable from those of normal embryos. These targetless neurons also project out of the cord as usual but, in the absence of target tissue, form a neuroma at a set point within the body wall. It is not until E5–E6, long after target removal, that neurons begin to die – a destruction which extends over the next few days and is nearly complete.

Neuronal Death and Normal Development

The apparent requirement by motoneurons for some target-derived factor has its effects during normal development as well. At day 5 of incubation, all of the approximately 50,000 motoneurons present in the chick lumbar lateral motor columns project to the hindlimbs. Then, on E5, these seemingly normal neurons begin to die. Thousands of motoneurons, inseparable in every way from their surviving brethren, begin suddenly to degenerate, and disappear completely within a matter of hours. By day 10–11, nearly half of the initial population has been lost, and those neurons which remain are those which will compose the motoneuron pool throughout the rest of life [16, 17, 19–21]. This phenomenon of naturally occurring cell death is not unique to the motoneuron pool, but has been described, with notable exceptions, in virtually every neuronal nucleus in which it has been investigated.

While cell death in various parts of the nervous system may serve a variety of functions and be under various means of control, that which has been most widely studied, and which occurs within motoneuronal nuclei, is of an epigenetic nature, involving interactions of the neurons with their targets and afferent contacts [20–22]. The mechanism for this attrition of an over-abundant neuronal population to one composed of a mature number of neurons is thought to be based on a competition among the projecting cells. This competition or trophic theory has evolved largely as an explanation for how neuronal targets may regulate the survival and maintenance of neurons, as seen above in response to axotomy and as demonstrated, as well, by events affecting naturally occurring cell death. In its most widely held form, the trophic theory holds that it is a neurotrophic substance for which neurons compete. Such a substance should be produced by the target in limiting amounts, taken up by innervating nerves, and retrogradely transported to provide trophic support to the neuron.

If, prior to the period of cell death, one alters this competition for trophic support by decreasing the number of neurons in competition, or increasing the size of the target for which the neurons compete, the loss of neurons during the cell death period is much reduced [23, 24]. If the competition is increased, by decreasing the target size, the resulting cell death is exacerbated [16, 25]. While the basis of this competition could, for example, be the formation of stable synaptic connections per se, we and others hypothesize that the competition is based upon the need of neurons to secure sufficient amounts of a diffusible trophic molecule produced by the target. Synaptic contacts may be the sites at which the factor is taken up by the motoneurons, and thereby necessary to its action. However, it is the regulated supply by muscle of the factor that most likely acts during development to govern the retrograde survival of innervating neurons.

Neuronal Death and Trophic Molecules

The work of Hamburger and Levi-Montalcini, begun nearly 50 years ago, provided the initial formulation of the competition hypothesis, and as well eventually culminated in the discovery and purification of the only known molecule which meets all criteria for a neurotrophic substance [26, 27]. Nerve growth factor (NGF) is produced in a variety of tissues [28–30] and it is from these tissues that the terminals of neurons of the sympathetic chain and dorsal root ganglia specifically incorporate and retrogradely transport the protein [30–32]. Both sympathetic and sensory neurons undergo a period of naturally occurring cell death during embryonic development, and when exogenous NGF is supplied during this period, neurons which would normally die are maintained [33 34,]. When antibodies specific to NGF deplete the endogenous supply, a drastic loss of susceptible neurons results [35, 36]. Thus, for these neurons,

NGF appears to be the diffusible trophic substance on which the competition underlying cell death is based.

Competition for and availability of NGF determine the functional state of these neurons, not only while immature but throughout life. Damage to the peripheral projections of sensory neurons in young animals results in a large percentage of these neurons dying, as is the case for motoneurons. Administration of NGF to the injured animals prevents this perinatal axotomy-induced death of a proportion of these cells [37, 38]. Also, many of the chromatolytic changes which occur after nerve crush of mature sympathetic neurons can also be prevented or ameliorated by supplying NGF to the affected cells [39–41].

For certain classes of neurons, then, naturally occurring cell death, perinatal axotomy-induced death, and chromatolytic changes in axotomized mature cells are under the control of, or are largely influenced by, NGF. These developmental and experimental responses of NGF-sensitive neurons are so similar to those of NGF-insensitive cells, including motoneurons, that the notion of separate and distinct target-derived trophic molecules as a common means of neuronal control is most compelling.

In tissue culture, NGF is capable of controlling the survival, neurite outgrowth, and phenotypic differentiation of a number of types of susceptible cells [42–44]. The primary strategy of search for motoneuronal analogues to NGF, therefore, has been one of demonstrating similar effects on motoneurons in culture, by extracts of various sources. A number of promising candidates have been identified. Notably, factors have been isolated or partially purified from skeletal muscle or muscle-conditioned media, which enhance the survival, cholinergic enzyme activity, and/or fibre outgrowth of motoneurons *in vitro* [45–51]. Requisite to any interpretation of *in vitro* results, however, is the awareness that factors acting in culture may be doing so by providing some essential component necessary to *in vitro* growth, but without relevance for control in the animal. As this work continues, cautionary tales accumulate of substances purified and characterized as having specific *in vitro* effects, only to have the material later identified as one which is normally in excess or acting non-specifically *in vivo* [52, 53]. It is inherent in the identification of a material as a neuronal trophic factor, therefore, that it be shown to have meaningful effect in a physiologically relevant context.

Despite their limitations, a number of *in vitro* studies have shown target-derived factors to act in culture in manners consistent with a possible role of controlling cell survival *in vivo*. Since, as we have argued above, cells are most sensitive to the influences of such target-derived factors during the period of naturally occurring cell death, we were led to conduct experiments on the possible role of such factors in cell death of limb motoneurons in the embryonic chick. We found that the *in ovo* administration of fractions of E9 chick-leg homogenate could rescue motoneurons from the death which normally occurs between E5 and E10 [54]. Control tissue extracts had no effect in this system, and the inactivation of muscle extract by heat and trypsin would indicate that a proteinaceous molecule is responsible. The observation that neither sympathetic, parasympathetic, sensory, nor cholinergic sympathetic preganglionic neurons are affected by such treatment would indicate that the factor may be specific to motoneurons. Furthermore, treatment with the extract can at least partially ameliorate the neuronal death resulting from complete absence of target tissue after early limb-bud removal. If, in fact, the effects we have observed are due to a motoneuron analogue to NGF, we may hope that, like NGF, it will effectively regulate motoneuron survival not only during embryonic development but also in response to the various traumas experienced by the mature cell.

Neuronal Death and Disease Sera

The traumatic insults which may affect motoneurons are, of course, not limited to mechanical injury to the axon, but may include, for example, viral infection, toxin exposure, metabolic malfunction, and immunologic attack. All of these, and other traumatic insults, have been considered as candidates for the cause of human motoneuron disease [55]. Extending the trophic factor hypothesis of motoneuronal maintenance, one can also postulate that an insult directed against some portion of this support system could result in neuronal pathology [56]. For example, the enhancement of motoneuron survival and differentiation which is brought about with extracts from muscle and muscle-conditioned media in culture might be inhibited by substances contained in sera from patients with motoneuron disease. The possibility that circulating toxins or antibodies in motoneuron disease act either against motoneurons directly or against some aspect of their trophic support has been repeatedly addressed by exposure of motoneurons in culture to disease sera. Unfortunately, while a number of such studies have reported that this treatment does, indeed, have deleterious effects, an equal number of studies have been unable to demonstrate any such serum activity, or else have shown that any adverse neuronal effects are not confined to sera from patients with motoneuron disease [57–63].

As noted above, cells which are responsive to NGF at any one developmental stage can be demonstrated responsive, under certain circumstances, at all stages of development. Sympathetic neurons, for example, appear most dependent upon NGF during the earliest stages of development, during their period of cell death. Withdrawal of NGF during embryonic development (through induction of anti-NGF antibodies) results in a nearly complete loss of all sympathetic cells. Similar administration of anti-NGF to adults results only in an acute decrease in transmitter-related enzymes [33, 64]. With the possibility of a single substance providing trophic support to neurons throughout life, we hypothesized that if material which interferes with this trophic support of motoneurons was present in the sera of motoneuron disease patients, as indicated by some of the *in vitro* work, effects of these blood-borne substances might be most severe and most readily observed in their *in vivo* effects during the motoneuron cell death period.

We therefore administered to chick embryos, during the period of LMC motoneuron cell death in the lumbar lateral motor column (LMC), sera from patients with amyotrophic lateral sclerosis (ALS) and other neurological diseases [65]. Sera were heat-inactivated and extensively dialysed, and then applied daily to the chick chorio-allantoic membrane from E6 through E9. On E10, the embryos' spinal cords were processed for histology and cell counts performed. Of the 10 ALS sera tested, 5 resulted in a significant *rescue* of motoneurons in the LMC. The active sera resulted in a range of 2500–6000 more motoneurons in serum-treated than in saline-injected controls (where the normal LMC motoneuron number on E10 is 12,000–13,000). The effects of the active sera appear specific to motoneurons. No effects were seen on the numbers of neurons in either the dorsal root ganglia or the sympathetic ganglia. However, medial motor neurons of the thoracic cord (which innervate axial skeletal musculature) were also increased in number.

This rescuing effect was not confined to sera from ALS patients, however. Of the 10 disease control sera tested, 3 also caused decreases in the extent of motoneuron cell death. These active, non-ALS sera were all from patients with potentially denervating disorders, including a denervating polyneuropathy and Guillain-Barre and post-polio syndromes.

All of the sera effective in reducing cell death were from patients exhibiting active muscle denervation, demonstrated by muscle biopsy and/or electromyography. Those sera from patients with denervating disease which were inactive in our *in vivo* system exhibited a denervation most often characterized in laboratory reports as 'mild' or 'early.' Two indirect measures of muscle denervation – serum creatine kinase levels and clinical measures of muscle weakness [see 66] – were directly correlated with the serum cell death rescuing effect.

What mechanism could account for this unexpected *saving* of cells, which would otherwise have died, by sera from patients with denervating disease? One possibility is that such sera contain a factor mimicking the effects of a naturally occurring survival trophic factor. If embryos are paralysed during the period of cell death through a pharmacologic block of neuromuscular transmission, naturally occurring cell death of motoneurons can be almost entirely prevented [21, 67]. It has been proposed that normal neuromuscular activity acts as a signal for the down-regulation of muscle-derived neurotrophic substance. With paralysis of the embryos, trophic factor production proceeds at an accelerated pace and sufficient amounts are available to support all innervating moto-neurons. While the application of patient sera to chick embryos had no direct effect upon embryonic motility, *in vitro* studies of muscle extract effects on motoneurons in culture have shown that such activity is greatly increased if the muscle is denervated prior to its extraction [46, 68, 69]. One possibility, therefore, is that the patients' muscles were producing increased quantities of trophic substance in response to dener-vation, such that amounts of the substance present in their sera were sufficient to result in an effect on chick embryo motoneuron death. It is of interest that sprouting of motoneurons, also indicative of response to production of trophic factor by denervated muscle [70], is a notable early sign of ALS, delaying the onset of symptomatic weakness [71].

Another possibility which cannot be discounted, however, is that of an immunologic basis for the effect. Application of the globulin faction of one serum which was active in this system also produced a reduction in motoneuron degeneration. Studies are currently under way to determine what portion of this cell survival effect resides in the immuno-globulin (Ig) fraction of other active sera. If significant effects of patient Ig are found, we can predict, at least, that the effect is not due to the presence of antibodies to the acetylcholine receptor (α-AChR), implicated in an earlier study of the effects on cell death of a pool of myasthenic Ig [72]. Of the 8 sera which we tested, for which levels of serum α-AChR were known, 7 had normal levels of α-AChR (4 of which resulted in decreased motoneuron death), and the one serum with elevated α-AChR was entirely without effect on cell death. Alternative scenarios for possible actions of patient Ig on embryonic cell death might include antibodies to a trophic factor receptor which act as agonists to that receptor, as are found to the thyrotropin receptor in Graves' disease [73], or antibodies somehow interfering with the normal down-regulation of a trophic substance which occurs with the onset of neuromuscular activity.

Conclusions

We have argued that motoneurons, like neurons of the sympathetic and dorsal root ganglia in response to NGF, show a decrease in sensitivity to target trophic factor support with maturation. This gradation of responsiveness may also be reflected in the severity and rapidity with which such infantile neuromuscular diseases as Werdnig-Hoffmann proceed in contrast to ALS and other diseases of the mature system [74, 75].

There exists no incontrovertible evidence, however, to implicate alterations of neurotrophic support molecules in the pathogenesis of any neurologic disease. The strong evidence that such trophic substances do exist, however, implies that they may be regarded as realistic candidates for a role in pathologic processes. The demonstration of substances in disease sera which have an effect on *in vivo* motoneuron survival does not, of course, indicate that these substances are related to a primary pathology. It does seem, however, that the courses of some denervating diseases, including ALS, are correlated with changes in these substances. The presence, in human sera, of factors demonstrated to effect chick embryonic cell death nourishes one of the premises under which we work, that this and other lab models may some day provide a better understanding of human neuromuscular disease.

In summary, we have reviewed evidence for the proposition that motoneurons, like other neurons, are sensitive to target-derived factors for their growth and maintenance. We extend this proposition to suppose that, like neurons sensitive to NGF, this sensitivity and support is present throughout the life of the neuron, taking different forms at different stages of maturation. Under the assumption of developmental changes in dependency, we propose that it is during the embryonic period of naturally occurring cell death that neurons are most sensitive to perturbations of these factors. Two examples of *in vivo* effects on naturally occurring motoneuron cell death are presented. First, extracts of the target organs (legs) of embryonic chick motoneurons are shown to rescue these neurons from degeneration. Second, sera from a proportion of patients with ALS and other denervating diseases produce a similar decrease of motoneuron death during embryonic development. The neuromuscular interactions which lead to, or result from, motoneuron disease may be under the control of those same mechanisms which govern aspects of normal development. By understanding the bases of these laboratory models of neuromuscular interactions, we may hope to gain rational approaches to the study of human neuropathology.

Acknowledgments

Portions of our research on chick motoneuron survival were supported by NIH grants NS20402, NS23058, the Muscular Dystrophy Association, and California Biotechnology, Inc. We wish to acknowledge the participation in some of these studies, as well as the advice and suggestions, of Stanley Appel, Jim McManaman, David Prevette, Sharen McKay, and Scott Stewart.

References

1 Lieberman AR. The axon reaction. A review of the principal features of perikaryal responses to axon injury. Int Rev Neurobiol 1971;14:49–124

2 Sumner BEH. A quantitative analysis of the response of presynaptic boutons to postsynaptic motor neuron axotomy. Exp Neurol 1975;46:605–615

3 Sumner BEH, Watson WE. Retraction and expansion of the dendritic tree of motor neurons of adult rats induced *in vivo*. Nature 1971;233:273–275

4 Mendell LM, Munson JB, Scott JG. Alternations of synapses on axotomized motoneurones. J Physiol (Lond) 1976;255:67–79

5 Romanes GJ. Motor localization and the effects of nerve injury on the ventral horn cells of the spinal cord. J Anat 1946;80:117–131

6 Schmalbruch H. Motoneuron death after sciatic nerve section in newborn rats. J Comp Neurol 1984;224:252–258

7 Lowrie MB, Krishan S, Vrbova G. Recovery of slow and fast muscles following nerve injury during early post-natal development in the rat. J Physiol (Lond) 1982;331:51–66

8 Krishnan S, Lowrie MB, Vrbova G. The effect of reducing the peripheral field on motoneurone development in the rat. Brain Res 1985;351:11–20

9 Lowrie MB, Krishnan S, Vrbova G. Permanent changes in muscle and motoneurones induced by nerve injury during a critical period of development of the rat. Dev Brain Res 1987;31:91–101

10 Prestige MC. The control of cell numbers in the lumbar ventral horns during the development of *Xenopus laevis* tadpoles. J Embryol Exp Morphol 1967;18:359–387

11 Prestige MC. Differentiation, degeneration and the role of the periphery: Quantitative considerations. In: Schmitt FO, ed. The Neurosciences, 2nd Study Program. New York, The Rockefeller University Press, 1970;73–82

12 Kashihara Y, Kuno M, Miyata Y. Cell death of axotomized motoneurones in neonatal rats, and its prevention by peripheral reinnervation. J Physiol 1987;386:135–148

13 Kawamura Y, Dyck PJ. Permanent axotomy by amputation results in loss of motor neurons in man. J Neuropathol Exp Neurol 1981;40:658–666

14 Feringa ER, Vahlsing HL. Spinal motor neurons after cord transection, limb amputation or both procedures. J Neuropathol Exp Neurol 1985;44:355

15 Houthoff HF, Drukker J. Changing patterns of axonal reaction during neuronal development. A study in the developing chicken nervous system. Neuropath Appl Neurobiol 1977;3:441–451

34 Amyotrophic Lateral Sclerosis

16 Chu-Wang IW, Oppenheim RW. Cell death of motoneurons in the chick embryo spinal cord. I. A light and electron microscopic study of naturally occurring and induced cell loss during development. J Comp Neurol 1978;177:33–58

17 Chu-Wang IW, Oppenheim RW. Cell death of motoneurons in the chick embryo spinal cord. II. A quantitative and qualitative analylsis of degeneration in the ventral root, including evidence for axon outgrowth and limb innervation prior to cell death. J Comp Neurol 1978;177:59–86

18 Oppenheim RW, Chu-Wang IW, Maderdrut J. Cell death of motoneurons in the chick embryo spinal cord. III. The differentiation of motoneurons prior to their induced degeneration following limb-bud removal. J Comp Neurol 1978;177:87–112

19 Hamburger V. Cell death in the development of the lateral motor column of the chick embryo. J Comp Neurol 1975;160:535–546

20 Hamburger V, Oppenheim RW. Naturally occurring neuronal death in vertebrates. Neurosci Comment 1982;1:39–55

21 Oppenheim RW, Chu-Wang I-W. Aspects of naturally occurring motoneuron death in the chick spinal cord during embryonic development. In: Burnstock G, Vrbova G eds. Somatic and Autonomic Nerve-Muscle Interactions. Amsterdam, Elsevier, 1983;57–107

22 Oppenheim RW. Neuronal cell death and some related regressive phenomena during neurogenesis: A selective historical review and progress report. In: Cowan WM, ed. Studies in Developmental Neurobiology: Essays in Honor of Viktor Hamburger. New York, Oxford Univ Press, 1981;75–133

23 Pilar G, Landmesser L, Burnstein L. Competition for survival among developing ciliary ganglion cells. J Neurophysiol 1980;43:233–254

24 Hollyday M, Hamburger V. Reduction of the naturally occurring motor neuron loss by enlargement of the periphery. J Comp Neurol 1976;170:311–320

25 Lanser ME, Fallon JF. Development of the brachial lateral motor column in the *wingless* mutant chick embryo: Motoneuron survival under varying degrees of peripheral load. J Comp Neurol 1987;261:423–434

26 Levi-Montalcini R. Developmental neurobiology and the natural history of nerve growth factor. Ann Rev Neurosci 1982;5:341–362

27 Levi-Montalcini R. The nerve growth factor 35 years later. Science 1987;237:1154–1167

28 Harper GP, Thoenen H. Target cells, biological effects, and mechanism of action of nerve growth factor and its antibodies. Ann Rev Pharmacol 1981;21:205–229

29 Korshing S, Thoenen H. Nerve growth factor in sympathetic ganglia and corresponding target organs of the rat: Correlation with density of sympathetic innervation. Proc Natl Acad Sci 1983;80:3513–3516

30 Davies AM, Bandtlow C, Heumann R, et al. Timing and site of nerve growth factor synthesis in developing skin in relation to innervation and expression of the receptor. Nature 1987;326:353–358

31 Stockel K, Schwab M, Thoenen H. Specificity of retrograde transport of nerve growth factor (NGF) in sensory neurons: A biochemical and morphological study. Brain Res 1975;89:1–14

32 Stockel K, Schwab M, Thoenen H. Comparison between the retrograde axonal transport of nerve growth factor and tetanus toxin in motor, sensory and adrenergic neurons. Brain Res 1975;99:1–16

33 Hamburger V, Brunso-Bechtold JK, Yip JW. Neuronal death in the spinal ganglia of the chick embryo and its reduction by nerve growth factor. J Neurosci 1981;1:60–71

34 Oppehneim RW, Maderdrut JL, Wells DJ. Cell death of motoneurons in the chick embryo spinal cord. VI. Reduction of naturally occurring cell death in the thoracolumbar column of Terni by nerve growth factor. J Comp Neurol 1982;210:174–189

35 Levi-Montalcini R, Booker B. Destruction of the sympathetic ganglia in mammals by an antiserum to a nerve-growth protein. Proc Natl Acad Sci 1960;46:384–391

36 Johnson EM, Gorin PD, Brandeis LD, Pearson J. Dorsal root ganglion neurons are destroyed by exposure in utero to maternal antibody to nerve growth factor. Science 1980;210:916–918

37 Miyata Y, Kashihara Y, Homma S, Kuno M. Effects of nerve growth factor on the survival and synaptic function of Ia sensory neurons in neonatal rats. J Neurosci 1986;6:2012–2018

38 Yip HK, Rich M, Lampe PA, Johnson EM. The effects of nerve growth factor and its antiserum on the postnatal development and survival after injury of sensory neurons in rat dorsal root ganglia. J Neurosci 1984;4:2986–2992

39 Hendry IA, Campbell J. Morphometric analysis of the rat superior cervical ganglion after axotomy and nerve growth factor treatment. J Neurocytol 1976;5:351–360

40 Hendry IA. The response of adrenergic neurons to axotomy and nerve growth factor. Brain Res 1975;94:87–97

41 Nja A, Purves D. The effects of nerve growth factor and its antiserum on synapses in the superior cervical ganglion of the guinea-pig. J Physiol 1978;277:53–75

42 Levi-Montalcini R, Angeletti PU. Essential role of nerve growth factor in the survival and maintenance of dissociated sensory and sympathetic nerve cells in vitro. Dev Biol 1963;7:653–659

43 Levi-Montalcini R, Hamburger V. Selective growth-stimulating effects of

mouse sarcoma on the sensory and sympathetic nervous system of the chick embryo. J Exp Zool 1951;116:321–362

44 Thoenen H, Barde YA. Physiology of nerve growth factor. Physiol Rev 1980;60:1284–1335

45 Bennet MR, Lai K, Nurcome V. Identification of embryonic motoneurons in vitro: Their survival is dependent on skeletal muscle. Brain Res 1980;190:537–542

46 Smith RG, McManaman JL, Appel SH. Trophic effects of skeletal muscle extracts on ventral spinal cord neurons *in vitro*: Separation of a protein with morphologic activity from proteins with cholinergic activity. J Cell Biol 1985;101:1608–1621

47 McManaman JL, Crawford F, Stewart SS, Appel SH. Purification of a skeletal muscle polypeptide which stimulates choline acetyltransferase activity in cultured spinal cord neurons. J Biol Chem (in press)

48 Dohrmann U, Edgar D, Thoenen H. Distinct neurotrophic factors from skeletal muscle and the central nervous system interact synergistically to support the survival of cultured embryonic spinal motor neurons. Dev Biol 1987;124:145–152

49 O'Brien RJ, Fischbach GD. Isolation of embryonic chick motoneurons and their survival in vitro. J Neurosci 1986;6:3265–3274

50 Crutcher KA. The role of growth factors in neuronal develoment and plasticity.. CRC Crit Rev Clin Neurobiol 1986;2:297–333

51 McManaman JL, Haverkamp LJ, Appel SH. Developmental discord among markers for cholinergic differentiation: *In vitro* time courses for early expression and responses to skeletal muscle extract. Dev Biol 1988;125:311–320

52 Markelonis GJ, Bradshaw RA, Oh TH, et al. Sciatin is a transferrin-like polypeptide. J. Neurochem 1982;39:315–320

53 Walicke P, Varon S, Manthrope M. Purification of a human red blood cell protein supporting the survival of cultured CNS neurons, and its identification as catalase. J Neurosci 1986;6:1114–1121

54 Oppenheim RW, Haverkamp LJ, Prevette D, et al. Reduction of naturally occurring motoneuron death in the chick embryo *in vivo* by a target-derived neurotrophic factor. Science 1988;240:919–922

55 Stewart SS, Appel SH. The treatment of amyotrophic lateral sclerosis. Curr Neurol 1987;7:51–90

56 Appel SH. A unifying hypothesis for the cause of amyotrophic lateral sclerosis, parkinsonism, and Alzheimer's disease. Ann Neurol 1981;10:499–505

57 Touzeau G, Kato AC. Effects of amyotrophic lateral sclerosis sera on cultured cholinergic neurons. Neurology 1983;33:317–322

58 Wolfgram F. Blind studies on the effect of amyotrophic lateral sclerosis sera

on motor neurons in vitro. In: Andrews JM, Johnson RT, Brazier MAB, eds. Amyotrophic Lateral Sclerosis Recent Research Trends. New York, Academic Press, 1976;145–149

59 Horwich MS, Engel WK, Chauvin PB. Amyotrophic lateral sclerosis sera applied to cultured motor neurons. Arch Neurol 1974;30:332–333

60 Liveson J, Frey H, Bornstein MB. The effects of serum from ALS patients on organotypic nerve and muscle tissue cultures. Acta Neuropathol (Berl) 1975;32:127–131

61 Digby J, Harrison R, Jehanli A, et al. Cultured rat spinal cord neurons: Interaction with motor neuron disease immunoglobulins. Muscle & Nerve 1985;8:595–605

62 Roisen FJ, Bartfield H, Dunnenfeld H, Baxter J. Neuron specific in vitro cytotoxicity of sera from patients with amyotrophic lateral sclerosis. Muscle & Nerve 1982;5:48–53

63 Doherty P, Dickson JG, Flanigan TP, et al. Effects of amyotrophic lateral sclerosis serum on cultured chick spinal neurons. Neurology 1986;36:1330–1334

64 Otten U, Goedert M, Schwab M, Thibault J. Immunization of adult rats against 2.5 S NGF: Effects on the peripheral sympathetic nervous sytem. Brain Res 1979;176:79-90

65 Haverkamp LJ, Oppenheim RW, Appel SH, et al. Reduction of naturally occurring motoneuron death by sera from patients with denervating disease. Soc. Neurosci Abstr 1987;13:923

66 Appel V, Stewart SS, Smith G, Appel SH. A rating scale for amyotrophic lateral sclerosis: Description and preliminary experience. Ann Neurol 1987;22:328–333

67 Pittman R, Oppenheim RW. Cell death of motoneurons in the chick embryo spinal cord. IV. Evidence that a functional neuromuscular interaction is involved in the regulation of naturally occurring cell death and the stabilization of synapses. J Comp Neurol 1979;187:425–446

68 Nurcombe V, Hill MA, Eagleson KL, Bennett MR. Motoneurone survival and neuritic extension from spinal cord explants induced by factors released from denervated muscle. Brain Res 1984;291:19–28

69 Henderson CE, Huchet M, Changeux JP. Denervation increases a neurite-promoting activity in extracts of skeletal muscle. Nature 1983;302:609–611

70 Brown M, Holland R, Hopkins W. Motor nerve sprouting. Ann Rev Neurosci 1981;4:17–42

71 Stalberg E. Electrophysiological studies of reinnervation in ALS. Adv Neurol 1982;36:47–59

72 Sohal GS, Lehner RT, Swift TR. Myasthenia gravis immunoglobulin augments motor neuron survival without producing muscle paralysis. Muscle & Nerve 1983;6:122–127

73 Rees-Smith B, Creagh FM, Hashim FA, et al. Thyrotropin receptor anti-bodies. Arzneimittelforschung 1985;35:1943–1948
74 Byers RK, Banker BQ. Infantile muscular atrophy. Arch Neurol 1961;5:140–164
75 Dyken P, Krawiecki N. Neurodegenerative dieseases of infancy and child-hood. Ann Neurol 1983;13:351–364
76 Bates CA, Stelzner DJ. Do corticospinal projection neurons die after spinal transection in the neonatal rat? Soc Neurosci Abstr 1987;13:921
77 Crews L, Wigston DJ. Fate of motorneurons after limb amputation in postnatal mice. Soc Neurosci Abstr 1987;13:921
78 McBride RL, Feringa ER, Pruitt JN, II. Prelabeled red nucleus and sensory-motor cortex neurons 10 weeks after spinal cord transection. Soc Neurosci Abstr 1987;13:920

Ganglioside G_{M2} and Motor Neuron Disease: Amyotrophic Lateral Sclerosis and β-Hexosaminidase Deficiencies with ALS-like Symptoms

GLYN DAWSON, LARRY W. HANCOCK,
AND NORAH R. McCABE

Amyotrophic lateral sclerosis (ALS) is typically a sporadic disease of unknown etiology, but with some suggestion of a viral or environmental toxin cause. Fewer than 5% of all ALS cases have even a suggestion of a familial origin and none of these pedigrees have yet been subjected to restriction fragment polymorphism analysis which would indicate linkage to a particular chromosome. Within this group, however, exists a small number of ALS-like cases where the biochemical defect and the cause of motor neuron degeneration are much better understood, and where the relatively slow progression of ALS-like symptoms offers some opportunity for remedial therapy. All of these 40 or more cases [1–3] are characterized by the early onset of mild neurological symptoms in the teenage years, progressing to locomotor incapacitation and upper motor neuron disease in the second and third decades, and death in the fourth decade or later. However, the phenotype is considered too variable to serve as a basis for genetic classification. Despite this, they are all characterized by an abnormality in the ability of the lysosomal hydrolase N-acetyl-β-hexosaminidase (β-Hex) to remove a terminal sugar (GalNAc) residue from the membrane glycosphingolipid G_{M2} ganglioside (GalNAc [NeuAc] Gal-Glc-Ceramide). Gangliosides are negatively charged glycolipids in which the lipid (ceramide) is part of the outer leaflet of the lipid bilayer and the sugar residues project outside of the cell. Gangliosides have been implicated as receptors (e.g., for cholera toxin) [4], modulators of cell recognition or adhesion, and agents which facilitate neuronal differentiation and regeneration [4]. Their high level of bioactivity makes them attractive candidates for a pivotal role in the pathogenesis of ALS. G_{M2} ganglioside is synthesized primarily by neurons, and has a much higher turnover rate in motor neurons than in sympathetic or other neurons [5]. Because of this, a defect in β-Hex appears to result in preferential storage of G_{M2} in motor neurons, leading to swelling of the neuron, abnormal meganeurite formation [6], dysfunction, and death. In this chapter, we will discuss the mechanism for the defect in β-Hex activity, and if there is any evidence that a defect in G_{M2} metabolism resulting from viral or environmental insult could contribute to some of the diseases we categorize as sporadic motor neuron disease or ALS.

N-acetyl-β-D-hexosaminidase (β-Hex)

Human β-Hex exists as two major isoenzymes termed Hex A and Hex B, which can be readily separated by charge (electrophoresis or ion-exchange chromatography) or the increased thermolability of Hex A. Hex A consists of one α-polypeptide subunit linked to two different β-subunits (βA and βB) by disulphide bonds and in association with a third gene product (activator protein) is required in order to catabolize G_{M2} ganglioside [7, 8]. The gene for the α-subunit is on chromosome 15 [9], whereas the genes for β-subunit and activator protein are on different portions of chromosome 5 [10]. Thus, mutations in any of the three gene products can give rise to a defective β-Hex and lead to neurological disease. Hex B consists of four β-subunits (two βA, two βB) linked by disulphide bonds and hydrolyses both neutral glycolipids and glycoproteins, but not ganglioside G_{M2}.

Both α- and β-chains are initially synthesized as high-molecular-weight peptides. (67 Kd and 63 Kd, respectively) which are partially degraded and glycosylated before being assembled and processed in the acidified lysosome, where all glycolipids and glycoproteins are finally degraded [5, 11]. A scheme for this is presented in Figure 1, which also shows that transport into the lysosome is inhibited if acidification is prevented by adding ammonium chloride or chloroquine to cultured cells (which causes secretion of precursors into the culture media). As we will see, this technique [11] has proved very useful in studying and distinguishing between the many differential human β-Hex mutants which cause varying degrees of neurologic dysfunction.

β-Hex Mutants

α-Chain Defect

The prototypic α-chain disease is Tay-Sachs disease in which failure to synthesize α-chain results in the absence of Hex A [12], increased

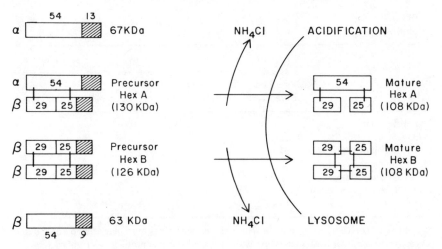

Figure 1. Schematic diagram of post-translational processing of β-Hex α- and β-chains. Hex A is a heteropolymer of $\alpha\beta_2$, is thermolabile, and requires a 22 Kd activator protein to hydrolyse G_{M2} ganglioside, but not to hydrolyse glycoprotein-associated oligosaccharides and neutral glycolipids. Hex B is a homopolymer (β_4) which is thermostable, and only hydrolyses glycoprotein-associated oligosaccharides and neutral glycolipids. Ammonium chloride (NH_4Cl) treatment prevents acidification of the post-Golgi lysosomal vesicle, resulting in the secretion of precursors of α- and β-chains.

amounts of Hex B, and the accumulation of G_{M2} in all neurons – leading to loss of vision by 6 months and loss of all neural function by 24 months of age. A partial deficiency of Hex A results in onset of milder neurological symptoms around age 6 years and slower onset of blindness and dementia [2]. A third type of partial Hex A deficiency involving an α-chain mutation results in muscle atrophy (with or without an encephalopathic course) and symptoms resembling those of ALS [2, 3] (Table 1). The clinical symptoms of this group have been summarized by Navon et al [3]. All are characterized by some degree of upper and lower motor neuron disease, overt cerebellar signs, normal mental status (but psychosis in 30% of cases), an Ashkenazi Jewish background, and lack of seizures or optic degeneration. In some of the cases there was a family history of Tay-Sachs disease, suggesting that α-chain β-Hex deficiency patients could be compound heterozygotes for the α-chain (that is, having one Tay-Sachs allele in combination with a second mutant α-chain allele).

TABLE 1
Adult-onset β-Hex deficiency with ALS-like symptoms

| | Patient age when studied (years) | Neuron involvement | | | Genetics |
Type		Lower motor	Sensory	Cerebellar	Ashkenazi
Hex A deficient					
(33 cases) [19]	11–67	+	−	+/−	+
Hex A deficient (Pr)*	64	−	−	+	+
Hex B deficient (KL)	25	+	−	−	−
Adult Sandhoff (Hex A and B partially deficient)					
(10 cases)	10–47	+	0	+	−

* Patient Pr is a 65-year-old female with progressive spinal muscular atrophy and overt cerebellar signs (ataxia). Her retina is normal and she has no history of visual problems.

β-Chain Defects

The prototypic β-chain disease is Sandhoff-Jatzkewitz disease, where an absent or defective β-chain results in the absence of both Hex A and Hex B [13]. Clinically, the patients resemble those with Tay-Sachs disease, but in addition exhibit visceromegaly caused by storage of globoside and oligosaccharide. A juvenile form of Sandhoff's disease has been attributed to partial Hex B deficiency and often presents as cerebellar ataxia with additional progressive decline in pyramidal tract function and, frequently, dementia [14]. The seizures and abnormalities of optic fundi typical of infantile Sandhoff are also absent. Of considerable interest have been reports of adult Sandhoff disease [14] (Table 1). Such patients present with progressive but severe spinocerebellar degeneration with motor neuron involvement but no dementia, seizures, or eye abnormalities. At autopsy, typical findings are loss of neurons, severe swelling of remaining neurons (resulting from lysosomal accumulation of G_{M2} ganglioside), especially in cerebellum and the motor nuclei of the spinal cord, together with demyelination of the posterior columns [14].

In contrast to these adult cases of Sandhoff's disease where both Hex A and Hex B are markedly deficient, we have described a patient KL [1, 5, 15] in which Hex A in fibroblasts was normal, as determined by synthetic substrate assay, and Hex B was completely deficient. In this case, the abnormal β-chain apparently combines poorly either with α-chain or with activator protein with the result that G_{M2} ganglioside is incompletely degraded and accumulates in motor neurons. This patient was initially evaluated at age 7 with speech problems and clumsy behaviour, but deteriorated slowly so that by age 24 a diagnosis of ALS could be made in the absence of her previous neurological history. She has a progressive upper and lower motor neuron disease with little evidence of tremor, sensory abnormalities, or cerebellar degeneration. Her major neurological findings are peripheral muscle atrophy, widespread fascic-ulations, and limb weakness without any intellectual or visual impair-ment and with almost normal speech. Biochemical studies, discussed below, suggested that her mother and one sibling are heterozygotes for β-chain deficiency, but her father and another sibling are normal for α- and β-chain as determined by simple thermal lability and electrophoretic assay of the type employed in Tay-Sachs screening tests. When the var-ious β-Hex mutants are taken together with additional cases of pseudo Hex B deficiency and the wide range of clinical variability, it is obvious that more detailed clinical tests are necessary to establish the biochemical defect, offer effective genetic counselling, and plan appropriate thera-peutic strategies. Recently available biochemical approaches include the use of antibodies specific for β-Hex to study the synthesis, processing, and turnover of α- and β-chain in fibroblasts cultured from skin biopsies and the use of cDNA probes for both α- and β-chains [8, 12, 16] to study the nature of the defect at the DNA and RNA level. This latter technique can use white cells rather than fibroblasts, and is therefore more ame-nable to family studies.

Processing and Assembly of Alpha and Beta Chains in β-Hex Mutants

Cells were grown in leucine/methionine-deficient culture medium and incubated with [^{3}H]leucine and [^{35}S]methionine as described previously [11, 15]. A 6-hour pulse was necessary to incorporate sufficient amounts of these labelled amino acids into α and β precursor polypeptides. Fol-lowing precipitation of β-Hex with antibody, the precursors can be seen (following exposure of the SDS gel-separated [^{3}H] and [^{35}S]-labelled pro-teins to x-ray film for 3 weeks) as a broad band encompassing the 63 and 67 Kd forms (Fig. 2, lanes 1-5). Normal cells (lanes 1 and 2), Tay-Sachs cells [5], and cells from adult patients deficient in Hex B (KL) (lane 3) and Hex A (lane 4) show different, characteristic patterns. Strikingly, it can be seen that Sandhoff fibroblasts (lane 6) synthesize neither α- nor β-chains, with most of the normally synthesized α-chain precursors being rapidly degraded in the absence of β-chains. After a 48-hour chase in unlabelled medium (lanes 7–12), the labelled hexosaminidase is pro-cessed in the lysosome and the initially synthesized α- and β-precursors are converted to 54 Kd (α) and 29 Kd (β) mature forms as seen in lanes

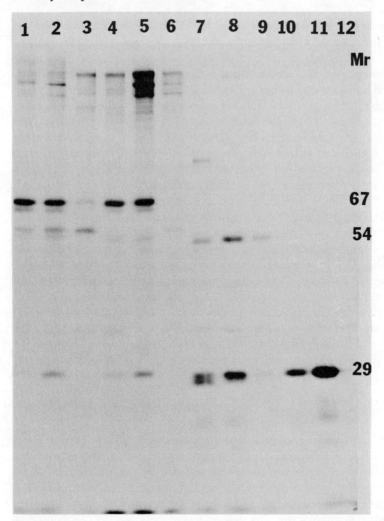

Figure 2. Synthesis of hexosaminidase polypeptide chains. Cultured fibroblasts were labelled for 6 hours with ³⁵S-methionine, and harvested immediately (lanes 1–6) or after a 48-hour chase period (lanes 7–12). Cells were harvested, extracted, and immunoprecipitated with polyclonal antibody to Hex B (from Drs Neufeld and Proia), which recognizes both α and β polypeptide chains. After sodium dodecyl sulphate polycrylamide gel electrophoresis, SDS-PAGE, immunoprecipitated polypeptides were visualized by fluorography. Molecular weights (Mr) are given on right (67 Kd, etc.). Lanes 1, 2, 7, 8, normal controls; 3, 9, patient KL; 4, 10, Hex A deficient adult (Pr); 5, 11, Tay-Sachs disease; 6, 12, Sandhoff disease.

TABLE 2
β-Hex α- and β-chain processing in adult Hex-deficient patients

Deficiency	α-chain		β-chain	
	Precursor 67 Kd peptide	Mature 54 Kd peptide	Precursor 63 Kd peptide	Mature 29/25 Kd peptide
Hex A (TSD)	A	A	N	N
Hex A (adult)*	N	R	N	N
Hex A and B (Sandhoff)	N	R	R	A
Hex A and B (adult)*	N	R	R	R
Hex B (KL)*	N	N	R	R

A, absent; R, reduced; N, normal
* ALS phenocopy

7 and 8. Tay-Sachs (lane 11) and adult Hex A deficiency patients (lane 10) accumulate no mature α (54 Kd), but more than normal β (29 Kd), whereas Hex B deficient patient KL synthesized normal α and reduced amounts of β-chain (lane 9). Sandhoff patients (Hex A and B deficient; lane 12) contain very little mature α and β. The results are summarized in Table 2 and form a useful diagnostic test for distinguishing the different β-Hex variants.

Unfortunately, such studies do not evaluate the ability of the patients' cells to degrade G$_{M2}$ ganglioside, which is the definitive test of any β-Hex deficiency. Since human skin fibroblasts do not synthesize G$_{M2}$ ganglioside, exogenous G$_{M2}$, preferably radioactive [^{3}H]G$_{M2}$, must be fed to cells and allowed to accumulate over a period of 4–8 days [5]. When this is done, it is possible to distinguish between the complete, partial, and pseudo deficiencies (Table 3).

Molecular Basis of β-Hex Deficiencies

Classical Ashkenazi Jewish Tay-Sachs disease appears to result from a mutant α-chain DNA which cannot be transcribed to a stable messenger RNA (mRNA) [12], whereas Sandhoff disease results from either deletions in the DNA for β-chain or a similar failure in transcription [8]. The adult onset forms with ALS-like symptoms pose a more complex biochemical challenge since in all cases studied thus far it appears that functional mRNA for α-chain is synthesized and small amounts of partially active α-chain (complexed with β-chain to form Hex A) are produced.

TABLE 3
Relative accumulation of unhydrolysed ^{3}H-G$_{M2}$ following feeding of exogenous [^{3}H]G$_{M2}$ to human skin fibroblasts

	Expt. 1	Expt. 2	Expt. 3
Control	1.0	1.0	1.0
Tay-Sachs disease	4.5	2.6	1.7
Sandhoff disease	4.2	2.6	1.3
Patient KL	2.2	1.8	1.5

Navon et al [3] concluded that most of their patients had one parent who was heterozygous for the Tay-Sachs allele and one parent who had a rare α-chain mutation – i.e., the patient was a compound heterozygote. Such families are important because they often give anomalous results in TSD carrier testing programs [3]. In studies on patients with adult Sandhoff disease resembling ALS and a clinical phenotype of Kugelberg-Welander disease [18], Bolhuis et al (14) concluded that initial synthesis of α- and β-chains was normal, but a destabilizing mutation in the β-locus caused very little mature β-chain to be present in cells. They could not rule out the possibility of an allelic compound mutation. A similar explanation could account for the findings in our patient KL, although the actual mutation must be different. To resolve these issues, it is necessary to probe the structure of the DNA and resulting mRNA using full-length cDNA probes for α [8, 12] and β [8] chains, labelled with ^{32}P, in Southern and Northern blot analysis [8, 12].

A typical Southern blot is shown in Figure 3, in which the DNA isolated from white cells of control, father, mother, and patient KL was digested with different restriction endonucleases (BamHI and HindIII). The digested DNA fragments were separated on gels by electrophoresis, transferred to nitrocellulose, and visualized by hybridization to ^{32}P-labelled β-chain (or α-chain) probe, followed by exposure to x-ray film for 6–24 hours. Similar digestions using restriction endonucleases EcoRI and TaqI indicated that there was no polymorphism evident in patient KL DNA. However, many other nucleases are available, and for other β-Hex mutants, this approach has yielded specific insights into the molecular defect.

A typical Northern blot is shown in Figure 4, in which the RNA isolated from human skin fibroblasts is separated by electrophoresis and hybridized with ^{32}P-labelled β-chain cDNA probe [8]. Isolated total RNA is initially electrophoresed on 0.8% agarose gel at 40 mV for 18 hours and then transferred to nitrocellulose prior to hybridization blotting. In both normal and patient KL a 2.2 kb transcript was seen, indicating that

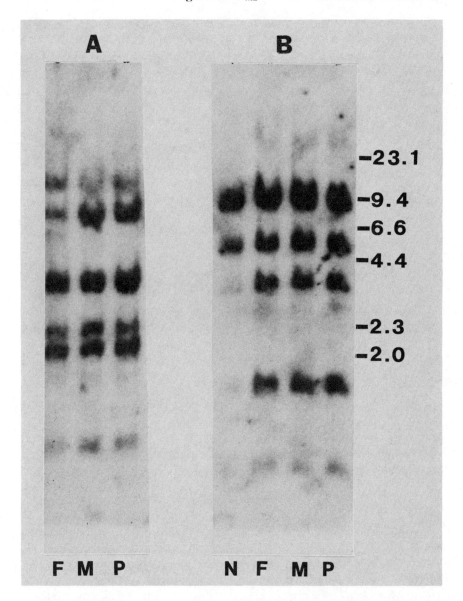

Figure 3. Southern blot of DNA isolated from leukocytes of normal (N), patient KL (P), father (F), and mother (M) of patient following digestion with restriction endonucleases *Hind*III (A) and *Bam*HI (B) hybridized with β-chain cDNA. The pattern of digested fragments in patient KL was similar to that of M, F, and N, indicating normal β-chain DNA.

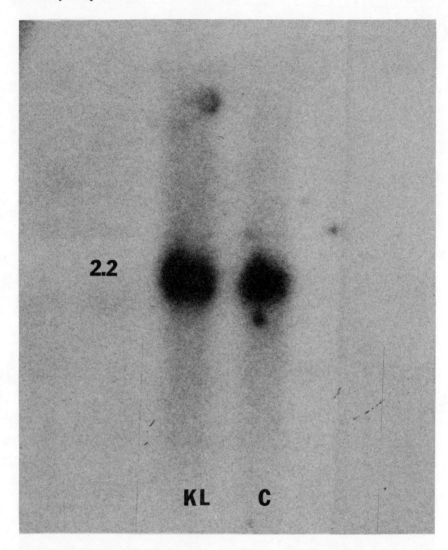

Figure 4. Northern blot analysis of RNA. Northern blot analysis (autoradiograph) of total RNA isolated from fibroblasts of the patient KL and a normal control. Total RNA (10 μg) was electrophoresed and transferred to nitrocellulose. Hybridization with the β-chain cDNA probe labelled with [32]P (5 × 10[6] dpm) was carried out at 42°C overnight. A single 2.2 kb RNA species is evident in both normal and patient RNA.

the diminished amount of β-chain observed after metabolic labelling must result from impaired translation of the RNA into polypeptide or instability of newly synthesized β-chain.

Ganglioside Abnormalities in Sporadic ALS

There is no microscopic or enzymatic evidence to suggest that ALS is a lysosomal storage disease with multilamellar cytosomal storage bodies of the type seen in patient KL (Fig. 5), but there have been a number of reports of ganglioside abnormalities greater than one would anticipate as secondary events related to neurological degeneration. Thus, Kundu et al [19] identified an abnormal neutral glycosphingolipid, sialosylglobotetraosylceramide, in ALS muscle, and we have confirmed this in five patients. However, the glycolipid also accumulates in other muscle-degenerative diseases and cannot be considered diagnostic for ALS.

Rapport et al [20] found a relative increase in simple gangliosides (G_{M2} and G_{M3}) and a relative decrease in complex gangliosides G_{D1b}, G_{T1b}, and G_{Q1b} (using the Svennerholm nomenclature for di (D) and tri (T) sialogangliosides) in 16 ALS post-mortem cortices with no similar switch in composition in 11 non-ALS pathological controls. This was somewhat in agreement with our own previous findings in ALS spinal cord [17] in which we found elevated G_{M2} and disialohematoside (G_{D3}) and abnormal sialosylglobotetraosylceramide (NeuAc-GalNAc-Gal-Gal-Glc-Ceramide), as well as L_{M1} ganglioside (Gal-GlcNAc(NeuAc)Gal-Glc-Ceramide). We have recently examined post-mortem cortex from ALS patients and do observe increased amounts of G_{M2} compared to other pathological conditions such as multiple sclerosis. This is obviously a provocative finding since G_{M2} accumulation in motor neurons in β-Hex deficiencies leads to motor neuron degeneration and ALS-like symptoms. However, EM studies have not revealed any lysosomal storage bodies in ALS, and at present there is no evidence as to the subcellular localization of the G_{M2} ganglioside.

Much attention has been given to the possibility that ALS is an autoimmune disease, and we have screened serum from over 50 ALS patients for evidence of anti-glycolipid antibodies. Apart from sporadic positive sera (especially against galactosylceramide) we find no evidence, within the limits of our technology, to suggest that ALS is an anti-ganglioside autoimmune disease. Such diseases do exist; for example the Waldenstrom macroglobulinemia-associated peripheral neuropathies result from circulating monoclonal IgM against sulphoglucuronyl-Gal-GlcNAc-Gal-Glc-Ceramide [21], but tend not to affect the CNS. In addition, we have recently followed two sisters, 27 and 32 years old, who

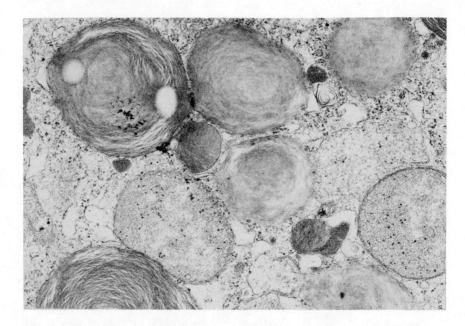

Figure 5. Electron micrograph of swollen submucosal nerve cell showing numerous secondary lysosomes filled with multilamellar bodies characteristic of ganglioside storage diseases. Photomicrograph courtesy of Dr R.L. Wollmann, University of Chicago.

had ALS preceded by Graves' disease, an autoimmune disease in which anti-ganglioside antibodies have been claimed to circulate [22]. The question of glycolipid autoimmune disease in ALS will only be resolved when we understand more about glycolipid metabolism in the motor neuron. Initial studies on sensory neurons [23] suggest that some unusual glycolipids are found, some of which could have terminal hexosamine residues and require β-Hex A for their catabolism. Another provocative area for future research centres around the many observations that gangliosides can cause sprouting of neurons in culture and might be of clinical value in treatment of degenerative diseases such as ALS [4]. However, ganglioside administration to ALS patients has not been successful in reversing the relentless neuromuscular degeneration, and new answers must be sought.

In summary, approximately 40 patients with early-onset, prolonged ALS-like symptoms have been shown to have a partial deficiency of the lysosomal hydrolase N-acetyl-β-D-hexosaminidase. Inherited defects have been associated with both alpha and beta chains of hexosaminidase and motor neuron death is the result of excessive accumulation of G_{M2} ganglioside over a period of 20–30 years. The accumulation of similar gangliosides has been observed in spinal cord and motor cortex from patients with typical ALS, but there is no evidence of a hexosaminidase deficiency, and the rapid course of ALS (3 years) is quite different from that of the partial hexosaminidase deficiencies. The cause of classic ALS is at present unknown, but the disease apparently results in impaired metabolism of gangliosides, which leads to rapid death of motor neurons.

Acknowledgments

Supported by USPHS Grants NS-23131, HD-06426, and HD-04583 and a Research Grant from the ALS Association. We gratefully acknowledge the receipt of clinical material from Dr J. Antel, Dr R. Roos, and Dr K. Stefansson, UCHC Neurology Department, and helpful discussions with Dr A.L. Horwitz and Dr N. Cashman.

References

1 Cashman, NR, Antel JP, Hancock LW, et al. N-acetyl-β-hexosaminidase β locus defect and juvenile motor neuron disease: a case study. Ann Neurol 1986;19:568–572

2 Kolodny EH, Raghaven SS. G_{M2}-gangliosidosis-hexosaminidase mutants. Trends in Neurol Sci 1983;6:16–20

3 Navon R, Argov Z, Frisch A. Hexosaminidase A deficiency in adults. Am J Med Genet 1986;24:179–196

4 Ledeen RW. Biology of gangliosides: Neuritogenic and neuronotrophic properties. J Neurosci Res 1984;12:147–159

5 Dawson G, Hancock LW, Vartanian T. Regulation of G_{M2} ganglioside metabolism in cultured cells. Chem Phys Lipids 1986;42:105–116

6 Purpura DP, Suzuki K. Distortion of neuronal geometry and formation of aberrant synapses in neuronal storage disease. Brain Res 1976;116:1–21

7 Myerowitz R, Piekarz R, Neufeld EF, et al. Human β-hexosaminidase α chain: Coding sequence and homology with β chains. Proc Natl Acad Sci (USA) 1985;82:7830–7834

8 O'Dowd B, Quan F, Willard HF, et al. Isolation of cDNA clones encoding the β-hexosaminidase gene. Proc Natl Acad Sci (USA) 1985;82:1184–1188

9 Fox MF, Dutoit DL, Warnich L, Retief AE. Regional localization of β-galactosidase (GAL) to Xpter-q22, hexosaminidase β (Hex β) to 5 q 13. Cytogenet Cell Genet 1984;38:45–49

10 D'Azzo A, Proia RL, Kolodny EH, et al. Faulty association of α- and β-subunits in some forms of β-hexosaminidase A deficiency. J Biol Chem 1984;259:11070–11074

11 Hasilik A, Neufeld EF. Biosynthesis of lysosomal enzymes in fibroblasts. Synthesis as precursors of higher molecular weights. J Biol Chem 1980;255:4937–4945

12 Myerowitz R, Proia RL. A cDNA for the α-chain of human β-hexosaminidase; deficiency of the α-chain in mRNA in Ashkenazi Tay-Sachs fibroblasts. Proc Natl Acad Sci (USA) 1984;81:5396–5398

13 Sandhoff K, Christomanou H. Biochemistry and genetics of gangliosides. Hum Genet 1979;50:107–143

14 Bolhuis PA, Oonk JGW, Kamp PE, et al. Ganglioside storage, hexosaminidase lability and urinary oligosaccharides in adult Sandhoff's disease. Neurology 1987;37:75–81

15 Hancock LW, Horwitz AL, Cashman NR, et al. N-acetyl-β-hexosaminidase B deficiency in cultured fibroblasts from a patient with progressive motor neuron disease. Biochem Biophys Res Comm 1985;130:1185–1192

16 Korneluk R, Mahuran DJ, Neole K, et al. Isolation of cDNA clones for the α-subunit of human β-hexosaminidase. J Biol Chem 1986;261:8407–8413

17 Dawson G, Stefansson K. Gangliosides of human spinal cord: Aberrant composition of cords from patients with amyotrophic lateral sclerosis. J Neurosci Res 1984;12:213–220

18 Barbeau A, Plasse L, Cloutier T, et al. Lysosomal enzymes in ataxia: Discovery of two new cases of late-onset hexosaminidase A and B deficiency (adult Sandhoff disease) in French Canadians. Can J Neurol Sci 1984;11:601–610

19 Kundu SK, Harati Y, Misra LK, Marcus DM. Sialosylaglobotetraosylceramide: A marker for amyotrophic lateral sclerosis. Biochem Biophys Res Comm 1983;118:82–89

20 Rapport MM, Donnenfeld H, Brunner W, et al. Ganglioside patterns in amyotrophic lateral sclerosis brain regions. Ann Neurol 1985;18:60–67

21 Chou KH, Ilyas AA, Evans JE, et al. Sulfated-glucuronic acid-containing glycolipid reacting with IgM M-proteins in patients with neuropathy. Biochem Biophys Res Comm 1985;128:383–388

22 Lacetti P, Grollman EF, Aloz SM, Kohn LD. Ganglioside-dependent return of TSH receptor function in a rat thyroid tumor with a TSH receptor defect. Biochem Biophys Res Comm 1983;110:772–778

23 Jessel T, Solter D, Dodd J. Monoclonal antibodies defining specific glycolipids on subsets of sensory neurons. Nature 1984;311:469–472

Retrovirus-Induced Lower Motor Neuron Disease in Mice: A Model for Amyotrophic Lateral Sclerosis and Human Spongiform Neurological Diseases

PAUL JOLICOEUR

A small number of human diseases are characterized by degeneration and loss of motor neurons from the anterior horn of the spinal cord and from the brain-stem. These include the motor neuron diseases, among which amyotrophic lateral sclerosis (ALS) is the most frequent, and acute poliomyelitis. The etiology of any of the motor neuron diseases and specifically of ALS has not yet been determined. Very few animal models of ALS exist. The neurotoxic models do not selectively induce motor neuron loss [1] and therefore are missing one of the major features of ALS. The wobbler (wr) [2, 3] and the motor neuron degeneration (Mnd) [4] mutant mice show motor neuron degeneration as a consequence of a genetic disorder transmitted, respectively, by an autosomal recessive and by an autosomal dominant gene. These genetic models appear relevant to ALS, but little is known about the pathophysiology of these diseases. The model most extensively studied, and probably quite relevant to ALS, remains the retrovirus-induced motor neuron disease of mice, discovered by Gardner's group in wild mice [5] and later by McCarter's group in laboratory animals [6]. We would like to review briefly the main features of this murine retrovirus-induced motor neuron disease and discuss the latest findings related to these unique viruses.

1. Characteristics of the Murine Motor Neuron Disease and Identification of Mouse Retroviruses

Retroviruses from Wild Mice

Excellent reviews on the identification of these viruses and on this murine model of motor neuron disease have previously been published

[7, 8]. In search of natural oncogenic retroviruses among feral mice, Gardner and collaborators trapped many wild mice (*Mus musculus domesticus*) from different areas in the Lake Casitas region of California. Some of these ageing mice spontaneously developed a progressive form of lower-limb paralysis [5]. This neurologic disease could be transmitted by cell-free extracts from brains of paralysed mice, as well as from filtered supernatants of infected tissue culture cells. These experiments strongly suggested that a virus was inducing this disease. Two classes of retroviruses could be isolated from tissues of these paralysed wild mice: amphotropic murine leukemia viruses (MuLVs) (able to replicate in mouse cells and in cell lines of several heterologous species) and N-tropic ecotropic MuLVs which replicate exclusively on $Fv-1^n$ mouse cells (see Section 3 for a discussion of Fv-1). Isolates of both viruses were cloned by cell culture techniques and only N-tropic ecotropic MuLVs were found to have a paralytogenic potential. These viruses could be propagated on mouse cells in culture without apparent loss of pathogenicity. One isolate (Cas-Br-E, also called Cas-Br-M) of these wild mouse ecotropic neurovirulent MuLVs has been used by most investigators and remains the best characterized to date.

The same ecotropic virus preparations could also induce various forms of leukemia (B-cell, T-cell, lymphoblastic, myelogenous, megakariocytic leukemia and erythroleukemia) in inoculated mice [7, 9]. Until the molecular cloning of the viral genome [10] (see below), it was unknown whether paralysis and leukemia were induced by two or more viruses or by a unique virus.

Clinically, the disease appearing spontaneously in wild mice is very similar to that induced experimentally by inoculation of viruses. Early in the disease, a fine rear-limb tremulousness and the appearance of rear-limb abduction reflex (when mice are suspended by the tail) are detected. These signs are followed by loss of splay and of extensor reflexes. This state is eventually followed by progressive (first proximal) bilateral, symmetric paralysis of lower limbs. A marked amyotrophy of the rear limbs and of the lumbar back region occurs, and a kyphosis is observed. The forelimbs are not affected. After the appearance of the first signs, 2–5 months post-inoculation, the course accelerates and the mouse dies usually rapidly (within a few weeks).

Experimentally, induction of the disease is very dependent on dose [11–13] and age [12, 13]. Only newborn mice are fully susceptible to the inoculated virus, older mice quickly developing a T-cell-mediated immune response to it [12, 14]. The same phenomenon occurs with leukemogenic non-paralytogenic MuLVs which can induce leukemia only if inoculated into newborn mice [15]. Inoculation of viruses can be done intraperitoneally, intravenously, or intracerebrally and all three routes are very efficient in inducing neurological disease in nearly 100% of susceptible mice within 2–5 months. The natural transmission of viruses among wild mice appears to be mainly through the milk, although it also occurs transplacentally [8, 16].

Little is known about the factors which modulate entry of the virus into the CNS. Viremia is required for the appearance of CNS pathology and the spleen appears the major organ of virus replication. Indeed, it has been found that splenectomy or passive immunization against MuLV prevents the appearance of paralysis [7, 17]. Whether the virus gains access to the CNS as free virus or through infected circulating hemato-poietic cells has not been studied rigorously. Most probably, brain cells remain sensitive to the deleterious effect of the virus later in life, as lesions appear 2–5 months following virus inoculation. However, fetal brain cells seem to be much more sensitive to the virus. A severe neu-rological disease has been observed within 25 days after birth in mice inoculated with the virus at day 8.75–9.0 of pregnancy [18]. Brain cells are still actively dividing in these embryos, presumably leading to higher virus replication and consequently to rapid neuronal degeneration.

Interestingly, no immune response was detected against the paraly-togenic ecotropic MuLV inoculated at birth. Serum-neutralizing anti-body activity was lacking and antibodies against various viral proteins could not be detected [19]. This immune tolerance appeared very specific to this paralytogenic MuLV strain and a normal humoral immune re-sponse against a non-viral antigen was detected. The absence of cellular inflammatory infiltration in the CNS lesions of paralysed mice inoculated with the virus at birth suggested that cellular immunity against the virus was absent. However, when the virus is inoculated later in life (10 days), no neurological disease develops and this resistance is mediated by a cellular immune response [14].

Laboratory-Derived Retroviruses

The Moloney strain of MuLV is a highly leukemogenic virus inducing T-cell leukemia [15]. Several temperature-sensitive mutants of Moloney MuLV were isolated *in vitro* [6]. They were subsequently assayed *in vivo* for their pathogenic potential. Unexpectedly, three of them (ts-1, ts-7, and ts-11) induced a lower-limb paralysis in 100% of the inoculated sus-ceptible mice within a very short latent period (34 days) [6]. Clinically, the disease was very similar to the one induced with wild-mouse retro-viruses. It is also age-dependent [6]. These three paralytogenic mutants were found to have a common defect in the processing of the *env* precursor protein Pr80^{eny}, at the restrictive temperature [20]. Recently, another ts mutant of Moloney MuLV (ts Mo BA-1) has been reported to induce a progressive neurodegenerative disease [21]. The clinical presentation was less severe and only a syndrome of tremor, weakness of the hindlimbs, and spasticity was observed. The processing of Pr80^{eny}, at the restrictive temperature, was normal in this mutant.

2. Pathology of the Retrovirus-Induced Neurological Disease

Detailed descriptions of the neuropathological changes observed in this retrovirus-induced lower motor neuron disease have been published [22–28]. In brief, the major alterations in the CNS are predominantly found in anterior horns of the lumbosacral spinal cord. In disease induced by ts-1 Moloney MuLV, lesions are also detected in cortex and cerebellum [28]. With ts Mo BA-1 MuLV, lesions were predominantly found in the cerebellar grey matter, brain-stem, and upper spinal cord [21, 29]. In disease induced experimentally by Cas-Br-E MuLV injection, dentate nucleus, brain-stem, and basal ganglia are also affected. Spongiform changes, predominant in grey matter, are the salient features of the disease. Cytoplasmic vacuolar changes are present both in neurons and in glial cells (astrocytes and mainly oligodendrocytes). Eventually, neuronal loss and gliosis occur. Typically, no inflammatory cells are present in the affected areas. Less severe spongiform changes also occur in myelinated tracts accompanied by loss of myelin. The onset of spongiform changes correlates with the maximum virus titre [30]. By electron microscopy, the vacuoles are found to be predominantly in the rough and smooth endoplasmic reticulum and seem to arise first in axonal and dendritic processes.

Early after infection, budding viruses are most frequently observed in vascular endothelial cells and in pericytes [24, 27, 30]. Both types of cells retain a normal morphology. Later, numerous typical type C viruses are seen in extracellular spaces in relation to capillaries. Rare virus particles have been seen in astrocytes [30], but no budding particles could be detected in these cells [27, 30]. Viral particles, with aberrant morphology, budding from rough endoplasmic reticulum cisternae can occasionally be observed in neurons, sometimes in great abundance, in mice inoculated with wild-mouse retrovirus [23, 25, 26, 30], but not in mice inoculated with ts-1 or ts BA-1 Moloney MuLV [6, 21, 28].

The budding viruses seen in endothelial cells and pericytes most likely represent the inoculated virus replicating in these cells in the absence of pathological changes. It is not clear whether viral particles seen in neurons and glial cells represent the replicating inoculated virus since

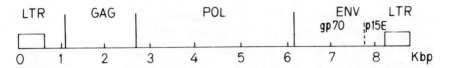

Structure of a retroviral DNA genome. The localization of the three viral genes, *gag*, *pol*, and *env*, is illustrated. The *env* gene encodes two distinct proteins, gp70 and p15E. LTR, long terminal repeat.

these particles exhibit an abnormal morphology and are not observed in mice inoculated with ts-1 Moloney MuLV. They might represent endogenous type C viruses induced by the pathological process. Such an explanation for the presence of these viral particles in neurons has been suggested before [23, 27, 30]. Most likely, the extracellular typical type C particles represent the inoculated viruses shed from the endothelial cells where they appear to replicate.

The histopathological lesions seen in this retrovirus-induced disease are similar to those observed in other transmissible spongiform encephalopathies, such as scrapie, Creutzfeldt-Jakob, Gerstmann-Sträussler, and Kuru [27, 31]. However, in human diseased tissues, type C particles are not found. Nevertheless, a similar underlying molecular mechanism might explain these two types of diseases.

3. Genetic Control of Retrovirus-Induced Lower Motor Neuron Disease

As soon as the disease was discovered, it became apparent that host factors were critical for its outcome [7, 8]. Indeed, not all trapped wild mice were susceptible to the neurological disease, strongly suggesting a role for host factors. Not surprisingly, the first gene to be identified as a major factor in the outcome of the paralysis was the Fv-1 gene [32]. This gene has two alleles, Fv-1^n and Fv-1^b, and almost every mouse strain harbours one or the other of these alleles, which were found to inhibit virus replication respectively of B-tropic and N-tropic MuLV [33]. This inhibition of virus replication prevents development of leukemia or lymphoma. The Fv-1 host range viral determinant has been mapped within *gag* p30 [34]. The Fv-1 gene product blocks virus replication at an early step of the virus cycle, by preventing supercoiled viral DNA formation [35, 36].

Crosses between wild mice (Fv-1^n) and C57BL/6 (Fv-1^b) mice revealed segregation of the resistance to paralysis with the Fv-1^b allele [32]. Further studies with inbred strains confirmed that the Fv-1 gene was critical in determining susceptibility to this disease, all the Fv-1^b mice tested

(A/ST, C57BL/6, BALB/C, BALB/ST, BALB/WEHI, and BALB/K, B10.D2) remaining free of disease after inoculation with the N-tropic Cas-Br-E MuLV [25, 26]. Together, these results on Fv-1 clearly indicated that virus replication was a prerequisite for the development of paralysis, an expected finding. A B-tropic (able to replicate in Fv-1^b mice) or NB-tropic (able to replicate in Fv-1^n and Fv-1^b mice) neurotropic MuLV would be needed to test the susceptibility of Fv-1^b mice to this neurological disease. We have recently constructed a chimeric NB-tropic virus whose genome harbours the NB-tropic p30 sequences from wild-type Moloney MuLV and the remaining sequences (*pol, env*, LTR) derived from the Cas-Br-E genome (Y. Paquette and P. Jolicoeur, unpublished). This chimeric virus should be instrumental in determining susceptibility of Fv-1^b mice to lower motor neuron disease. These studies would also be feasible with the NB-tropic paralytogenic ts Moloney MuLV [6, 21]. No complete genetic study on mouse susceptibility to ts-1 Moloney MuLV has been reported: the CFW/D, CBA/H, C3H/Bi/Ka, NIH/Swiss mice were found to be highly susceptible to the neurological disease [6]. However, the C57BL/6 mouse was found to be totally resistant to the paralysis-inducing potential of ts-1 MuLV, despite the fact that virus replication occurred in these mice [6]. Similarly, NFS, SJL, and CBA mice were susceptible to ts BA-1 MuLV, but C57BL/10 mice were resistant [21]. Such results strongly suggest that C57BL/6 mice harbour one or several genes of resistance which do not affect virus replication but affect the disease process itself.

Although most wild mice are N-tropic, only a fraction (10%) of the virus-positive mice developed paralysis [7, 8]. Much of this restriction could be attributed to another gene, Akvr-1^r [37]. This gene is unique to wild mice and apparently identical to the Fv-4 gene identified in Japanese wild mice (*Mus molossinus*) and some Japanese inbred mice (FRG strain) [38]. The gene appears to be unique [39] and confers a dominant restriction to virus replication in wild mice. The gene product is an *env* glycoprotein (gp70) which occupies the cell-surface receptor for ecotropic MuLV, thus blocking penetration of infecting ecotropic MuLV [40, 41].

Several Fv-1^n inbred mouse strains have been tested for susceptibility to Cas-Br-E MuLV–induced paralysis [25, 26, 42, 43]. Substantial variation in susceptibility to the disease has been observed, the most susceptible mice being SWR/J and NFS, closely followed by SIM.S and various strains of C3H, DBA/2, CBA, C57BR/cd, and HAICR mice appeared to be less susceptible, developing disease after a longer latency and/or at a lower frequency. Three Fv-1^n strains, AKR, NZB, and C58, were found to be resistant to Cas-Br-E MuLV–induced paralysis, most likely as a consequence of their high endogenous viremic state which prevents infection by newly inoculated ecotropic MuLV [43]. Breeding experiments between NFS and DBA/2 mice suggested that the long-latency phenotype was a semidominant trait, possibly determined by two or more independently assorting loci [43].

No other gene affecting the outcome of this neurological disease has yet been identified. The H-2 locus has been studied and was found to be not involved [25, 26]. Whether the gene controlling the latency of scrapie in mice [44] will also be involved in controlling the appearance of MuLV-induced spongiform degeneration is not known. Since the pathological features of both diseases are quite similar (non-inflammatory spongiform changes), it might be possible to identify a gene affecting this apparently similar process in both diseases.

Inducing disease with the Cas-Br-E or ts-1 Moloney MuLV in other species has been attempted. Among several species tested, only the rat was found to be slightly susceptible to the Cas-Br-E MuLV–induced disease [8], but not to the ts-1 Moloney MuLV–induced disease [6]. These results indicate a requirement for a specific interaction of the viral sequences and/or the viral gene products with specific mouse target factors not highly conserved in other species. Probably this species specificity reflects the replication potential of the virus in each species.

When considering the genetic control of this disease, the most interesting genes to identify would be genes affecting the pathological process itself. These genes would not be expected to control virus replication, and would be expected to be conserved and operating in other species, including man. Developing a model to identify such genes in the mouse appears to be important.

4. Molecular Cloning of the Etiological Agent of the Disease

Gardner's group identified the etiologic agent as being a retrovirus of the ecotropic family. However, since the virus was only cloned biologically, another passenger virus could have remained undetected and been responsible for this novel disease [23]. This hypothesis was especially plausible in view of the spongiform nature of the CNS degeneration which resembles lesions found in scrapie. To rule out this possibility, we therefore decided to clone molecularly the genome of the ecotropic MuLV present in a culture supernatant able to induce paralysis when inoculated into susceptible mice [10]. Our cloned viral DNAs were microinjected into NIH 3T3 cells and were tested for their ability to generate the production of infectious viral particles. Viruses derived from these DNAs were found to have the same biological characteristics as the parental MuLV and induced paralysis and leukemia if inoculated to newborn animals [10]. This work demonstrated conclusively that the virus responsible for paralysis belonged indeed to the retrovirus class. Additionally, the requirement of other agents for the propagation of the disease was excluded: i.e. agents which could have eluded detection and separation from N-tropic MuLV by the biological technique available at the time of the isolation of the virus.

Subsequently, the genomes of the paralytogenic ts-1 and ts-7 Moloney MuLVs were also molecularly cloned [45]. The viruses recovered from these clones were also shown to induce paralysis as the parental virus [45]. The availability of infectious molecular clones of the paralytogenic viral genomes enables their further characterization. A physical restriction map of the genomes could be derived [10, 45]. In our laboratory, we could also start sequencing important regions of Cas-Br-E MuLV genome, and derive probes specific to this neurotropic viral genome [46].

Isolation and Characterization of Env-Specific and U3 LTR–Specific Probes from Cas-Br-E MuLV

Two reasons motivated us to develop probes which would be specific to the neurotropic Cas-Br-E MuLV genome [46]. The first was the prospect that such probes would allow detection of specific Cas-Br-E viral mRNA or DNA sequences without detecting other homologous sequences from the endogenous mouse viral sequences. These endogenous viral sequences are quite abundant in the mouse genome and constitute a serious background problem for the detection of newly acquired viral sequences of an infectious retrovirus. Availability of such probes should be instrumental in the study of different aspects of the virus cycle in various tissues. The second reason to derive these probes was to determine the origin of the 'neurotropic' gp70 sequences. We reasoned that these probes would be required to determine whether these viral sequences were endogenous to normal murine cells and whether they were homologous to other known sequences, such as neurotoxins or neuronal growth factors.

We first chose to investigate the *env* region, which appeared to be unique by restriction analysis [46, 47]. The probes NE-8A and NE-8B were derived from the *env* region and they both hybridized exclusively to homologous Cas-Br-E DNA at high stringency and not to any other MuLV DNA genomes tested, namely amphotropic, Moloney, BALB/c endogenous ecotropic, and non-ecotropic MuLVs, or radiation leukemia viruses [46].

The U3 LTR region of each MuLV is unique and has been shown to determine the tissue [48] and disease [49–51] specificity of these viruses.

Using this LTR region, we derived a probe specific to the Cas-Br-E MuLV U3 LTR [46]. At high stringency, it hybridized to homologous Cas-Br-E MuLV DNA, as expected, but not to other endogenous MuLV LTRs. However, it also hybridized to amphotropic 4070-A and Moloney MuLV DNAs, strongly suggesting that these three viruses are part of the same family (see below).

5. Origin of the Cas-Br-E Neurotropic Wild Mouse Retrovirus

The Cas-Br-E MuLV and other similar paralytogenic MuLVs were isolated from the brains of paralysed wild mice. Among the mammalian retroviruses, the ability to induce a neurological disease is a rare characteristic. Therefore, knowledge of their origin appears important. Using the *env*-specific probes, which encompass a large portion of the region known to harbour the determinant of paralysis, we could not detect any fragment hybridizing with these probes in several mouse strain DNAs tested [46], suggesting the these *env* sequences were not part of the normal genome of *M. musculus*. Therefore, these neurotropic *env* sequences were unlikely to have been captured by recombination with endogenous mouse sequences, unless such sequences were present in the genome of some wild mice. An indication of the origin of these viruses was obtained when a good restriction map became available. Clearly, the paralytogenic MuLV genome had a restriction map quite similar to those of amphotropic and Moloney MuLVs. Derivation of our U3 LTR–specific probe also indicated that amphotropic, neurotropic, and Moloney MuLV U3 LTR were homologous [46]. Moreover, sequencing of the Cas-Br-E LTR [46] showed a remarkable similarity to that of Moloney MuLV. Together, these results suggested that these three viruses belong to the same family.

Interestingly, amphotropic non-paralytogenic MuLVs were isolated from the same wild mice from which paralytogenic MuLVs were discovered [7]. These paralytogenic viruses have probably emerged by successive additions of point mutations, small insertions, and deletions within the *pol-env* region of the genome of amphotropic MuLV. Amphotropic MuLVs appear to be present in the population of wild mice as exogenous retroviruses, since their genome was previously found to be absent from the normal mouse genome [52]. Our data tend to confirm these findings. Indeed, the Cas-Br-E MuLV U3 LTR probe, whose sequence is identical (except for five non-clustered point mutations) to the corresponding U3 LTR sequences from amphotropic MuLV (Friedrich, personal communication), could not detect homologous endogenous viral sequences at high stringency. It appears that amphotropic MuLV, the putative progenitor of Cas-Br-E MuLV, is not endogenous to *M. musculus*. Its origin remains unknown. It could have originated from another species and established itself in some wild mice. Alternatively, an endogenous provirus could have sustained multiple genetic alterations and evolved to the point of appearing as an exogenous genome.

This last hypothesis of an evolving virus which acquires new biological properties is quite plausible and is strengthened by the isolation of the paralytogenic ts-1 and ts-7 Moloney MuLVs from a stock of wild-type Moloney MuLV [6]. The genomes of the mutants and wild-type Moloney MuLVs are highly homologous by restriction endonuclease mapping [45].

6. Physical Mapping of the Primary Determinant of the Spongiform Neurological Degeneration

Since these paralytogenic MuLVs induce disease in susceptible mice, we expected that some viral sequences were responsible for the paralysis-inducing potential of these viruses. These sequences could code for protein or could be non-coding. We thought that the identification of these sequences would help in understanding the molecular basis of this disease. To map the paralysis-inducing sequences on the viral genome, we constructed chimeric viruses whose genomes were derived from parental paralytogenic and non-paralytogenic MuLVs [42]. We took advantage of the diversity of MuLVs found in nature and of the similarity of their restriction maps.

We chose the non-paralytogenic 4070-A amphotropic MuLV and the paralytogenic Cas-Br-E MuLV. These two viruses have very distinct paralysis-inducing potential and have similar restriction endonuclease maps. Therefore, these two parental MuLVs appeared suitable to identify the viral sequences responsible for the spongiform degeneration, by constructing chimeric viruses. The first three recombinants (pNEA-1, pNEA-2, and pNEA-3) helped us to identify which region of the genome was critical for the appearance of the disease. Indeed only the first chimeric pNEA-1 MuLV induced paralysis. It was constructed with the *pol-env* fragment from Cas-Br-E MuLV and the LTR-*gag-pol* region from amphotropic MuLV. Therefore these results indicated that the *pol-env* fragment of Cas-Br-E MuLV was sufficient and necessary to transfer the paralysis-inducing potential to chimeric MuLVs.

Using a similar approach, the determinant of paralysis of the ts-1 paralytogenic Moloney MuLV was first mapped within a 1.6 kbp *pol-env*-fragment. [53]. The same region was found to control the processing of Pr80[eny] (impaired in this mutant) and the temperature sensitivity of the virus. The construction of additional recombinants, however, revealed that, in fact, two functionally distinct regions of the ts-1 genome were responsible for its paralytogenic ability [54]. One of the regions comprises the end of *pol* and the 5' half of *env*, while the other, comprising the two-thirds carboxy terminal of *env*, the LTR, and 5' leader sequences, determined the enhanced neurotropism of ts-1.

We [108] have constructed additional chimeric viruses to narrow down the region of the Cas-Br-E viral genome harbouring the determinant of paralysis. All chimeric viral genomes were constructed with the LTR and *gag-pol* regions derived from the amphotropic MuLV and with the *env* region from Cas-Br-E MuLV. Biological assays of these recombinant viruses have allowed us to map the determinant of paralysis within a single region, the gp70. We could exclude the *pol* gene in its entirety, most of the leader peptide of the *env* gene product, as well as most of *env* p15E region, as contributing to the paralytogenic phenotype. Therefore, the gp70, which is found at the surface of the virion anchored in its membrane, and which is responsible for the binding of the virus to its cellular receptor, harbours the determinant of neurovirulence of Cas-Br-E MuLV.

Sequencing of this region [46] revealed the structure of a typical retroviral gp70 quite homologous to other gp70 molecules from Moloney, ecotropic AKR, or Friend MuLVs. All the cysteine residues and most of the glycosylation sites have been conserved. However, several amino acid differences (mutations and small deletions) could be observed all along the molecule unlike the corresponding sequences from other non-paralytogenic MuLVs. These numerous changes precluded the precise mapping of the determinant of spongiform degeneration by simple analysis of the sequences. The construction of finer recombinants within the gp70 region will be needed to map this determinant within a specific domain of gp70.

Whether the same region of ts-1 Moloney MuLV is responsible for its paralytogenic potential is not clear at the moment, since at least two distinct regions of its genome appear to be required to induce paralysis [54]. Nor is it known if these two viruses, Cas-Br-E and ts-1 MuLVs, induce disease by the same mechanism.

7. Physical Mapping of the Determinant Involved in the Preferential Targeting of the Virus to Motor Neurons of the Anterior Horn

That the primary determinant of neurovirulence mapped within the *env* region and not within the LTR was unexpected. Indeed, previous work in our and other laboratories had demonstrated that the U3 LTR enhancer sequences played a critical role in targeting the virus into specific cell populations such as thymocytes [48], and in determining the leukemogenic potential [55, 56] and the disease specificity [49–51] of several strains of MuLVs. We were not detecting such a role for the LTR with Cas-Br-E/amphotropic chimeric viruses. The amphotropic LTR sequences used in the construction of our chimeric viruses could have been functionally similar to those of Cas-Br-E MuLV, thus masking the detection of secondary determinants of paralysis within these sequences in our previous study. To test this hypothesis and to determine whether the tropism of Cas-Br-E MuLV for anterior horn cells was determined by its LTR, we constructed another chimeric MuLV (pNEMO-1) harbouring the primary determinant of neurovirulence (the *gag-pol-env* sequences of Cas-Br-E MuLV) and the LTR-containing fragment from the strongly T-cell tropic leukemogenic non-paralytogenic Moloney MuLV [57]. We chose this LTR for several reasons: it is known to be a highly efficient promotor; it was found to harbour determinants of disease specificity (T-cell leukemia) [49–51]; it belongs to the same family of LTR as do Cas-Br-E and amphotropic MuLVs, as found by hybridization and sequencing [46]; it had some convenient restriction sites to construct the chimeric molecules easily.

Infectious pNEMO-1 viruses were recovered from the supernatant of microinjected NIH 3T3 cells, titrated, and appropriately characterized by restriction enzyme analysis of their unintegrated viral DNA.

Leukemogenic Potential and Novel Tissue Tropism of pNEMO-1 MuLV

To determine whether pNEMO-1 MuLV had a different tissue tropism than the parental Cas-Br-E MuLV and to assess the target lymphoid cells being transformed, we first studied its leukemogenic potential [57]. As expected, the parental Moloney MuLV was found to be highly leukemogenic and the majority (53/59) of the Moloney MuLV-induced leukemias were of the thymic form. The true incidence of leukemia with Cas-Br-E MuLV was difficult to ascertain because most of the inoculated mice died early from neurological disease before getting leukemia. Nevertheless, leukemia developed in some of the mice inoculated intraperitoneally or intrathymically and, in contrast with those observed with Moloney MuLV, most (10/13) of the Cas-Br-E MuLV–induced leukemias were of the non-thymic form.

The pNEMO-1 chimeric MuLV induced leukemia in most NIH/Swiss mice inoculated intraperitoneally. Half of these were of the thymic form. It was also leukemogenic but to a lesser degree for SIM.S and SWR/J mice. Intrathymic inoculation of pNEMO-1 MuLV induced early neurological disorders in a large proportion of the inoculated mice. Nevertheless, leukemia developed early enough to be detected in nearly half of the inoculated mice of the three strains. The majority of these leukemias (13 of 19) were of the thymic form. These results indicated that pNEMO-1 MuLV had a different lymphoid tissue tropism than Cas-Br-E MuLV and that the *Pvu* I–*Cla* I LTR-containing fragment of Moloney MuLV was responsible for this new tissue tropism. This fragment harbours sequences determining this disease specificity, in confirmation of previous results [49–51].

Low Incidence of Neurological Disorders Induced by pNEMO-1 MuLV Inoculated Intraperitoneally

Surprisingly, the chimeric pNEMO-1 MuLV induced only a low incidence of neurological disease in susceptible mice [57]. However, of the few mice that developed neurological disorders with this virus, most did not have a typical hindlimb paralysis but exhibited a neurological disorder usually not seen with the parental Cas-Br-E MuLV. These mice had no hindlimb paralysis, were excessively tremulous and spastic, and tended to remain immobile for a long period of time. These results indicated that pNEMO-1 MuLV was less pathogenic for the CNS than the parental Cas-Br-E MuLV when inoculated intraperitoneally. They also showed that the virus induced a different form of neurological disease in the few mice that were affected. Somehow, the 1.0 kbp *Cla*I–*Pvu*I Moloney fragment was responsible for this new phenotype.

Effect of Intrathymic Inoculation on the Incidence of Neurological Disorders Induced by pNEMO-1 MuLV

To determine the effect of the route of injection on the CNS pathogenicity, pNEMO-1 MuLV and control parental MuLVs were inoculated intrathymically. Intrathymic inoculation of the parental Cas-Br-E MuLV was very effective in inducing a typical hindlimb paralysis in most mice [57]. After intrathymic inoculation, the chimeric pNEMO-1 MuLV induced neurological disorders in a large proportion of the inoculated mice after shorter latent periods than those seen with parental Cas-Br-E MuLV. The majority (21/28) of these neurological disorders were, however, atypical, and of the same type as those described above, showing no hindlimb paralysis. These results indicated that the incidence of neurological disease induced by pNEMO-1 MuLV was significantly enhanced, in the three mouse strains studied, if the virus was inoculated intrathymically. More interesting, these data showed that pNEMO-1 MuLV had the propensity to induce a different form of neurological disease, not usually seen with the parental Cas-Br-E MuLV.

Distribution of CNS Lesions in Cas-Br-E and pNEMO-1 MuLV–Induced Neurological Disorders

Since Cas-Br-E and pNEMO-1 MuLVs induced clinically distinct neurological disorders, the distribution of the lesions in brains of mice developing each clinical form of the disease was studied [57]. We found that both viruses induced spongiform degeneration. In both clinical forms, both viruses extensively destroyed the brain-stem and deep cerebellar nuclei, but hippocampi and cerebellar cortex were always spared. The pontine and medullary tegmental nuclei were most severely involved in brain-stem structures. Mild extension into adjacent white matter was noted. In the atypical syndrome (tremulousness, spasticity, immobility) caused by pNEMO-1 MuLV, lesions were multifocal and more extensive in fronto-temporo-parietal cortices, striatum, and thalamus than those found in the paralytic syndrome induced by Cas-Br-E MuLV. These results suggested that the different topography of the spongiform lesions correlated with the specific clinical manifestations seen after inoculation of these two viruses.

Together, these results indicate that the 1 kbp *Cla* I–*Pvu*-I LTR-containing fragment of Cas-Br-E MuLV harbours a determinant of target cell specificity which results in the induction of lesions preferentially in anterior horns. We know that the target specificity is conserved even when the virus is inoculated intraperitoneally or intracerebrally. Interestingly, the Cas-Br-E MuLV LTR is remarkably similar to the Moloney MuLV LTR [46, 58]. Only one small addition and few point mutations distinguish the two sequences. Nevertheless, these few changes are sufficient to change the specificity of the virus within the lymphoid system and within the CNS when the LTR are exchanged. Presumably, factors in cortical cells can distinguish the LTR sequences from these two MuLVs.

The paralytogenic ts-1 Moloney MuLV has a strong tropism for the anterior horns [6, 28]. A 2.3 kbp fragment which includes the LTR has been reported to be necessary for induction of the disease [54]. It would therefore be interesting to find out whether its LTR differs from that of the wild-type Moloney MuLV and whether it has acquired a specificity for anterior horns.

8. What Are the Target Cells for the Neurovirulent Retroviruses in the Anterior Horn?

A good understanding of the pathophysiology of the retrovirus-induced spongiform degeneration of the CNS will require the identification of the target cells for virus replication as well as the target cells which sustain the pathological process and degeneration. The two populations are not necessarily the same. One of the target cell populations, known to be affected by the pathological process, is certainly the motor neurons from the anterior horn which sustain spongiform changes, as shown by light and electron microscopic examination. The question remains whether virus replicate in the anterior horn motor neurons. Particles and budding type-C virions with aberrant morphology have been seen in neurons of mice inoculated with Cas-Br-E MuLV, an observation which led some investigators to suggest that Cas-Br-E MuLV replicates in neurons [26]. This was a very provocative suggestion in view of the fact that retroviruses are known to require at least one cell mitosis to integrate their proviruses into host chromosomal DNA [59], and that mammalian neurons are thought to be non-dividing after birth. However, since every mouse species harbours several copies of endogenous proviruses, an alternative possibility would be that the viral particles observed in neurons represent endogenous retroviruses and not the inoculated neurovirulent MuLV. Such endogenous retroviruses have been found to be induced in various conditions [60]. *In situ* hybridization with probes specific to the neurovirulent viral genome (such as the ones we derived [46]) or immunohistochemistry with antibodies specific to Cas-Br-E MuLV will be needed to identify the cell type(s) replicating the inoculated MuLV.

In contrast to what was observed with Cas-Br-E MuLV, no virus particles were seen in anterior horn motor neurons from mice inoculated with the paralytogenic ts-1 Moloney MuLV [6, 28], suggesting that neurons do not replicate the inoculated neurovirulent MuLV. Further studies are required to clarify this point and to understand why virus particles are seen in neurons from mice inoculated with one virus (Cas-Br-E) and not with the other one (ts-1). Virus particles have also been observed in glial cells of Cas-Br-E–inoculated mice. In fact, the virus is thought to get into the CNS first through endothelial cells. Whether these are the primary target cells for the virus remains unknown.

Our study with the chimeric pNEMO-1 MuLV (harbouring Moloney MuLV LTR and *gag-pol-env* from Cas-Br-E MuLV) indicated that the ability of the virus to induce lesions in the anterior horn was determined by the Cas-Br-E MuLV LTR. By exchanging this LTR for the Moloney

LTR, the virus induced lesions in a different CNS area, not affected by the wild-type Cas-Br-E MuLV, namely cortex, striatum, and thalamus [57]. It seems that we have modified the virus so that it replicates in a novel class of target cells. Therefore, target cells present in the anterior horn are functionally different from the target cells in other CNS areas, such as cortex. The most likely explanation for their differences is the presence of factor(s) in anterior horn cells that are able to recognize specifically the Cas-Br-E LTR enhancer/promotor region, thus increasing replication of the virus. Identifying these target cells is of great importance. If they are neurons, it would confirm and extend the notion that these motor neurons form a functionally distinct class of neurons, being specifically selected as a target by an incoming virus over other neurons, such as cortical neurons. It will remain to find out whether proviruses integrate into these presumably non-dividing cells. If the target cells replicating the virus in the anterior horn are not the motor neurons themselves, then our experiment indicates that non-neuronal cells have functional specificity within the CNS (able to replicate Cas-Br-E MuLV preferentially over pNEMO-1 MuLV), a concept with wide implications. It would also indicate that the degeneration of neurons is caused by an indirect mechanism through viral replication within surrounding non-neuronal cells. The identification of the target cells replicating these neurovirulent MuLVs might lead to concepts applicable to a wide range of problems in the neurosciences.

9. Proposed Model for Retrovirus-Induced Lower Motor Neuron Disease

At present, little is known regarding retrovirus-induced lower motor neuron disease in mice. However, progress made in the last few years with the molecularly cloned chimeric viruses has provided sufficient information to formulate novel hypotheses. We would like to propose a model to explain this disease. The main feature of the model rests on the observation that the primary determinant of neuronal degeneration mapped within the *env* gp70 sequences. We have shown that this region is necessary and sufficient to induce specific spongiform changes in CNS [42, 108]. Another important aspect of the model is the presence of a second determinant of neurological disease identified within the LTR region of Cas-Br-E MuLV genome. These sequences determine in which region of the CNS (cortex, striatum, anterior horn) the spongiform degeneration will occur [57], but are not sufficient by themselves to induce a neurological disease.

We propose that, following viremia which occurs soon after inoculation, the neurovirulent virus infects many different types of cells in different areas of the CNS. However, replication of viruses, largely determined by their LTR, will occur significantly only in CNS cells encoding cell-specific factors able to recognize these LTR sequences. These cells could be neuronal or non-neuronal. With the Cas-Br-E MuLV LTR, these target cells are localized preferentially in the anterior horn of the spinal cord. Of course, this virus replication alone would be insufficient to induce neuronal degeneration: expression of a specific neurotoxic gp70 molecule is required. Neuronal degeneration might be induced by gp70 present on the virions or by free gp70. Free gp70 has indeed been found in mouse serum [61] and can presumably bind to the virus receptor. The deleterious effect of gp70 might occur in the target infected cells replicating the virus. Since neurons are the degenerating cells, this will indicate that neurons replicate the virus. Alternatively, free or virion-associated gp70, shed outside the cell, might affect other surrounding cells (paracrine model). In other words, the infected target cells replicating the virus need not necessarily be the cells degenerating. This would be compatible with the numerous type C particles seen in the extracellular spaces.

The only well-known function of gp70 of retroviruses is to recognize a cellular receptor to initiate infection. We propose that the Cas-Br-E MuLV gp70 produces its deleterious effect through binding to a neuron-specific cellular receptor. Obviously, this receptor would have a normal function in neuron metabolism. It would also have a normal physiological ligand, possibly a trophic factor, essential for neuron function and/or survival. The gp70 could compete for this trophic factor on the receptor, thus preventing its action. Since virions are probably too large to occupy all the receptors on a cell surface, free gp70 would be more likely to be involved in such competition. Alternatively, the gp70 (free or virion-associated) could occupy a fraction of the receptors on the cell surface and interfere with their normal function.

The spongiform degeneration of neurons might be the consequence of an electrolyte imbalance [27]. Therefore likely candidate receptors with which gp70 might interfere would be the ion-channel receptors. Binding of Cas-BR-E MuLV gp70 could inappropriately lead to opening of such receptors, ion movements, and water entry into the cell. Interestingly, the neuronal spongiosis induced by ouabain [62], a specific inhibitor of Na^+-K^+-activated ATPase, was thought to resemble the retroviruses-induced vacuolization [27] in its similar disruption of Golgi apparatus and of rough endoplasmic reticulum. Alternatively, if the early lesions leading to spongiform changes are the 'synthesis of large amount membrane constituents (multilaminated membranes)' [63], the receptor might be a growth factor receptor. Under abnormal stimulation, this receptor might lead to inappropriate synthesis of membranes or to synthesis of abnormal membranes, both conditions presumably eventually leading to a change in plasma membrane permeability [63].

This model assumes that Cas-Br-E gp70 has evolved to the point of recognizing a normal physiologically important receptor. This concept is not novel and several viral proteins have been shown to recognize such receptors [64, 65]. The Epstein Barr gp350/220 viral protein has been found to recognize and use the B lymphocyte C3d complement receptor for infection [66, 67]; the rabies glycoprotein appears to bind to the acetylcholine receptor [68, 69]; the HIV-1 utilizes the CD4 receptor [70–72]; cytomegalovirus can use class I HLA molecules as a virus receptor [73]; the Semliki forest virus uses the H-2K or H-2D histocompatibility antigens as receptors [74]; the lactate dehydrogenase virus uses the Ia antigen as receptor [75]; the vaccinia virus encodes a polypeptide related to epidermal growth factor (EGF) which can bind the cell EGF receptor and stimulates its autophosphorylation [76, 77]; the neuronal or lymphoid reovirus type 3 receptor seems similar to the β-adrenergic hormone receptor [78] and the same virus has been shown to use the M-N blood group antigen, glycophorin, as its receptor on erythrocytes [79].

We know very little about the role of the *env* gene products of retroviruses. The primary determinant of pathogenicity has been mapped within *env* on only three retroviruses: SFFV, HIV-1, and Cas-Br-E MuLV. The spleen focus-forming virus (SFFV) induces erythroleukemia in mice and the *env* gp55 molecule, responsible for erythroblast transformation, needs to bind to a cell receptor to exert its transforming action [109], probably by mimicking an erythroblast growth factor. The HIV-1 *env* gene product binds to the normal CD4 receptor [70–72] and this binding is required for cell fusion [72, 80] and appears an important component of the disease process. In addition, the gp70 of highly leukemogic MuLVs, including Cas-Br-E MuLV [81], have been shown to contribute to leukemogenesis [51, 82]. They may do this by stimulating a specific receptor on target cells (lymphoid or other hematopoietic cells).

Since some retrovirus *env* gene products have been shown to exert their action through a cell receptor, it is not unreasonable to suggest that Cas-Br-E gp70 might act through a similar process. If correct, this model could help to identify this receptor and its physiological ligand in the CNS. Also, the proposed model has the advantage of being consistent with one major feature of the pathological process, the absence of inflammation. Many hypotheses formulated here are experimentally testable.

10. Is Retrovirus-Induced Lower Motor Neuron Disease a Good Model for ALS?

Clinically, this mouse model is quite good, and it resembles human ALS especially because of prominent amyotrophy. This clinical presentation reflects the preferential degeneration of anterior horn motor neurons found in these mice and in ALS. In both the mouse disease and human ALS, the pathology is non-inflammatory and the immunological reactions are minimal.

The major difference between these two diseases resides in the type of pathological changes. In contrast to the extensive spongiform lesions found in murine anterior horns, the most frequent pathology found in classical ALS is a loss of neurons with some gliosis, in the absence of spongiform changes. However, vacuolar changes have been observed in rare cases of human infantile motor neuron disease [83, 84], and more frequently in the cortices of patients with ALS-dementia [85], suggesting that the mouse model might be relevant to these syndromes. Moreover, the extent of vacuolar changes might be a reflection of the acuteness of the neuronal degeneration. We recently observed significantly less spongiform change in mice expressing only low level of Cas-Br-E MuLV gp70 (unpublished results). In these mice, neuronal loss with some gliosis was the main characteristic of the lesions, as in ALS.

In summary, the targeting of anterior horn motor neurons with Cas-Br-E MuLV represents a good model for the specific destruction of motor neurons seen in ALS. Whether the different pathological changes seen in both diseases reflect different etiologic agents and a different molecular mechanism of cell death remain to be determined.

11. Is Retrovirus-Induced Spongiform Myeloencephalopathy a Good Model for Other Neurological Degenerative Diseases?

We have shown that the exchange of a short LTR-containing region on Cas-Br-E MuLV genome is sufficient to induce a different clinical disease [57]. Pathologically, the distribution of spongiform lesions was found in novel areas of the CNS (such as cortex, striatum, and thalamus), not usually affected by the wild-type Cas-Br-E MuLV. This experiment provided evidence that the same etiological agent has the ability to induce a wide variety of clinical syndromes if appropriately modulated.

Creutzfeldt-Jakob, Gerstmann-Sträussler Syndrome and Kuru

With the evidence that spongiform lesions could be generated in cortical areas, this retrovirus-induced neurological disease represents an attractive model for the human spongiform encephalopathies (Creutzfeldt-Jakob, Gerstmann-Sträussler syndrome and Kuru) [31]. In both diseases, the vacuolar pathological lesions appear identical. These specific vacuolar changes, in absence of inflammation, are a rare neuropathological finding. Furthermore, the underlying molecular mechanisms of neuronal vacuolar degeneration might be similar in man and mouse. The etiological agent of the human spongiform encephalopathies was found to be transmissible [86] and does not appear to be a retrovirus [87, 88]. Nevertheless, the prion itself or another putative protein (not yet identified) of this unusual agent might also interact with a neuronal receptor and induce this vacuolar degeneration, as we hypothesized in the previous section for the mouse retrovirus-induced disease. Interestingly, variants of Cruetzfeldt-Jakob disease with motor neuron involvement have been described [85, 89]. Such syndromes appear to present great resemblance to the mouse model.

AIDS

AIDS is frequently associated with a neurological disease [90]. The AIDS-dementia complex is thought to be induced by HIV-1. A significant inflammatory component is part of most AIDS encephalopathies. In this regard, they appear quite distinct from the mouse model. However, spongiform lesions, in absence of inflammatory cells, are characteristics of the AIDS myelopathies [91, 92] which occur in about 20% of the AIDS neurological diseases, and of some cases of AIDS encephalopathy [93]. For these specific AIDS myelopathies, the mouse model might be very relevant. Both human and mouse myelopathies show spongiform degeneration without inflammation. In AIDS myelopathies, spongiform changes in the spinal cord are predominantly in the white matter, most severe in lateral and posterior columns. Although the spongiform lesions induced by the murine retrovirus are predominantly in the grey matter in the anterior horns, spongiform lesions have also frequently been seen in the white matter and in lateral columns. Moreover, both diseases are presumably induced by a retrovirus and both viruses (Cas-Br-E and HIV-1) appear to harbour the determinant of pathogenicity within their *env* gene. Interestingly, the HIV-1 gp120, which shows some homology with a neurotrophic factor, neuroleukin, has been found to inhibit some of its biological actions [94].

Alzheimer's Disease

Anterior horn dysfunction [95] and spongiform changes [96, 97] have been detected in rare cases of Alzheimer's disease. However, the typical lesions (neurofibrillary tangles and senile plaques) found in Alzheimer's disease are notably absent in the murine disease. Interestingly, however, the major protein subunit (A4) of the amyloid fibril of tangles resembles a glycosylated cell-surface receptor [98]. Whether the Cas-Br-E MuLV–induced disease will be instrumental in understanding some aspects of Alzheimer's disease remains an open question.

12. Is a Retrovirus the Etiological Agent of ALS?

The etiology of ALS remains unknown and may be multifactoral. Because of the epidemiological features of the disease and its clinical course, an infectious agent has long been considered to be a good candidate for its etiology [99–101]. Charcot, who first described the disease, apparently thought it was 'infectious.' Today, despite the numerous failures to find a virus in ALS patients, viruses remain high on the list of putative etiological agents. And the negative results of the last decades cannot be used as an argument against the viral hypothesis. What we have learned in virology during this time emphasizes the point. (1) The absence of viral particles in the diseased tissues does not indicate absence of viral infection. Several viruses, including retroviruses, can infect cells and remain in a latent form, expressing only part of their viral genes, thus preventing the formation of virus particles. (2) The absence of an inflammatory reaction seen in ALS lesions can no longer be used as an indication of absence of viral infection. The Cruetzfeldt-Jakob/Kuru transmissible agent and the neurovirulent murine retroviruses induce neurological diseases in the absence of inflammatory reactions in the affected lesions and even in the absence of a general immune response. (3) Likewise, the failure to transmit ALS to primates or other mammals [99, 100] does not indicate that viruses are not involved, like any negative result. Viral infection might be present but infectious particles might be absent. Or the host range of the virus might be very restricted. For example, AIDS has not yet been transmitted to other species, despite the fact that several animal species have been inoculated with very high titres of pure virus (HIV-1) preparations. Only chimpanzees have been reported to replicate the virus, but they do not develop the disease [102].

ALS is characterized by a very specific degeneration of the motor neurons. Can viruses have such specific target cells? The answer is 'yes.' The polio virus specifically attacks human anterior horn motor neurons. The neurovirulent mouse retroviruses (Cas-Br-E, ts-1 and ts-7 Moloney MuLVs) also have this strict tropism for anterior horn motor neurons. Indeed, viruses endowed with strong tropism for motor neurons do exist.

Many known viruses have been considered as putative etiologic agents of ALS [103]. None of them has been convincingly shown to be involved in ALS. In view of recent findings, retroviruses should be considered good candidates for inducing ALS. (a) The human retrovirus HTLV-I or a related viral strain has now been shown to be involved in the development of myelopathies in man (HTLV-I–associated myelopathy (Ham)) [104, 105]. (b) Another human retrovirus, HIV-I, is now recognized as having a strong tropism for the CNS and many neurological abnormalities are associated with AIDS [90, 106], including a vacuolar myelopathy [91, 92] and vacuolar encephalopathy [93]. (c) A syndrome, indistinguishable from classical ALS, has been reported in an AIDS patient, and an HIV-I isolate was recovered from this patient [107]. Although the presence of these two syndromes in the same patient might be coincidental, this association remains quite suggestive. (d) Mice spontaneously develop a lower motor disease induced by retroviruses, a model mimicking many features of ALS. Since at least four different human retrovirus strains (HTLV-I, HTLV-II, HIV-I, HIV-2) have now been isolated, it would not be surprising to identify another one having the properties of the mouse neurovirulent retroviruses and inducing ALS.

13. Conclusions

Very few animal models perfectly mimic a human disease. The retrovirus-induced motor neuron disease in mice represents a model which presents several interesting features of different human neurological degenerative diseases, including some apparently not induced by retroviruses. This model can be instrumental in understanding different aspects of these diseases. In the future, novel human neurovirulent retroviruses might be identified and isolated. We hope that the information gathered on this murine model would then be directly applicable to these human retrovirus-induced diseases.

Because of their intimate genetic parasitism, retroviruses have evolved with the cell and tend to use cell machinery and mimic some of its components. For this reason, we believe that a significant understanding of the molecular basis of the retrovirus-induced motor neuron disease in mice will teach us a lot about the normal neurophysiology of motor neurons, and we hope will help to find new ways to prevent and treat these terrible, debilitating human neurological diseases.

Acknowledgments

I am grateful to Dr Neil Cashman and Yves Robitaille (Montreal Neurological Institute) for reviewing the manuscript and for their helpful comments and stimulating discussions. I also thank Dr Dennis Kay for reading the manuscript and for his helpful suggestions. The work performed in my laboratory was funded by grants from the Medical Research Council of Canada and from the Amyotrophic Lateral Sclerosis Association (USA) to the author.

References

1 Spencer PS, Schaumburg HH. The pathogenesis of motor neuron disease: Perspectives from neurotoxicology. In: Rowland LP, ed. Human Motor Neuron Disease. New York, Raven Press, 1982;249–266 (Adv Neurol 36)

2 Andrews JM, Gardner MB, Wolfgram FJ, et al. Studies on a murine form of spontaneous lower motor neuron degeneration. The wobbler (wr) mouse. Am J Pathol 1974;76:63–78

3 Duchen LW, Strich SJ, Falconer DS. An hereditary motor neuron disease with progressive denervation of muscle in the mouse: The mutant 'wobbler.' J Neurol Neurosurg Psychiat 1968;31:535–542

4 Messer A, Flaherty LA. Autosomal dominance in a late-onset motor neuron disease in the mouse. J Neurogenet 1986;3:345–355

5 Gardner MB, Henderson BE, Officer JE, et al. A spontaneous lower motor neuron disease apparently caused by indigenous type-C RNA virus in wild mice. J Natl Cancer Inst 1973;51:1243–1254

6 McCarter JA, Ball JK, Frei JV. Lower limb paralysis induced in mice by a temperature-sensitive mutant of Moloney leukemia virus. J Natl Cancer Inst 1977;59:179–183

7 Gardner MB. Type-C viruses of wild mice: Characterization and natural history of amphotropic, ecotropic and xenotropic murine leukemia viruses. Cur Top Microbiol Immunol 1976;79:215–239

8 Gardner MB. Retrovial spongiform polioencephalomyelopathy. Rev Infect Dis 1985;7:99–110

9 Frederickson TN, Langdon WY, Hoffman PM, et al. Histologic and cell surface antigen studies of hematopoietic tumors induced by Cas-Br-M murine leukemia virus. J Natl Cancer Inst 1984;72:447–454

10 Jolicoeur P, Nicolaiew N, DesGroseillers L, Rassart E. Molecular cloning of infectious viral DNA from ecotropic neurotropic wild mouse retrovirus. J Virol 1983;45:1159–1163

11 Brooks BR, Swarz JR, Narayan O, Johnson RT. Murine neurotropic retro-

virus spongioform polioencephalomyelopathy: Acceleration of disease by virus inoculum concentration. Inf Immun 1979;23:540–544

12 Hoffman PM, Ruscetti SK, Morse HC III. Pathogenesis of paralysis and lymphoma associated with a wild mouse retrovirus infection. Part 1. Age- and dose-related effects in susceptible laboratory mice. J Neuroimmunol 1981;1:275–285

13 Officer JE, Tecson N, Estes JD, et al. Isolation of a neurotropic type C virus. Science 1973;181:945–947

14 Hoffman PM, Robbins DS, Morse HC III. Role of immunity in age-related resistance to paralysis after murine leukemia virus infection. J Virol 1984;52:734–738

15 Gross L. Oncogenic Viruses. Elmsford, New York, Pergamon Press Inc, 1970

16 Gardner MB, Chiri A, Dougherty MF, et al. Congenital transmission of murine leukemia virus from wild mice prone to the development of lymphoma and paralysis. J Natl Cancer Inst 1979;62:63–70

17 Gardner MB, Estes JD, Casagrande J, Rasheed S. Prevention of paralysis and suppression of lymphoma in wild mice by passive immunization to congenitally transmitted murine leukemia virus. J Natl Cancer Inst. 1980;64:359–364

18 Sharpe AH, Jaenisch R, Ruprecht RM. Retroviruses and mouse embryos: A rapid model for neurovirulence and transplancental antiviral therapy. Science 1987;236:1671–1674

19 Klement V, Gardner MB, Henderson BE, et al. Inefficient humoral immune response of lymphgoma-prone wild mice to persistent leukemia virus infection. J Natl Cancer Inst 1976;57:1169–1173

20 Wong PKY, Soong MM, MacLeod R, et al. A group of temperature-sensitive mutants of Moloney leukemia virus which is defective in cleavage of env precursor polypeptide in infected cells and also induces hind-limb paralysis in newborn CFW/D mice. Virology 1983;125:513–518

21 Bilello JA, Pitts OM, Hoffman PM. Characterization of a progressive neurodegenerative disease induced by a temperature-sensitive Moloney Murine leukemia virus infection. J Virol 1986;59:234–241

22 Andrews JM, Andrews RL. The comparative neuropathology of motor neuron diseases. In: Andrews JM, Johnson RT, Brazier MAB, eds. Amyotrophic Lateral Sclerosis. New York, Academic Press, 1976;181–216

23 Andrews JM, Gardner MB. Lower motor neuron degeneration associated with type C RNA virus infection in mice: Neuropathological features. J Neuropathol Exp Neurol 1974;33:285–307

24 Brooks BR, Swarz JR, Johnson RT. Spongioform polioencephalomyelopathy caused by a murine retrovirus. Lab Invest 1979;43:480–486

25 Oldstone MBA, Jensen F, Dixon FJ, Lampert PW. Pathogenesis of the slow

disease of the central nervous system associated with wild mouse virus. Virology 1980;107:180–193

26 Oldstone MBA, Lampert PW, Lee S, et al. Pathogenesis of the slow disease of the central nervous system associated with WM 1504 E virus. I. Relationship of strain susceptibility and replication to disease. Am J Pathol 1977;88:193–212

27 Swarz JR, Brooks BR, Johnson RT. Spongiform polioencephalomyelopathy caused by a murine retrovirus. II. Ultrastructural localization of virus replication and spongioform changes in the central nervous system. Neuropathol Appl Neurobiol 1981;7:365–380

28 Zachary JF, Knupp CJ, Wong PKY. Noninflammatory spongiform polioencephalopathy caused by a neurotropic temperature-sensitive mutant of Moloney murine leukemia virus TB. Am J Pathol 1986;124:457–468

29 Hoffmann PM, Pitts OM, Bilello JA, Cimino EF. Retrovirus-induced motor neuron degeneration. Rev Neurol (Paris) 1988;144:676–679

30 Johnson RT. Selective vulnerability of neural cells to viral infections. In: Rowland LF, ed. Human Motor Neuron Disease. New York, Raven Press, 1982;331–337 (Adv Neurol 36)

31 Gardner MB, Rasheed S, Klement V, et al. Lower motor neuron disease in wild mice caused by indigenous type C virus and search for a similar etiology in human amyotrophic lateral sclerosis. In: Andrews JM, Johnson RT, Brazier MAB, eds. Amyotrophic Lateral Sclerosis. New York, Academic Press, 1976;217–234

32 Gardner MB, Klement V, Henderson BE, et al. Genetic control of type C virus of wild mice. Nature 1976;259:143–145

33 Jolicoeur P. The Fv-1 gene of the mouse and its control of murine leukemia virus replication. Curr Top Microbiol Immunol 1979;86:67–122

34 DesGroseillers L, Jolicoeur P. Physical mapping of the Fv-1 tropism host range determinant of BALB/c murine leukemia viruses. J Virol 1983;48:685–696

35 Jolicoeur P, Baltimore D. Effect of Fv-1 gene product on proviral DNA formation and integration in cells infected with murine leukemia viruses. Proc Natl Acad Sci (USA) 1976;73:2236–2240

36 Jolicoeur P, Rassart E. Effect of Fv-1 gene product on synthesis of linear and supercoiled viral DNA in cells infected with murine leukemia virus. J Virol 1980;33:183–195

37 Gardner MB, Rasheed S, Pal BK, et al. Akvr-1, a dominant murine leukemia virus restriction gene, is polymorphic in leukemia-prone wild mice. Proc Natl Acad Sci (USA) 1980;77:531–535

38 O'Brien SJ, Berman EJ, Estes JD, Gardner MB. Murine retroviral restriction genes Fv-4 and Akvr-1 are alleles of a single locus. J Virol 1983;47:649–651

39 Kozak CA, Gromet NJ, Ikeda H, Buckler CE. A unique sequence related to

the ecotropic murine leukemia virus is associated with the Fv-4 resistance gene. Proc Natl Acad Sci (USA) 1984;81:834–837

40 Ikeda H, Odaka T. A cell membrane 'gp70' associated with Fv-4 gene: Immunological characterization, and tissue and strain distributions. Virology 1984;133:65–76

41 Rasheed S, Gardner MB. Resistance of fibroblasts and hematopoietic cells to ecotropic murine leukemia virus infection: An Akvr-1[R] gene effect. Int J Cancer 1983;31:491–496

42 DesGroseillers L, Barrette M, Jolicoeur P. Physical mapping of the paralysis-inducing determinant of a wild mouse ecotropic neurotropic retrovirus. J. Virol 1984;52:356–363

43 Hoffman PM, Morse HC III. Host genetic determinants of neurological disease induced by Cas-Br-M murine leukemia virus. J Virol 1985;53:40–43

44 Carlson GA, Kingsbury DT, Goodman P, et al. Linkage of prion protein and scrapie incubation time genes. Cell 1986;46:503–511

45 Yuen PH, Malehorn D, Nau C, et al. Molecular cloning of two paralytogenic, temperature-sensitive mutants ts-1 and ts-7, and the parental wild-type Moloney murine leukemia virus. J Virol 1985;54:178–185

46 Rassart E, Nelbach L, Jolicoeur P. Cas-Br-E murine leukemia virus: Sequencing of the paralytogenic region of its genome and derivation of specific probes to study its origin and the structure of its recombinant genomes in leukemic tissues. J Virol 1986;60:910–919

47 Chattopadhyay SK, Oliff AI, Linemeyer DL, et al. Genomes of murine leukemia viruses isolated from wild mice. J Virol 1981;39:777–791

48 DesGroseillers L, Rassart E, Jolicoeur P. Thymotropism of murine leukemia virus is conferred by its long terminal repeat. Proc Natl Acad Sci (USA) 1983;80:4203–4207

49 Chatis PA, Holland CA, Hartley JW, et al. Role of the 3' end of the genome in determining disease specificity of Friend and Moloney murine leukemia viruses. Proc Natl Acad Sci (USA) 1983;80:4408–4411

50 Chatis PA, Holland CA, Silver JE, et al. A 3' end fragment encompassing the transcriptional enhancers of nondefective Friend virus confers erythroleukemogenicity on Moloney leukemia virus. J Virol 1984;52:248–254

51 DesGroseillers L, Jolicoeur P. Mapping the viral sequences conferring leukemogenicity and disease specificity in Moloney and amphotropic murine leukemia viruses. J Virol 1984;52:448–456

52 Barbacid M. Robbins KC, Aaronson SA. Wild mouse RNA tumor viruses. A nongenetically transmitted virus group closely related to exogenous leukemia viruses of laboratory mouse strains. J Exp Med 1979;149:254–266

53 Yuen PH, Malehorn D, Knupp C, Wong PKY. A 1.6-kilobase-pair fragment in the genome of the ts1 mutant of Moloney murine leukemia virus TB that is associated with temperature sensitivity, nonprocessing of Pr80[env], and paralytogenesis. J Virol 1985;54:364–373

54 Yuen PH, Tzeng E, Knupp C, Wong PKY. The neurovirulent determinants of ts1, a paralytogenic mutant of Moloney murine leukemia virus TB, are localized in at least two functionally distinct regions of the genome. J Virol 1986;59:59–65

55 DesGroseillers L, Jolicoeur P. The tandem direct repeats within the long terminal repeat of murine leukemia viruses are the primary determinant of their leukemogenic potential. J Virol 1984;52:945–952

56 Lenz J, Haseltine WA. Localization of the leukemogenic determinant of SL3-3, an ecotropic, XC-positive murine leukemia virus of AKR mouse origin. J Virol 1983;47:317–328

57 DesGroseillers L, Rassart E, Robitaille Y, et al. Retrovirus-induced spongiform encephalopathy: The 3'-end long terminal repeat-containing viral sequences influence the incidence of the disease and the specificity of the neurological syndrome. Proc Natl Acad Sci (USA) 1985;82:8818–8822

58 Shinnick TM, Lerner RA, Sutcliffe JG. Nucleotide sequence of Moloney murine leukemia virus. Nature 1981;293:543–548

59 Temin HM. The RNA tumor viruses – Background and foreground. Proc Natl Acad Sci (USA) 1972;69:1016–1020

60 Coffin J. Endogenous viruses. In: Weiss R, Teich N, Varmus H, Coffin J, eds. Molecular Biology of Tumor Viruses: RNA Tumor Viruses. Cold Spring Harbor, Cold Spring Harbor Laboratories, 1982;1109–1203

61 Lerner RA, Wilson CB, Del Villano BC, et al. Endogenous oncornaviral gene expression in adult and feral mice: Quantitative, histological and physiologic studies of the major viral glycoprotein, gp70. J Exp Med 1976;143:151–166

62 Towfighi J, Gonatas NK. Effect of intracerebral injection of ouabain in adult and developing rats: An ultrastructure and autoradiographic study. Lab Invest 1973;28:170–180

63 Beck E, Daniel PM, Davey AJ, et al. The pathogenesis of transmissible spongioform encephalopathy: An ultrastructural study. Brain 1982;105:755–786

64 Crowell RL. Cellular receptor in virus infections. ASM News 1987;53:422–423

65 Mims CA. Virus receptors and cell tropisms. J Infect 1986;12:199–203

66 Fingeroth J, Weiss J, Tedder T, et al. Epstein-Barr virus receptor on human B lymphocytes is the C3d receptor CR2. Proc Natl Acad Sci (USA) 1984;81;4510–4516

67 Tanner J, Weis J, Fearow D, et al. Esptein-Barr virus gp350/220 binding to the B lymphocyte C3d receptor mediates absorption, capping and endocytosis. Cell 1987;50:203–213

68 Burrage TC, Tignor GH, Smith AL. Rabies virus binding at neuromuscular junctions. Virus Res 1985;2:273–279

69 Lentz TL, Wilson PT, Hawrot E, Speicher DW. Amino acid sequence

similarity between rabies virus glycoprotein and snake venom curami-
metic neurotoxins. Science 1984;222:847–848

70 Dalgleish AG, Beverley PCL, Clapham PR, et al. The CD4 (T4) antigen is
an essential component of the receptor for the AIDS retrovirus. Nature
1984;312:763–767

71 Klatzmann D, Champagne E, Chamaret S, et al. T-lymphocyte T4 molecule
behaves as the receptor for human retrovirus LAV. Nature 1984;312:767–
768

72 Maddon PJ, Dalgleish AG, McDougal JS, et al. The T4 gene encodes the
AIDS virus receptor and is expressed in the immune system and the brain.
Cell 1986;47:333–348

73 Grundy JE, McKeating JA, Ward PJ, et al. β_2 microcrobulin enhances the
infectivity of cytomegalovirus and when bound to the virus enables Class
I HLA molecules to be used as a virus receptor. J Gen Virol 1987;68:793–
803

74 Helenius A, Morein B, Fries E. Human (HLA-A and HLA-B) and murine
(H-2K and H-2D) histocompatibility antigens are cell surface receptor for
Semliki Forest virus. Proc Natl Acad Sci (USA) 1979;75:3846–3850

75 Inada T, Mims CA. Mouse la antigens are receptors for lactate dehydrogenase virus. Nature 1984;309:59–61

76 Stroobant P, Rice AP, Gullick WJ, et al. Purification and characterization of
vaccinia virus growth factor. Cell 1985;42:383–393

77 Twardzik DR, Brown JP, Ranchalis JE, et al. Vaccinia virus-infected cells
release a novel polypeptide functionally related to transforming and
epidermal growth factors. Proc Natl Acad Sci (USA) 1985;82:5300–5304

78 Co MS, Gaulton GN, Tominga A, et al. Structural similarities between the
mammalian β-adrenergic and reovirus type 3 receptors. Proc Natl Acad
Sci (USA) 1985;82:5315–5318

79 Paul RW, Lee PWK. Glycophorin is the reovirus receptor on human
erythrocytes. Virology 1987;159:94–101

80 Lifson JD, Feinberg MB, Reyes GR, et al. Induction of CD-4 dependent
cell fusion by the HTLV-III/LAV envelope glycoprotein. Nature
1986;323:725–728

81 Jolicoeur P, DesGroseillers L. Neurotropic Cas-Br-E murine leukemia virus
harbors several determinants of leukemogenicity mapping in different
regions of the genome. J Virol 1985;56:639–643

82 Holland CA, Hartley JW, Rowe WP, Hopkins N. At least four viral genes
contribute to the leukemogenicity of murine retrovirus MCF 247 in AKR
mice. J Virol 1985;53:158–165

83 Kohn R. Clinical and pathological findings in an unusual infantile motor
neuron disease. J Neurol Neurosurg Psychiat 1971;34:427–431

84 Reif-Kohn R, Mundel G. Second case of an infantile motor neuron disease.
Confin Neurol 1974;36:23–32

85 Hudson, AJ. Amyotrophic lateral sclerosis and its association with dementia, parkinson and other neurological disorders. A review. Brain 1981;104:217–247

86 Gibbs CJ, Gajdusek DC. Infection as the etiology of spongioform encephalopathy (Creutzfeldt-Jakob disease). Science 1969;165:1023–1025

87 Gajdusek DC. Unconventional viruses and the origin and disappearance of kuru. Science 1977;197:943–960

88 Prusiner FB. Prions and neurodegenerative diseases. New Eng J Med 1987;317:1571–1581

89 Tyler R. Nonfamilial amyotrophy with dementia or multisystem degeneration and other neurological disorders. In: Rowland LP, ed. Human Motor Neuron Disease. New York, Raven Press, 1982;173–180 (Adv Neurol 36)

90 Snider WD, Simpson DM, Nielsen S, et al. Neurological complications of acquired immune deficiency syndrome. Analysis of 50 patients. Ann Neurol 1983;14:403–418

91 Goldstick L, Mandybur TL, Bode R. Spinal cord degeneration in AIDS. Neurology 1985;35:103–105

92 Petito CK, Navia BA, Cho ES, et al. Vacuolar myelopathy pathologically resembling subacute combined degeneration in patients with the acquired immunodeficiency syndrome. New Eng J Med 1985;312:874–879

93 De La Monte SM, Moore T, Hedley-Whyte ET. Vacuolar encephalopathy of AIDS. New Eng J Med 1986;315:1549–1550

94 Lee MR, Ho D, Gurnery ME. Functional interaction and partial homology between human immunodeficiency virus and neuroleukin. Science 1987;237:1047–1051

95 Thomas M, Ballantyne JP, Hansen S, et al. Anterior horn cell dysfunction in Alzheimer's disease. J Neurol Neurosurg Psychiat 1982;45:378–381

96 Brown P, Salazar AM, Gibbs CJ, Gajdusek DC. Alzheimer's disease and transmissible virus dementia (Creutzfeldt-Jakob disease). Ann NY Acad Sci 1982;396:131–143

97 Flament-Durant J, Couck AM. Spongioform alterations in brain biopsies of presenile dementia. Acta Neruopathol (Berlin) 1979;46:159–162

98 Kang J, Lemaire HG, Unterbeck A, et al. The precursor of Alzheimer's diseae amyloid A4 protein resembles a cell-surface receptor. Nature 1987;325:733–736

99 Gibbs CJ Jr, Gajdusek DC. Amyotrophic lateral sclerosis, Parkinson's disease and the amyotrophic lateral sclerosis-parkinsonism-dementia complex on Guam. A review and summary of attempts to demonstrate infection as the etiology. J Clin Pathol 1972;25:(Suppl 6)132–140

100 Gibbs CJ, Gajdusek DC. An update on long-term in vivo and in vitro studies designed to identify a virus as the cause of amyotrophic lateral sclerosis, parkinsonism dementia and Parkinson's disease. In: Rowland

LP, ed. Human Motor Neuron Disease. New York, Raven Press, 1982;343–353 (Adv Neurol 36)

101 Johnson RT. Virological studies of amyotrophic lateral sclerosis: An overview. In: Andrews JM, Johnson RT, Brazier MAB, eds. Amyotrophic Lateral Sclerosis. New York, Academic Press, 1976;173–180

102 Alter HJ, Eichberg JW, Masur H, et al. Transmission of HTLV-III infection from human plasma to chimpanzees: An animal model for AIDS. Science 1984;226:549–552

103 Harter DH. Viruses other than poliovirus in human amyotrophic lateral sclerosis. In: Rowland LP, ed. Human Motor Neuron Disease. New York, Raven Press, 1982;339–342 (Adv Neurol 36)

104 Osame M, Matsumoto M, Usuku K, et al. Chronic progressive myelopathy associated with elevated antibodies to human T-lymphotropic virus type I and adult T-cell leukemia like cells. Ann Neurol 1987;21:117–122

105 Verant JC, Maurs L, Gessain A, et al. Endemic tropical spastic paraparesis associated with human T-lymphotropic virus type I: A clinical and sero-epidemiological study of 25 cases. Ann Neurol 1987;21:123–130

106 Navia BA, Cho ES, Petito CK, Price RW. The AIDS dementia complex: II Neuropathology Ann Neurol 1986;525–535

107 Hoffman PM, Festoff BW, Giron LT et al. Isolation of LAV/HTLV-III from a patient with amyotrophic lateral sclerosis. New Eng J Med 1985;313:324–325

108 Paquette Y, Hanna Z, Savard P, et al. Retrovirus-induced murine motor neuron disease: Mapping the determinant of spongiform degeneration within the envelope gene. Proc Natl Acad Sci (USA) 1989;86:3896–3900

109 Li JP, Bestwick RK, Spiro C, Kabat D. The membrane glycoprotein of Friend spleen focus-forming virus: Evidence that the cell surface component is required for pathogenesis and that it binds to a receptor. J Virol 1987;61:2782–2792

Immunologic Aspects of Motor Neuron Disease

JACK P. ANTEL, KARI STEFANSSON,
AND MARK GURNEY

Amyotrophic lateral sclerosis (ALS) remains a disorder of unknown etiology. Whether immune-mediated mechanisms contribute to the pathogenesis of at least some subtypes of motor neuron diseases (MNDs) remains to be determined. In this chapter, we will (a) review some of the principal epidemiologic, clinical, and pathologic features of human disorders considered to be 'autoimmune' in nature, describe the immunologic mechanisms mediating these clinical disorders, and discuss experimental animal disorders which serve as models of these diseases; (b) based on the above considerations, examine whether any available data derived from study of patients suggest involvement of immune-mediated mechanisms in any form of currently recognized MNDs; (c) summarize data regarding experimental antibodies which may provide insight into the unique properties of motor neurons which in turn may make them specifically susceptible to a disease process.

Clinical and Experimental 'Autoimmune' Disorders

Autoimmune disorders can be defined as those in which a host's immune system induces injury to self-tissue. Understanding of the mechanisms whereby such autoimmune processes may be triggered has progressed in parallel with expanding knowledge regarding the organization of the immune system itself. The effector arm of the immune system can be subdivided into T-cell–mediated responses (cell-mediated immunity) and B-cell or antibody-mediated responses (humoral immunity). As will be discussed, both forms of response together with other mediators of inflammation such as macrophages may contribute to the overall extent of tissue injury in chronic autoimmune disorders.

The prototype of uniphasic cell-mediated autoimmune neurologic disorder is the syndrome of acute disseminated encephalomyelitis (ADEM), a syndrome which occurs following vaccination with neural tissue or exposure to particular viral infections, most commonly measles [1, 2]. The occurrence of neuroparalytic accidents in patients receiving the original Pasteur vaccine for prevention of rabies was recognized soon after its introduction in the late 19th century [3]. During the 1930s, Rivers and Schwentker demonstrated that recurrent injection of central nervous system tissue into monkeys resulted in a pathologic disorder characterized by perivascular inflammation and demyelination [4]. These original observations initiated the development of the model disorder 'experimental allergic encephalomyelitis' (EAE), which can now be produced in either an acute or chronic form by active immunization of a genetically susceptible host with the defined myelin antigens, myelin basic protein (MBP) or proteolipid protein, or by passive transfer of T-cells specifically sensitized to these myelin antigens [5, 6]. The pathologic findings are again those of perivascular inflammation and demyelination. Recent data suggest that administration of specific antibodies to myelin antigens in animals developing EAE can enhance the extent of demyelination, thus illustrating that multiple immune mechanisms can contribute to overall disease severity [7]. The genetic factors influencing susceptibility to EAE include those encoded by major histocompatibility complex (MHC) gene loci as well as non–MHC-loci including those determining properties of the blood/brain barrier. The clinical and pathological severity of EAE can be significantly reduced by a variety of immunosuppressive therapies, providing a foundation for utilizing response to therapy as an indicator that a given disease may be autoimmune.

The features common to multiple sclerosis (MS) and the EAE, experimental prototype T-cell–mediated disease – namely the pathologic findings of perivascular and intraparenchymal inflammation at the sites of central nervous system (CNS) demyelination, heightened frequency of disease in immunogenetically predisposed populations, and probable response of the disorder to immunotherapy – have strengthened the postulate that MS may also be an example of a cell-mediated autoimmune disease. The pathologic features of inflammation and the development of a T-cell–mediated animal model, termed experimental allergic neuritis, suggest that the acute (Guillain-Barré syndrome) and chronic forms of inflammatory demyelinating peripheral neuropathies also represent examples of cell-mediated autoimmune disorders. The putative antigens to which T-cells may be specifically sensitized have, however, not been identified in either MS or Guillain-Barré syndrome. The features of the currently recognized MNDs will be examined in the context of the above properties, which characterize cell-mediated autoimmune disorders, as well as in the context of the properties described below, which characterize antibody-mediated disease.

The clinical disorder usually considered as a prototype of a humoral or B-cell–mediated disorder is myasthenia gravis (MG). In a large majority of patients with MG, their sera contain antibodies which react with the nicotinic acetylcholine receptor (Achr) on the post-synaptic side of the neuromuscular junction. Passive transfer of MG patient sera into mice induces a uniphasic disease which clinically and physiologically mimics MG. Experimental anti-Achr monoclonal antibodies (mcAbs) can also be used to induce MG in recipient animals [8, 9]. A single injection of mcAb induces a transient disease (acute experimental autoimmune [EA] in MG) which is pathologically characterized by presence of antibody, complement, and macrophages at the neuromuscular junction. Chronic injection of mcAb results in the histologic, biochemical, and physiologic abnormalities characteristic of MG, namely persistent simplification of the motor end-plate, reduction in Achr content of the muscle, and reduced miniature end-plate potentials. There is no inflammation. The animals are, however, not clinically weak, a finding which may relate to the use of mcAb rather than polyclonal antibody [9]. Active immunization of animals with purified Achr protein can also induce experimental MG either as an acute uniphasic disorder physiologically and pathologically similar to that induced by passive transfer of antibody or as a more chronic disorder. Anti-Achr antibody can be detected in animals subsequent to the active immunization protocols. Achr-specific T-helper cell lines have been derived from MG patients, suggesting that immune regulatory T-cells contribute to the level of immune reactivity [10]. In this regard, anti-T helper cell antibody therapy has been shown to inhibit the development of experimental MG [11].

Although an immune-mediated basis for MG has long been suspected, no direct antibody-mediated activity could be demonstrated when whole or crude muscle preparations were used as 'targets.' Only when the specific antigen was serendipitously identified in the early 1970s was the antibody effect clearly demonstrated [12]. The more recent detection of antibodies that bind to calcium channels in the presynaptic neuromuscular junction in the Lambert-Eaton syndrome and the demonstration that one can passively transfer the disorder provide yet another precedent for the existence of antibody-mediated autoimmune disease [13].

The detection of target-directed antibodies against the tissue component affected in a disease is per se an insufficient criterion to establish that the disorder is an autoimmune one. Tissue-directed autoantibodies can be demonstrated in multiple pathologic conditions as well as in 'normal' individuals. With regard to the latter, as discussed later, a large majority of 'normal' human sera will react with neurofilament proteins when tested with an immunoblot technique. Thus, for any pathologic condition in which characteristic antibodies are detected, one need establish a cause/effect relationship between the antibody and the disease, a task which can be difficult. Perhaps passive transfer of the disease is the most rigid requirement.

The precise sequence of events underlying the development of autoimmune disorders continues to be explored. The demonstration, in both normal humans and animals, that one can recover T-cells specifically sensitized to autoantigens, as for example MBP-specific T-cells [14], suggests that potential autoaggressive immunoeffector cells may exist normally; disruption of immune regulatory mechanisms would result in their activation and expansion. Speculations regarding the events underlying initial immune sensitization to a specific antigen target include exposure of a normally sequestered antigen to the immune system, or alteration of an endogenous antigen by exogenous agents such as viruses. A more recent postulate suggests that such sensitization may result from the existence of shared antigenic properties between endogenous neural structures and exogenous agents. This concept, termed molecular mimicry, has gained credence from the demonstrations of (a) sequence homologies between neural structures and viruses as, for example, between MBP and mouse hepatitis virus [15], and (b) antibody cross-reactions between target organs and exogenous agents. The latter is illustrated by experimentally generated monoclonal antibodies (mcAbs) reacting with the nicotinic acetylcholine receptor and cross-reacting with selected bacterial antigens [16].

Susceptibility to most established immune-mediated diseases is influenced by genetic factors encoded by MHC-region genes [17]. Class II MHC gene products are shown to be critical requirements for presentation of antigen to T-cells by accessory cells. The class II MHC gene repertoire of the host can determine the epitope of a specific antigen to which the host responds. As an example, the MHC class II repertoire will determine the capability of a specific mouse strain to respond to the encephalitogenic portion of the MBP molecule. Non–MHC-region gene products, such as those which comprise the T-cell receptor, also, however, determine immune responsiveness.

Motor Neuron Diseases and the Immune System

EPIDEMIOLOGIC FEATURES

Studies have been undertaken to determine whether the prevalence of 'autoimmune' phenomena is increased in MND patients or in their families. These are based on observations in putative 'autoimmune' disorders such as myasthenia gravis which demonstrate not only the presence of tissue-specific disease-relevant autoantibodies but also an increased prevalence of multiple-tissue reactive autoantibodies and other 'autoimmune' disorders in patients as well as their families. Such studies require particular rigour with regard to selection of 'control' subjects, in that the incidence of 'anti-tissue antibodies' tends to increase as a function of ageing. Appel et al [18] examined a series of individuals and controls with respect to 'autoimmunity' and found that the overall incidence of 'autoimmune' phenomena in family members in the ALS population was increased, as was the incidence of thyroid disease associated with presence of microsomal and/or thyroglobulin antibodies (20–25% compared to expected values of <10%). Kiessling [19], however, found no apparent increase in anti-thyroid antibodies in a German ALS population living in an endemic goitre belt. Cashman et al [20] reported the development of rapidly progressive ALS in two sisters, with disease onset in their late 20s, following Graves' disease with marked hyperthyroidism and presence of anti-thyroid antibodies. Their father had developed ALS in his 40s without documented evidence of thyroid dysfunction. Whether a direct common pathogenic link exists in these cases or whether the hyperthyroid state precipitated the manifestations of ALS is uncertain.

The relationship between motor neuron syndromes and the co-occurrence of plasma cell dyscrasias, either malignant or benign, remains a subject of great interest, particularly in view of reports that in some such cases the neurologic disorder is responsive to immunotherapy. A summary of reported cases of motor neuron disease associated with IgM and IgG paraproteinemias is presented in Table 1 [21–38]. Shy et al [21] have reported an incidence of paraproteins in almost 5% of patients with motor neuron disease, which is higher than the expected incidence rate of 1–2% in the population age 50–80. In about 50% of reported cases of MND associated with paraproteinemia, the paraprotein has been of the IgM class, though the predicted frequency is only 10–20%. Among the IgM-MND cases for which adequate clinical data are available, about 80% feature lower motor neuron dysfunction as the major clinical feature. These cases seemingly cannot be distinguished from cases of progressive spinal muscular atrophy (PSMA) not associated with

TABLE 1

Motor neuron disease and paraproteinemia

	IgM		IgG	
	LMN signs	LMN + UMN signs (ALS)	LMN signs	ALS
Number of cases	15 [21–29]	4 [21, 30, 31, A]	3 [21, 32, B]	12 [21, 34, 37, C]
Mean patient age (years)	53	64	51	59
NCV				
normal	3 [24, 25, 28]	N/A	1 [B]	4 [34–37, C]
slow	3 [22, 26, 27]	N/A	1	
CSF protein				
< 80 mg%	6 [21, 24–27]	2 [19, A]	3 [21, 32]	5 [21, 35, 36, C]
> 80 mg%	2 [21]	1 [21]		
Pathology	Axonopathy [22], axonopathy with lymphatic infiltration of roots [28]	Neuronopathy, lymphatic infiltration of meninges [28]	Myeloma, neuropathy	ALS-neuronopathy [35]
Response to treatment				
+	4 [23, 25, 26, 28]			2 [36]
−	1 [22]	1 [21, A]	1 [B]	2 [36, C]

NOTE This table summarizes data from cases of motor neuron disease associated with paraproteinemia. Data are derived from published cases (cited by reference) or unpublished cases (A, B, C) observed at the Montreal Neurological Hospital (see below). Cases are divided on the basis of presence of IgM or IgG paraproteins (the cases associated with IgA or light-chain restricted dysproteinemias are not given) [33, 21], and whether only lower motor neuron (LMN) signs or combined LMN and upper motor neuron (UMN) signs were present; the latter cases are labelled as ALS. The numbers regarding studies of nerve conduction velocity (NCV), CSF protein, and therapeutic response indicate the number of cases in each category. The numbers are inconstant as all parameters are not available for all patients.

A 66-year-old male with 3-year course to death of progressive bulbar and limb muscle amyotrophy plus hyperreflexia and a serum IgM_k monoclonal paraprotein. No evidence of malignancy in bone-marrow aspirate. No response to plasmapheresis, prednisone, or melphalan.

B 61-year-old female with 3-year duration of progressive muscle amyotrophy with hyporeflexia leading to respiratory dependency. IgG_λ monoclonal paraprotein without reduction of serum IgG, IgM, or IgA. No response to plasmapheresis or azathioprine.

C 64-year-old male with 2-year duration of limb-muscle amyotrophy and hyperreflexia. IgG_k serum paraprotein. No response to melphalan, prednisone.

gammopathy on the basis of age of onset, male predilection, or rate of disease progression. Progression rates vary from subacute (complete quadriplegia developing within four months) [28] to chronic (patients followed for more than 5 years) [21]. Insufficient detail is contained within available case reports to be certain whether apparently minor sensory dysfunction is more frequently observed in the gammopathy-associated cases than the PSMA cases. Slowing of peripheral nerve conduction velocities seemingly is more frequent in the paraprotein-associated cases than in classical ALS. In most reported cases, however, data on proximal nerve conduction (F-waves) are not presented, nor is there specific information regarding multiple peripheral conduction blocks (see below). The limited number of pathologic studies suggests the disorder represents a primary neuropathic one, in that central chromatolysis of motor neurons (MNs) in the spinal cord is a prominent feature. The proportion of surviving spinal MNs exceeds those found in classical ALS or PSMA. The response of the above cases to treatments such as plasma exchange, corticosterioid, azathioprine, and alkeran has been variable, with significant response being the exception. The more precise clinical, pathologic, and immunologic characterization of these cases likely will result in more definable therapeutic strategies.

Progress has now been made with regard to documenting the finding that the paraprotein in some of the above cases of IgM-associated MND or motor neuropathy recognizes specific epitopes expressed on peripheral nerve. Freddo et al [39] found that the IgM$_\lambda$ paraproteins from two patients with lower motor neuron syndromes reacted with the gangliosides G$_{M1}$ and GD$_{1b}$ and asialo G$_{M1}$, which share the Gal(B1-3)GalNAc as their terminal structure. Nardelli et al [40] have also found the same pattern of reactivity using the IgM M-protein from an additional patient with lower MND. One does note that the epitopes recognized by the IgM antibody are distributed widely in the CNS as well as the peripheral nervous system (PNS), raising the issue of what determines the topography of this syndrome.

Recent data indicate that a similar antibody may arise in cases of lower MND or motor neuropathy without apparent serum paraproteins [41–43]. Shy et al have reported a case of 'motor neuropathy' manifesting as progressive (3-year course) lower motor neuron dysfunction in a 26-year-old male, in which they detected serum IgM antibodies binding to G$_{M1}$ and GD$_{1b}$. In this case, there was no evidence of a monoclonal paraprotein. Treatment with cyclophosphamide and plasma exchange resulted in almost complete recovery [42]. Pestronk et al [44, 45] have described patients with progressive limb weakness, which clinically mimics lower motor neuron forms of ALS, but in which one observes multifocal conduction blocks on nerve conduction testing. Such findings are compatible with patchy demyelination of motor axons. This syndrome, termed multifocal motor neuropathy, is characterized by presence of anti-G_{M1} antibodies and is seemingly responsive to cyclophosphamide therapy, but not to a regimen of prednisone and plasmapheresis. The above-described clinical cases help establish the syndrome of motor neuropathy-neuronopathy associated with IgM antibody. The cause/effect relation between the antibody and disease is not yet clearly demonstrated, although the response to immunotherapy of selected cases does support this postulate. As with IgM-associated mixed motor-sensory demyelinating neuropathies [41], species restrictions of the antibody complicate use of passive transfer experiments to establish the cause/effect relationship.

The existence of a classic ALS-IgM paraproteinemia syndrome is less well established. We have studied serum IgM from four patients with IgM monoclonal gammopathy and ALS (combined upper and lower motor neuron dysfunction). In our hands they have not differed from serum IgM from patients with IgM monoclonal gammopathy unassociated with neurologic disease, inasmuch as no difference has been found with binding to (a) immunoblots containing proteins from isolated anterior horn cells, unfractionated spinal cord, peripheral nerves, or striated muscles or (b) thin-layer chromatography plates containing glycolipids from peripheral nerves or the central nervous system. We did not find antibodies against G_{M1} and GD_{1b} in these patients [46].

The incidence of IgG and IgA paraproteinemias in any form of MND is not convincingly increased over that in age-matched controls. In the IgG paraproteinemia-associated ALS cases reported to date, the clinical, electrophysiologic and pathologic features are identical to those of classic ALS. Before dismissing all cases of IgG paraprotein-associated ALS cases as chance occurrence, one need note that some of these cases are reported to have been at least partially responsive to immunotherapy. Scattered cases of ALS or lower motor neuron dysfunction associated with IgA paraproteinemia [21] and the light-chain variant of myeloma are on record [33].

That MND occurs as a 'paraneoplastic' disorder in association with solid malignancy is suggested but not established by epidemiologic data. No specific solid tumour has been linked with ALS however, in contrast to the characteristic associations found in more clearly established syndromes such as subacute cerebellar degeneration with small cell carcinoma of the lung. A remitting lower motor neuron clinical syndrome, which likely represents a neuropathy, occurs in patients with lymphomas [47].

IMMUNOGENETICS AND MND

Diseases associated with immunogenetically determined susceptibility usually feature an increased incidence in specific populations, some increase in family members, and significant but not invariable concordance between monozygotic twins. The postulate is that susceptibility is inherited but that additional factors are required to trigger the disease. For surveys of populations with regard to immunogenetic predisposition to disease, a convenient approach has been to utilize serologic techniques to identify characteristic HLA phenotypes present in a given population. The HLA antigens, which are encoded within the MHC region, if not directly acting as immune-response gene products, serve as markers for genetically linked immune-response gene products. HLA linkage studies in ALS patients have at best produced equivocal results, several studies suggesting an over-representation of HLA antigens A3 and B35 [48]. Use of restriction fragment length polymorphism techniques will permit more detailed analysis of individual HLA gene structures in diseased populations.

IMMUNOLOGIC STATUS OF MND PATIENTS

The immune status of MND patients has been assessed both with respect to (a) whether generalized or 'non-specific' immune parameters in this disease state differ from control values (such data could suggest either a defect in overall immune status which may predispose to the development of an infectious disorder or provide evidence of ongoing immune reactivity as has been variably detected in prototype autoimmune diseases) and (b) the presence of a specific immune-mediated process directed against a selective target, either the motor unit itself or factors postulated to interact with motor neurons. The lack of the characteristic inflammatory pathology associated with cell-mediated immune responses has focused the studies on humoral mediators (antibody).

'Non-specific' Immune Parameters

With regard to cell-mediated responses, *in vitro* lymphocyte proliferative responses in MND patients are overall comparable to those of age-matched controls, although some reports of hyporeactivity do exist [48, 49]. With regard to the latter, one need consider the potential effects of circulating plasma factors such as proteases on lymphocyte responses. Lymphocyte T-cell subsets as currently defined by monoclonal antibodies follow the expected distribution [48, 49]. Any elevation in the proportion of T-cells bearing Ia or other activation antigens is seemingly minor [49]. Only a single case of ALS has to date been reported in an individual with acquired immunodeficiency syndrome. Scattered cases of ALS in immunodeficient individuals are reported [50]. Lymphocyte hyporeactivity to mitogen stimulation is reported in some ALS cases in Guam [51, 52].

With the exclusion of patients with monoclonal IgM paraproteinemias and motor neuropathy, no characteristic abnormality of serum or cerebral spinal fluid (CSF) Ig profiles is observed in the overall ALS patient population, particularly when age-matched controls are considered. Low levels of circulating immune-complexes can be detected in some ALS patients, with levels of reactivity generally being much below those encountered in systemic lupus erythematosus [48, 49]. The nature of the antigen and antibody being detected in these cases is not yet resolved. Serum complement levels are normal [53]. Donnenfeld et al demonstrated deposits of IgG and complement in astrocytes in motor cortex and spinal cord tissue sections obtained from ALS patients [54]. Similar findings were, however, observed in patients with MS and Alzheimer's disease, although not in patients with Parkinson's syndrome. In summary, the currently available data do not suggest significant generalized immune derangements in the usual cases of ALS.

Target-Directed Immunity in MND

Spinal Motor Neuron
The postulate that ALS sera or plasma contain factors potentially injurious to motor neurons continues to be explored. A repeatedly used approach to explore this issue has been to assess the effects of ALS plasma or serum (or Ig) on the survival and growth of spinal motor neurons derived from fetal or neonatal tissues and maintained in tissue culture systems [55–66]. As indicated in Table 2 the results of these studies have not produced a consensus. Wolfgram and Myers [55] initially observed a toxic effect of ALS sera (not specifically Ig) on monolayer spinal cord cultures prepared from 3-day-old mice. Roisen et al [56] also observed a toxic effect on neonatal but not on embryonic mouse monolayer spinal cord cultures and attributed the effect to the Ig fraction of the serum. Liveson et al [58] and Ecob et al [60] did not observe such an effect when using organotypic spinal cord cultures derived from mouse embryos. Horwich et al [59] also noted no specific effect of ALS sera using a culture system that was not precisely identical to that of

TABLE 2
ALS: effects of *serum* on neural tissue

Assay	Positive results	Negative results
Tissue culture studies		
Cytotoxic effects on cultured non-human spinal neurones	Wolfgram and Myers [55] Roisen et al [56] Ronnevi et al [57]	Liveson et al [58] Horwich et al [59] Ecob et al [60] Doherty et al [61]
Neurofilament protein content of spinal neurons – decreased by non-Ig serum factor		
Cytotoxic effect on parasympathetic ganglia		Touzeau and Kato [62]
Cytotoxic effect on neuroblastoma		Lehrich and Couture [63]
Cytotoxic effect on cultured fetal spinal neurons		Touzeau and Kato [64]
Immunohistochemical studies		
Ig binding to neurons	Digby et al [66]	Weiner et al [65]
Immunoblot analysis		
Ig binding to spinal cord homogenates		Brown et al [67] Kletti et al [68]
Functional assays		
Inhibition of botulinum toxin–induced terminal axonal sprouting	Gurney et al [80]	
Inhibition of neurite-promoting activity		Henderson et al [86]

NOTE This table presents a summary of studies which have evaluated the interaction between sera from ALS patients and either motor neurons, other cholinergic neurons (parasympathetic), or neuroblastoma cells. Assay systems used are divided into those using tissue culture, immunohistochemistry, and immunoblotting. Positive or negative results are based on whether results using ALS sera differed from those obtained using control sera.

Wolfgram and Myers. Touzeau et al [62] did not detect a toxic effect of ALS sera on fetal human spinal cord explant cultures.

Doherty et al [61] attempted to quantitate effects of ALS sera on cultured embryonic chick spinal neurons by using an ELISA to measure neurofilament protein expression in the cultures. ALS sera were found to lower the levels of neurofilament proteins below those produced by control and other neurological disease (OND) donor sera. The effect, however, was not due to a complement-mediated antibody activity and, indeed, the activity did not fractionate with the Ig component of the serum. Doherty et al could not demonstrate selectivity of the toxic effect to putative motor neurons in that there was no apparent selective toxicity for neurons which were responsive to muscle-derived survival factors. They concluded that their study showed no evidence of cytotoxic antineuronal antibodies in any ALS serum.

The effects of ALS sera have also been examined on neuronal populations other than motor neurons. Lehrich and Couture [63] found no evidence that ALS sera were cytotoxic to neuroblastoma cells in tissue culture. Touzeau and Kato [64] applied ALS sera to primary cultures of chick embryonic ciliary ganglia and observed a non-significant decrease in neuronal survival, choline acetyltransferase (CAT) activity, and acetylcholine synthesis compared to results obtained with control sera.

Immunohistochemical studies have also not clearly established the presence of specific Ig binding to motor nerve cells in cases of ALS. Weiner et al found no evidence of Ig bound to the surface of motor neurons isolated from the spinal cords of patients dying of ALS [65]. Digby et al [66], using dissociated spinal neuronal cultures derived from fetal rats, found enhanced binding of ALS sera (Ig) to such neurons compared to control Ig.

The possible existence of autoantibodies in ALS sera reactive with spinal cord constituents has also been explored in several studies using immunoblot analysis. Brown et al [67] concluded that no overall consistent differences existed in immunoblot profiles between ALS and control sera, using either mouse or human spinal cord as the antigen preparation and sera dilutions of 1:10 to 1:50. They did note, however, that reactivity of ALS sera with antigens of 50,000 and 70,000 daltons was possibly more frequent than for controls. These antigens were not CNS-specific and likely represented intermediate filaments.

We have also looked for antibodies in the serum of ALS patients using immunoblots. Our initial study [68] has been extended to include sera from 125 ALS patients and 125 age- and sex-matched controls. The controls included patients with various neurological diseases, including multiple sclerosis, Parkinson's disease, stroke, and Alzheimer's disease. We used as targets electrophoresed polypeptides from ventral grey matter of human spinal cord, isolated bovine anterior horn cells, isolated bovine Purkinje cells, human lymphocytes, human peripheral nerve, human striated muscle, and human kidney. The sera were used at 1:100 dilution. All of the sera used in this study had antibodies that bound to neurofilaments in all of the neural tissues used. All of the sera also had antibodies against many polypeptides in striated muscle. However, there was no difference in seroreactivity between ALS patients and controls. Hence, in our experience, ALS is not characterized by serum antibodies directed against epitopes on the polypeptides from the above-listed tissues that are accessible in our immunoblot system.

We also searched for autoantibodies against lipids from human spinal cord in the same ALS sera. The method we used was separation of lipids on thin-layer chromatography plates, followed by application of the test sera. Again, we found no difference between the ALS patients and controls. The ALS sera included those from four patients with ALS and IgM monoclonal gammopathy as previously mentioned, and two with angiofollicular hyperplasia and motor neuron disease. On balance, our results do not support the idea that autoantibodies play a role in the pathogenesis of the usual case of ALS or motor neuron disease. However, our results do not exclude the possibility that there are cases of the clinical syndrome of motor neuron disease that have autoantibodies participating in their pathogenesis.

Trophic-Factor–Directed Immune Factors

An appealing hypothesis regarding the pathogenesis of ALS concerns the role of specific soluble factors as essential elements required for maintaining MN survival (neuronotrophic) or, with specific regard to spinal motor neurons, inducing process outgrowth and innervation of skeletal muscle (neurotrophic). The postulate that motor neuron survival and function may be dependent on putative 'trophic' factors was initially derived from studies of the prototype neuronotrophic factor, nerve growth factor (NGF). NGF is an essential factor required for survival of sensory and sympathetic neurons during development. Research on NGF established a principle that the target tissue of a given neuronal population is likely to be a source of putative trophic factor, although other sites for the factor are found, such as the salivary glands. NGF extends its effect to more than sensory and sympathetic neurons. The most profound effects of the defined neuronotrophic factors are found in the developing rather than adult neuronal population. The existence of a molecule with the properties of NGF seems to raise the possibility that other molecules exist which play a similar role for other neuronal populations. In recent years, other trophic factor molecules have been purified, including the ciliary neuronotrophic factor found within intra-ocular muscle tissue which is innervated by the parasympathetic ciliary ganglion neuron [69, 70]. To date, no human disease state is identified in which a convincing abnormality of NGF or other neuronotrophic factor is the basic defect.

Neurite extension, as opposed to neuronal survival, can be promoted by a number of distinct molecules [71]. Both *in vitro* and *in vivo* axonal growth are promoted by factors which enhance adhesion of axons to substrate. These factors promote neurite extension of all neuronal types. Whether abnormalities of such factors influence the extent of reinner-vation remains under investigation in human neuronopathic-neuro-pathic diseases. With specific regard to MND, abnormality of the matrix proteins at the neuromuscular junction could result in defective nerve-muscle interactions [72].

Skeletal-muscle–derived growth factors Support for the existence of such factors comes from classic studies demonstrating that limb ablation or conversely implantation of supernumerary limb buds in developing tad-poles results in either enhanced or reduced programmed cell death re-spectively. In adult humans, amputation of a limb does not result in a dramatic reduction of the segmental MN pool, although lesser changes, such as chromatolysis of neurons, do occur. Embryonic spinal motor neurons do survive in culture in the absence of either their target organ or exogenous growth factor supplement, if the cells are maintained in an environment which includes the normal glial cells; the role of glial cells as trophic factor sources is considered later. This survival of MNs in isolation of target tissue contrasts with embryonic dorsal root ganglia cells, which have an absolute requirement for NGF.

The functional existence of skeletal-muscle–derived soluble factors has been demonstrated by *in vitro* assays evaluating cell survival, expres-sion of cholinergic activity (CAT), and neurite outgrowth using embry-onic spinal neuron cultures [73–79]. The lack of techniques to maintain adult spinal neurons dissociated in culture under any conditions has prevented similar studies on these cells. Similar biologic assays have also been used to assess experimental antisera, disease sera, or tissue extracts for inhibitory effects.

Smith et al [73, 74] showed that multiple skeletal muscle proteins, separated on the basis of molecular weight (MWT), act upon motor neu-rons contained within embryonic rat ventral spinal cord cultures. MNs could be identified in culture by pre-labelling the MNs *in vivo* with a lectin, wheat germ agglutinin (WGA) which was tagged with a fluores-cent marker, using a technique whereby the lectin is injected into skeletal muscle and retrogradely transported into MNs prior to dissecting the spinal cord. This labelling technique, supplemented by immunohisto-chemical studies of CAT content of spinal neurons, indicates that 5–10% of ventral spinal cord cells are motor neurons. Smith et al found that two-MWT protein species from muscle augmented CAT neuron survival and ACh synthesis; a 55,000-MWT glycoprotein induced ACh synthesis and MN-neurite extension but did not promote survival; a 35,000-MWT factor promoted neurite outgrowth but was not selective for CAT neurons. No specific inhibitory effects of human sera were detected in this system.

Doherty et al [75] found that human-muscle–conditioned media increased neurofilament protein expression within spinal but not sensory neuronal cultures using 7-day chick embryos as the source of neuronal cultures. The factor activity could not be adsorbed onto adhesive substrates, indicating that it was not one of the neurite-promoting factors which in general are not selective for motor neurons. The factor also was shown to act on fetal human neurons [75]. Identification of the entire spectrum of muscle-derived trophic factors has not yet been accomplished.

The capacity of ALS sera to inhibit the activity of putative muscle-derived neurotropic-trophic factors has been assessed in several assay systems. We found that 40% of ALS sera inhibit terminal axonal sprouting which follows botulinum-toxin–induced muscle paralylsis by more than 2 standard deviations of the mean effect of control sera (spouses of ALS patients, diabetics with neuropathy) [80]. Previously, Gurney [81] had demonstrated that antibodies which were raised against supernatants of denervated rat diaphragm muscle grown in organ culture could also inhibit the terminal axonal sprouting in this system. In the several ALS cases tested, the Ig fraction of the sera retained the inhibitory activity. Immunoblotting studies, using crude muscle-derived supernatant as antigen, suggested that an increased proportion of ALS sera compared to controls recognized a 56 Kd protein. Gurney et al purified and molecularly cloned this protein, termed neuroleukin, and demonstrated its neuronotrophic effects on spinal and sensory neurons [76]. The deduced nucleotide gene-encoding sequence of recombinant neuroleukin is identical to that of the glycolytic pathway enzyme glucose-6-phosphate isomerase (GPI) [82, 83].

Using the recombinant protein, we could not demonstrate a difference in reactivity of ALS sera from control sera on immunoblots; however, an increased proportion of ALS sera did react with the recombinant protein in an ELISA assay. Other control groups which reacted in the assay included patients with liver disease, CMV/EBV infection, leukemia/myeloma, and AIDS. These 'control' groups all feature increased serum Ig levels. When the individual ALS-sera–induced values of sprouting inhibition in the original botulinum toxin bioassay were correlated with reactivity in the ELISA assay, a significantly positive correlation was observed. How the biologic effects of neuroleukin can be ascribed to GPI remains speculative [84]. To date, the clinical significance, if any, of the anti-sprouting effect of ALS sera is not established. We observed no clinical effects of plasma-exchange and azathioprine therapy in the individual whose sera demonstrated the highest initial inhibitory activity, even though this activity was reduced after 4–6 weeks of therapy.

Hauser et al [85] evaluated the hypothesis that ALS serum factors interfere with survival and growth of lower motor neurons via an affect on muscle-derived trophic factors by testing ALS sera for reactivity against three muscle-derived preparations: a soluble extract from denervated chick skeletal muscle, conditioned media from organ culture of rat diaphragm muscle, and homogenized human muscle. They found no bands unique to ALS sera, although all sera reacted against a series of bands. IgG prepared from ALS sera also failed to inhibit chick-muscle–derived neurite-promoting activity. Henderson et al have found, however, that some muscle extracts from children with spinal muscular atrophy inhibit neurite outgrowth in this system [86].

Doherty et al, although finding that ALS sera were possibly toxic to spinal cord neuronal cultures, could not detect any inhibitory effect of ALS serum IgG on the neuronal survival enhancing factor released by G8-1 muscle cells [87]. As mentioned, neurite promoting and neuronal survival factors need not be identical molecules.

Glial-cell–derived trophic factors Growth of MNs *in vitro* is sharply inhibited if MNs are maintained in isolation rather than in the presence of glia. Whether this effect of glia is mediated via a single specific crucial MN-soluble factor remains to be resolved. C-6 glioma supernatant promotes survival with neurite extension by ventral spinal neurons, but this cell line seemingly secretes multiple soluble factors [88]. Whether ALS sera perturb glial function is speculative.

Neurohormone-neurotransmitter effects on MNs An array of soluble factors derived from sources other than skeletal muscle or glia may promote MN survival or function. Numerous hormones and neurotransmitter peptides have been shown to affect neurons either during development of *in vitro*. Androgens are shown to modify neuronal development, and the regional distribution of androgen receptors on motor neurons somewhat parallels the regional susceptibility of neurons involved in ALS [89]. Peptidergic transmitters reaching ventral spinal cord via descending brain-stem–spinal cord pathways, particularly thyrotropin-releasing hormone (TRH), are shown to enhance CAT levels in cultured spinal neurons [90]. Munsat et al report clinical cases of lower motor neuron syndromes with onset after cervical cord trauma, speculating that the trauma has interrupted these pathways [91]. One need also consider that excess neurotransmitter influences may induce neuronotoxic effects. This is suggested by known deleterious effects of an excess of excitatory transmitters on selected spinal non-motor neuronal populations. The existence of isolated lower or upper motor neuronal syndromes suggests that failure of trans-synaptic influences from upper to lower motor neurons does not inevitably result in degeneration of the corresponding lower motor neuron segment.

Effects of ALS Sera on Other Neural and Non-neural Tissues

ALS sera effects have been evaluated on a number of other target tissues. ALS sera seemingly exert a greater myelinotoxic effect on myelinated neural tissue cultures than do control sera; again one questions whether this represents an antibody-mediated effect. ALS sera will inhibit the ventral root response of frogs to an extent greater than control sera but to a lesser extent than sera from MS patients [92]. These observations have not been correlated with clinical parameters such as extent or tempo of disease progression.

ALS plasma has been reported to exert a toxic effect on red blood cells (RBCs) as measured by heightened degree of hemolysis [68, 93]. The effect is more apparent in classic ALS cases than in cases of progressive spinal muscular atrophy. Ronnevi et al [94] have found that the IgG and IgA fractions of ALS sera can induce the cytotoxic activity and that the effect is partially complement-dependent. Of note, RBCs from ALS patients are reported to show increased fragility in response to hypo-osmolality or mechanical force. Ronnevi et al suggest that putative 'noxious circulating substances' could directly affect the lower motor neuron at the motor end-plate region, which is outside the blood/brain barrier.

Less direct evidence regarding a role (or lack thereof) of immune factors in ALS is derived from the to-date negative results of passive transfer studies in which ALS sera were injected into animals [95]. The published data on immunosuppressive and plasma-exchange therapy for treatment of ALS, with the exclusion of the previously described IgM paraprotein motor neuropathy cases, suggest lack of efficacy of these modalities.

Characterization of MNs Using Monoclonal Antibodies (mcAbs)

Although the above-reviewed data indicate a failure as yet to detect unique antibodies interacting with motor neurons in ALS, these studies are greatly restricted by current lack of knowledge regarding the basic properties of motor neurons, which make them unique relative to other neuronal populations. Such knowledge may provide insight into the selectivity of the disease process ALS, for the motor neuron population. Even within the MN population, apparent selective vulnerability or resistance to the ALS disease process exists, such as in motor neurons within extraocular nerve nuclei and within selected sacral cord nuclei. Possible MN structures which might be recognized by antibody with subsequent functional cell disturbance could include surface receptors for transmitters or trophic factors, receptors for extracellular matrix molecules, structural proteins involved in axon transport or ion channel function, and internal organelles.

Epitopes on or in MNs have been defined by monoclonal antibodies raised using spinal cord or isolated MNs as initial immunogens. One cautions that the mcAbs derived by immunization of rats or mice, species not known to develop ALS, may be recognizing epitopes other than those which the human immune system may recognize and which may be relevant to the human disease. Human mcAbs recognizing neuronal elements, using ALS B-cells as the antibody-producing source, have not yet been developed.

An array of data suggest that specific neuronal populations, including motor neurons, possess specific epitopes either on their membrane surface or intracellularly. Note that retrograde axonal transport would provide a mechanism whereby an antibody could seek an intracytoplasmic determinant. Fabian and Petroff have documented retrograde Ig transport into motor neurons whose processes extend outside the CNS [96]. Among epitopes characteristic of particular neuronal subsets, as defined by mcAbs, many are shown to be preserved through a wide evolutionary spectrum. For example, mcAbs derived from immunization with *Drosophila* have been shown to recognize human spinal neurons [97]. Panels of mcAbs recognizing pre-synaptic motor neuron membranes cross-react widely across species, including humans [98]. Other neuron-directed mcAbs have been shown to be restricted in species specificity, as for example mcAbs which have been used to define mouse, leech, and cat spinal neurons [reviewed in 99]. Our experience with mouse-rat hybriodoma secreting Abs suggests that human-specific determinants do exist [100]. For example, we generated mcAbs recognizing human spinal neurons but not cerebral cortical neurons; these mcAbs did not stain murine tissue nor did most react with proteins on immunoblots. Increasingly, the concept is emerging that Ab directed against lipid or carbohydrate moieties and not just protein-directed Ab may be important in immune-mediated disorders. To date, no absolutely specific MN mcAb has been defined. This immunologic approach combined with molecular biologic studies searching for MN-specific genes holds promise for identification of MN-specific structures which, if defective, could directly result in disease, particularly familial ALS, or which may possibly become the target of an immune-mediated process.

References

1 Cohen JA, Lisak RP. Acute disseminated encephalomyelitis. In: Behan P and Aarli J, eds. Neuroimmunology for the Clinician. Oxford, Blackwell Scientific (in press)

2 Johnson RT, Griffin DE, Hirsch RL, et al. Measles encephalomyelitis – clinical and immunologic studies. New Eng J Med 1984;310:137–141

3 Pasteur L. Méthode pour prévenir la rage après morsure. C R Acad Sci 1885;101:765–747

4 Rivers TM, Schwentker FF. Encephalomyelitis accompanied by myelin destruction experimentally produced in monkeys. J Exp Med 1935;61:689–701

5 Sun D, Wekerle H. Ia-restricted encephalitogenic T lymphocytes mediating EAE lyse autoantigen-presenting astrocytes. Nature 1986;320:70–72

6 Endoh M, Tabira T, Kunishita T, et al. DM-20, a proteolipid apoprotein, is an encephalitogen of acute and relapsing autoimmune encephalomyelitis in mice. J Immunol 1986;137:3832–3835

7 Fierz W, Heininger K, Schaefer B, et al. Synergism in the pathogenesis of EAE induced by MBP-specific T cell line and monoclonal antibodies to galactocerebroside or to a myelin oligodendroglial glycoprotein. J Neuroimmunol 1987;16(1):55–56

8 Corey AL, Richman DP, Agius MA, Wollmann RL. Refractoriness to a second episode of experimental myasthenia gravis: Correlation with AChR concentration and morphologic appearance of postsynaptic membrane. J Immunol 1987;138:3269–3275

9 Gomez CM, Richman DP. Chronic experimental autoimmune myasthenia gravis induced by monoclonal antibody to acetylcholine receptor: Biochemical and electrophysiologic criteria. J Immunol 1987;139:73–76

10 Hohlfeld R, Toyka KV, Heininger K, et al. Autoimmune human T lymphocytes specific for acetylcholine receptor. Nature 1984;310:244–246

11 Christadoss P, Dauphinee MJ. Immunotherapy for myasthenia gravis: A murine model. J Immunol 1986;136:2437–2440

12 Patrick J, Linstrom J. Autoimmune response to acetylcholine receptor. Science 1973;180:871–872

13 Fukuoka T, Engel AG, Lang B, Newson-Davis J, Prior C, Wray DW. Lambert-Eaton myasthenic syndrome: I. Early morphological effects of IgG on the presynaptic membrane active zones. Ann Neurol 1987;22:193–199

14 Burns J, Rosenweig A. Zweiman B, et al. Isolation of myelin basic protein-reactive T-cell lines from normal human blood. Cellular Immunol 1983;81(2):435–440

15 Fujinami RS, Oldstone MBA. Amino acid homology between the ence-

phalitogenic site of myelin basic protein and virus: Mechanism for autoimmunity. Science 1985;230:1043–1045

16 Stefansson K, Dieperink ME, Richman DP, et al. Sharing of antigenic determinants between nicotinic acetylcholine receptor and proteins in *Escherichia coli, Proteus vulgaris* and *Klebsiella pneumoniae*. Possible role in the pathogenesis of myasthenia gravis. New Eng J Med 1985;312:221–225

17 Bach FH, Sachs DH. Transplantation immunology. New Eng J Med 1987;317:489–492

18 Appel SH, Stockton-Appel V, Stewart SS, Kerman RH. Amyotrophic lateral sclerosis. Arch Neurol 1986;43:234–238

19 Kiessling WR. Thyroid function in 44 patients with amyotrophic lateral sclerosis. Neurology 1982;39:241–242

20 Cashman N, Antel JP, Wissmann G, Bader P. Hyperthyroidism and familial amyotrophic lateral sclerosis (ALS). Ann Neurol 1983;14:117

21 Shy ME, Rowland LP, Smith T, et al. Motor neuron disease and plasma cell dyscrasia. Neurology 1986;36:1429–1436

22 Rowland LP, Defendini R, Sherman W, et al. Macroglobulinemia with peripheral neuropathy simulating motor neuron disease. Ann Neurol 1982;11:532–536

23 Peters HA, Clatanoff DV. Spinal muscular atrophy secondary to macroglobulinemia. Neurology (Minneap) 1968;18:101–108

24 Boyer M, Barat M, Mazaux JM, et al. Myélopathies non compressives et dysglobulinémies. Association fortuite? Discussion de trois nouveaux cas. Sem Hop (Paris) 1984;60:1109–1112

25 Donofrio PH, Greenberg HS, Albers JW, et al. IgM monoclonal protein binding to spinal cord and peripheral nerve glycolipids in a patient with motor neuron disease. Ann Neurol 1985;18:114

26 Engel WK, Hopkins LC, Rosenberg BJ. Fasciculating progressive muscular atrophy (F-PMA) remarkably responsive to antidysimmune treatment (ADIT): A possible clue to more ordinary ALS? Neurology 1985;35(Suppl 1):72

27 Rudnicki S, Chad DA, Drachman DA, et al. Motor neuron disease and paraproteinemia. Neurology 1987;37:335–337

28 Parry GJ, Holtz SJ, Ben-Zeev D, Drori JB. Gammopathy with proximal motor axonopathy simulating motor neuron disease. Neurology 1986;36:273–276

29 Bauer M, Bergstrom R, Ritter B, Olsson Y. Macroglobulinemia Waldenström and motor neuron syndrome. Acta Neurol Scand 1977;55:245–250

30 Chazot G, Berger B, Carrier H, et al. Manifestations neurologiques des gammopathies monoclonales. Rev Neurol (Paris) 1976;132:195–212

31 Solomon A. Neurological manifestations of macroglobulinemia. In: Brain

W, Norris FH, eds. The Remote Effects of Cancer on the Nervous System. New York, Grune & Stratton, 1965;112

32 Siden A, Kjellin KG. Isoelectric focusing of CSF and serum proteins in neurological disorders combined with benign and malignant proliferations of reticulocytes, lymphocytes and plasmacytes. J Neurol 1977;216: 251–264

33 Case records of the Massachusetts General Hospital. Case 31-1977. New Eng J Med 1977;297:266–274

34 Brownell B, Oppenheimer DR, Hugues JT. The central nervous system in motor neuron disease. J Neurol Neurosurg Psychiat 1970;33:338–357

35 Krieger C, Melmed K. A case of amyotrophic lateral sclerosis and paraproteinemia. Neurology 1982;32:617–621

36 Patten BM. Neuropathy and motor neuron syndromes associated with plasma cell disease. Acta Neurol Scand 1984;70:47–61

37 Poloni M, Rochelli R, Pinelli P, Scelsi R. Neuromuscular diseases associated with benign monoclonal gammopathy: Study of CSF and serum proteins by isoelectric focusing. Acta Neurol Scand 1982;65:154–159

38 Hobbs JR, Carter PM, Cooke KB, Foster M, Oon CJ. IgM paraproteins. J Clin Pathol 1975;28(suppl 6):54–64

39 Freddo L, Yu RK, Latov N, et al. Gangliosides G_{M1} and GD_{1b} are antigens for IgM M-protein in a patient with motor neuron disease. Neurology 1986;36:454–458

40 Nardelli E, Steck AJ, Barkas T, Schluep M, Jerusalem F. Motor neuron syndrome and monoclonal IgM with antibody activity against gangliosides G_{M1} and GD_{1b}. Ann Neurol 1988;23:524–528

41 Hays PH, Latov N, Takatsu M, Sherman WH. Experimental demyelination of nerve induced by serum of patients with neuropathy and an anti-MAG IgM M-protein. Neurology 1987;37:242–256

42 Shy ME, Heiman-Patterson T, Parry GJ, et al. Motor neuronopathy in patients with autoantibodies against gangliosides G_{M1} and GD_{1b}: Improvement following immunotherapy. Neurology 1988;38(suppl 1):252

43 Thomas FP, Hays AP, Latov N. Immunostaining of spinal cord, nerve, and the motor point of muscle with serum from patients with lower motor neuron disease and observed species differences. Neurology 1988;38(suppl 1):327

44 Pestronk A, Cornblath DR, Ilyas AA, et al. A treatable chronic, multifocal motor polyneuropathy associated with antibodies to a defined neural antigen. Ann Neurol 1987;22:119

45 Pestronk A, Adams RN, Clawson L, et al. Multifocal motor neuropathy: Clinical features of patients with anti-G_{M1} ganglioside antibodies. Neurology 1988;38(suppl 1):251

46 Shy ME, Evans VA, Lublin FD, et al. The presence of antibodies reacting with G_{M1} in motor neuron disease patients without plasma cell dyscrasia. J Neuroimmunol 1987;16(1):161

47 Schold SC, Cho E-S, Somasundaram M, Posner JB. Subacute motor neuronopathy: A remote effect of lymphoma. Ann Neurol 1979;5:271–287

48 Cashman NR, Gurney ME, Antel JP. Immunology of amyotrophic lateral sclerosis. Springer Sem Immunopathol 1985;8:141–152

49 Bartfeld H, Dham C, Donnenfeld H, et al. Immunological profile of amyotrophic lateral sclerosis patients and their cell-mediated immune responses to viral and CNS antigens. Clin Exp Immunol 1982;48:137–147

50 Maida E, Kristoferitsch W. Amyotrophic lateral sclerosis following herpes zoster infection in a patient with immunodeficiency. Eur Neurol 1981;20:330–333

51 Nemo GJ, Brody JA, Cruz M. Lymphoctye transformation study of Guamanian patients with amyotrophic lateral sclerosis and parkinsonism-dementia. Neurology 1974;24:579–581

52 Hoffman PM, Robbins DS, Nolte MT, et al. Cellular immunity in Guamanians with amyotrophic lateral sclerosis and parkinsonism-dementia. New Eng J Med 1978;299:680–685

53 Whitaker JN, Sciabbarrasi BS, Engel WK, et al. Serum immunoglobulin and complement (C3) levels. Neurology 1973;23:1164–1173

54 Donnenfeld H, Kascsak R:, Bartfeld H. Deposits of IgG and C_3 in the spinal cord and motor cortex of ALS patients. J Neuroimmunol 1984;6:51–57

55 Wolfgram F, Myers L. Amyotrophic lateral sclerosis: Effect of serum on anterior horn cells in tissue culture. Science 1973;179:579–580

56 Roisen FJ, Bartfeld H, Donnenfeld H, et al. Neruon specific in vitro cytotoxicity of sera from patients with amyotrophic lateral sclerosis. Muscle & Nerve 1982;5:48–53

57 Ronnevi L-O, Conradi S, Karlsson E. Cytotoxic effect of immunoglobulins in amyotrophic lateral sclerosis (ALS). Acta Neurol Scand 1984;98:182–183

58 Liveson J, Frey H, Bornstein MB. The effect of serum from ALS patients on organotypic nerve and msucle tissue culture. Acta Neuropathol (Berl) 1975;32:127–131

59 Horwich MS, Engel WK, Chauvin PB. Amyotrophic lateral sclerosis sera applied to cultured motor neurons. Arch Neurol 1974;30:332–333

60 Ecob MS, Brown AE, Young C, et al. Is there a circulating neurotoxic factor in motor neurone disease? In: Clifford Rose F, ed Research Progress in Motor Neurone Disease. London, Pitman, 1984;249–254

61 Doherty P, Dickson JG, Flanigan TP, et al. Effects of amyotrophic lateral sclerosis serum on cultured chick spinal neurons. Neurology 1986;36:1330–1334

62 Touzeau G, Kato AC. ALS serum has no effect on three enzymatic activities in cultured human spinal cord neurons. Neurology 1986;36:573–576

63 Lehrich JR, Couture J. Amyotrophic lateral sclerosis sera are not cytotoxic to neuroblastoma cells in tissue culture. Ann Neurol 1978;4:384

64 Touzeau G, Kato AC. Effects of amyotrophic lateral sclerosis sera on cultured cholinergic neurons. Neurology (Cleveland) 1983;33:317–322

65 Weiner LP, Stohlman SA, Davis RL. Attempts to demonstrate virus in amyotrophic lateral sclerosis. Neurology 1980;30:1319–1322

66 Digby J, Harrison R, Jehanli A, et al. Cultured rat spinal cord neurons: Interaction with motor neuron disease immunoglobulins. Muscle & Nerve 1985;8:595–605

67 Brown RH, Johnson D, Ogonowski M, Weiner HL. Antineural antibodies in the serum of patients with amyotrophic lateral sclerosis. Neurology1987;37:152–155

68 Kletti NB, Marton LS, Antel JP, Stefansson K. Antibodies against neural antigens in sera of pateints with amyotrophic lateral sclerosis. Neurology 1984;34(Suppl. 2):278

69 Manthrope M, Davis GE, Varon S. Purified proteins acting on cultured chick embryo ciliary ganglion neurons. Fed Proc 1985;44:2753–2759

70 Barbin G, Manthorpe M, Varon S. Purification of the chick eye ciliary neuronotrophic factor. J Neurochem 1984;43:1468–1478

71 Wagner JA. NIF (neurite-inducing factor): A novel peptide inducing neurite formation in PC12 cells. J Neurosci 1986;6(1):61–67

72 Festoff BW. Occurrence of reduced alpha$_2$-macro-globulin and lowered protease inhibiting capacity in plasma of amyotrophic lateral sclerosis patients. Ann NY Acad Sci 1983;421:369–376

73 Smith RG, Appel SH. Extracts of skeletal muscle increase neurite outgrowth and cholinergic activity of fetal rat spinal motor neurons. Science 1983;219:1079–1081

74 Smith RG, Vaca K, McManaman J, Appel SH. Selective effects of skeletal muscle extract fractions on motoneuron development in vitro. J Neurosci 1986;6(2):439–447

75 Doherty P, Dickson JG, Flanigan TP, Walsh FS. Human muscle cell conditioned media stimulate neurofilament protein expression in primary cultures of human and chick spinal cord. J Physiol (London) 1985;360:43P

76 Gurney ME, Heinrich SP, Lee MR, Yin H-S. Molecular cloning and expression of neuroleukin, a neurotrophic factor for spinal and sensory neurons. Science 1986;234:566–574

77 Henderson CE, Huchet M, Changeux JP. Denervation increases a neurite-promoting activity in extracts of skeletal muscle. Manture 1983;302:609–611

78 Bonyhady RE, Hendry IA, Hill CE, Watters DJ. An analysis of peripheral

neuronal survival factors present in muscle. J Neurosci Res 1985;13:357–367

79 Weber MJ, Raynaud B, Delteil C. Molecular properties of a cholinergic differentiation factor from muscle-conditioned medium. J Neurochem 1985;45(5):1541–1547

80 Gurney ME, Belton AC, Cashman N, Antel JP. Inhibition of terminal axonal sprouting by serum from patients with amyotrophic lateral sclerosis. New Eng J Med 1984;311:933–939

81 Gurney ME. Suppression of sprouting at the neuromuscular junction by immune sera. Nature 1984;307:546–548

82 Faik P, Walker IH, Redmill AAM, et al. Mouse glucose-6-phosphate isomerase and neuroleukin have identical 3' sequences. Nature 1988;332:455–456

83 Chaput M, Claes V, Portetelle D, et al. Neurotrophic factor neuroleukin is 90% homologous with phosphohexose isomerase. Nature 1988;332:454–455

84 Gurney ME. Gurney replies. Letter to the Editor. Nature 1988;332:456–457

85 Hauser SL, Cazenave P-A, Lyon-Caen O, et al. Immunoblot analysis of circulating antibodies against muscle proteins in amyotrophic lateral sclerosis and other neurological diseases. Neurology 1986;36:1614–1618

86 Henderson CE, Huchet M, Changeux JP. Neurite-promoting activities for embryonic spinal neurons and their developmental changes in the chick. Dev Biol 1984;104:335–347

87 Doherty P, Dickson JG, Flanigan TP, Walsh FS. Human skeletal muscle cells synthesise a neuronotrophic factor reactive with spinal neurons. J Neurochem 1986;46:133–139

88 Amico L, Yu R, Antel JP, Arnason BGW. Growth-promoting effect of C-6 glioma conditioned media on spinal cord cells. Trans Am Neurol Assoc 1981;106:1–3

89 Weiner LP. Possible role of androgen receptors in amyotrophic lateral sclerosis: A hypothesis. Arch Neurol 1980;37:129–131

90 Schmidt-Achert KM, Askanas V, Engel WK. Thyrotropin-releasing hormone enhances choline acetyltransferase and creatine kinase in cultured spinal ventral horn neurons. J Neurochem 1984;43:586–589

91 Munsat TL, Sloan M, Van den Bergh P, Baquis G. Motor neuron disease after cervical spinal cord trauma. J Neuroimmunol 1987;16(1):127

92 Schauf CL, Antel JP, Arnason BGW, et al. Neuroelectric blocking activity and plasmapheresis in amyotrophic lateral sclerosis. Neurology 1980;30:1011–1013

93 Ronnevi L-O, Conradi S. Increased fragility of erythrocytes from amyotrophic lateral sclerosis (ALS) patients provoked by mechanical stress. Acta Neurol Scand 1984;69:20–26

94 Ronnevi L-O, Conradi S, Karlsson E, Sindhupak R. Nature and properties

of cytotoxic plasma activity in amyotrophic lateral sclerosis. Muscle & Nerve 1987;1:240.1–240.10

95 Denys EH, Jackson JE, Aguilar MJ, et al. Passive transfer experiments in amyotrophic lateral sclerosis. Arch Neurol 1984;41:161–163

96 Fabian RH, Petroff G. Intraneuronal IgG in the central nervous system: Uptake by retrograde axonal transport. Neurology 1987;37:1780-1784

97 Zipursky SL, Venkatesh TR, Benzer S. From monoclonal antibody to gene for a neuron-specific glycoprotein in *Drosophila*. Proc Natl Acad Sci (USA) 1985;82:1855–1859

98 Kushner PD, Stephenson DT, Sternberg H, Weber R. Monoclonal antibody Tor 23 recognizes a determinant of a presynaptic acetylcholinesterase. J Neurochem 1987;48:1942–1953

99 Reichardt LF. Immunological approaches to the nervous system. Science 1984;225:1294–1299

100 Antel JP, Kuchibhotla J, Stefansson K. Generation of monoclonal antibodies recognizing neuronal elements in formalin-fixed paraffin-embedded human tissue. J Neuropathol Exp Neurol 1985;44:533–545

Amyotrophic Lateral Sclerosis: Clinical Evidence for Differences in Pathogenesis and Etiology

ARTHUR J. HUDSON

The practice of medicine depends largely on physicians recognizing the different clinical patterns of disease. Increased diagnostic and therapeutic expertise, however, has brought an awareness that even highly skilled clinical pattern recognition can be unreliable because etiologically different disorders can sometimes have remarkably similar appearance. This has been demonstrated, most recently and dramatically, in cases of idiopathic and drug-induced forms of parkinsonism that are clinically indistinguishable. It is axiomatic, therefore, that diseases of identical clinical appearance can have different causes. Included among the apparently single clinical entities with potentially multiple causes is amyotrophic lateral sclerosis (ALS).

ALS is a relentlessly progressive and fatal wasting disease of skeletal muscle that in the *classical sporadic form* has focal onset and is accompanied by fasciculation and spasticity. To complete this triad of signs there are the corresponding characteristic pathological changes of lower and upper motor neuron degeneration. There is a tendency to view ALS as a single entity but in addition to clinically identical disorders with distinctly different pathological findings there are a number of conditions that more or less resemble the classical sporadic form because they share one or more of the triad of ALS signs. Classical sporadic ALS constitutes by far the larger proportion of all ALS cases throughout the world. In the following presentation the various disorders that are identical to or closely resemble classical ALS are described (Table 1). It is important to recognize that while much attention is given to them a number of the motor neuron diseases that will be described are rare. Also, some conditions with resemblance to ALS have sometimes been

TABLE 1
Classification of syndromes with resemblance to classical amyotrophic lateral sclerosis

1 Classical sporadic amyotrophic lateral sclerosis

2 Syndromes that are clinically indistinguishable from classical sporadic amyotrophic lateral sclerosis
   (a) Familial amyotrophic lateral sclerosis
   (b) Western Pacific amyotrophic lateral sclerosis
   (c) Post-encephalitic amyotrophic lateral sclerosis
   (d) Presumably infective amyotrophic lateral sclerosis
   (e) Juvenile neuronal inclusion-body amyotrophic lateral sclerosis

3 Distinct but clinically similar disease states that may be confused with classical amyotrophic lateral sclerosis
   (a) Post-poliomyelitis progressive amyotrophy
   (b) Lipid disorder and motor neuron disease
   (c) Mercury poisoning
   (d) Motor neuropathy accompanying Hodgkin's disease
   (e) Autoimmune disease and amyotrophic lateral sclerosis
   (f) Other uncommon motor neuron diseases

4 Combined motor neuropathy and corticospinal tract disease resembling classical sporadic amyotrophic lateral sclerosis
   (a) Thyrotoxicosis
   (b) Hyperparathyroidism
   (c) Other metabolic disorders
   (d) Lead poisoning
   (e) Radiation neuromyelopathy
   (f) Motor neuropathy and unrelated corticospinal tract disease

5 Probable coincidental occurrence of classical sporadic amyotrophic lateral sclerosis with other unrelated disease
   (a) Cancer and amyotrophic lateral sclerosis
   (b) Irreversible amyotrophic lateral sclerosis and other disease

called ALS whereas the proper designation is 'ALS-like' or, simply, motor neuron disease in its broadest sense.

Classical Sporadic ALS

Classical sporadic ALS is a bench-mark to which all other amyotrophic syndromes are compared. While this form of ALS is the condition most of us see and recognize as ALS it is important to appreciate the difficulties which can arise in distinguishing with certainty 'classical' ALS from clinically similar syndromes. ALS is not exclusively a disease of the upper and lower motor neurons; a variety of other neuronal structures can be affected. While such diversity of findings is largely based on pathological evidence, nevertheless, clinical signs other then those due to corticospinal and lower motor neuron degeneration may be present. For example, about 3.5% of ALS patients show dementia, 1.5% have parkinsonism, and approximately 25% have minor sensory symptoms and signs [1–3].

Epidemiology

The average life expectancy of a patient with classical ALS is about 2.7 years from the time of diagnosis, with a range of approximately 6 months to 20 years [2, 4, 5]. Survival data, based on all patients living and deceased in a 5-year (1978–82) epidemiological study [2] of southwestern Ontario, Canada, were compared with data gathered by Rosen [4] in the United States. The data are remarkably close. At the end of a 5-year period the Ontario study showed an overall 35.5% (Rosen, 31.5%) survival. Survival by the end of the 5th year for patients under the age of 50 was 56% (Rosen, 62.5%) and for patients over the age of 50 only 31% (Rosen, 31.5%). In agreement with Rosen's study, younger patients have a significantly better prognosis ($p < 0.002$). In both studies the prognosis in men and women was similar.

There is a male to female preponderance ranging from 1.2:1 to 1.6:1. ALS is an age-related disease that increases in incidence throughout life but because the elderly population progressively diminishes with age the peak non-age-related incidence occurs between 55 and 66 years [2, 4, 6–8]. The estimated crude incidence of ALS world-wide is not more than 2.4 per 100,000 and in our study of southwestern Ontario it was 1.6 [2]. We found that the incidence of ALS in the 5th decade of life was 1.7 – about the same as the overall incidence – whereas in the 6th, 7th, and 8th decades it was 3.9, 6.3, and 7.4, respectively. Estimates are difficult beyond the 8th decade because of the common tendency to regard all infirmity in the elderly as due to 'old age.' Thus, it is not possible to say whether the disease steadily increases with age. Older patients, certainly those over 50 years of age, have shorter survival times than those under 50. With bulbar ALS there is generally a shorter life expectancy than for ALS affecting the limbs because of a propensity to upper airway obstruction and aspiration. Early diaphragmatic involvement leads to a very short survival time.

Conditions such as the environment, diet, and trauma have been explored by many researchers and it is recognized that living and working conditions play a role in the pathogenesis of ALS [2]. Occasionally, clusters of three or so ALS patients are found within a fairly small geographic area which increases such concerns but the significance of clusters, if any, is never clear. A high male to female ratio suggests the influence of physical and occupational factors relating to the largely male role in heavy industry and agriculture but these differences may be evening out. Kurtzke and Beebe [9] found that ALS patients more often gave a history of trauma, especially fractures of limbs or surgical operations. However, not all investigators are agreed that trauma is important [10].

Clinical Features

The lower and upper motor neuron features of ALS are relentlessly progressive but, from time to time, a case may show very slow deterioration or apparent plateauing. Although sustained reversal of illness has been described, such cases are likely not true ALS. The disorder is usually focal in onset with mild weakness and wasting or spasticity. Lower motor neuron signs occur in all ALS patients while corticobulbar and/or corticospinal signs (mild spasticity with hyperreflexia and a Babinski sign) are present in 85% of cases. When the first sign of disease is weakness and wasting of an extremity, especially if accompanied by fasciculation, the diagnosis is not difficult. Fasciculation varies from one case to the next and is sometimes negligible. Onset with spastic dysarthria is more difficult since fasciculation and muscular wasting may not be initially apparent. As the disease spreads, often spottily, weakness and wasting become generalized. Eventually, the diaphram atrophies and when this becomes severe the patient dies from pulmonary failure. Upper motor signs usually appear early, adding spasticity and 'pyramidal' weakness to the picture of established lower motor neuron muscular weakness and wasting, but their presence alone – i.e. in the absence of some wasting – is unusual except in cases with spastic dysarthria at onset. The diagnosis of ALS should be made cautiously in cases that present exclusively with spasticity. Onset in different regions has given rise to the concept of different disease states, such as progressive bulbar palsy (onset in the bulbar region) or progressive muscular atrophy (onset in the limbs or trunk). Amyotrophic lateral sclerosis (ALS) refers to a type with both upper and lower motor neuron signs, but since these are eventually present in most patients, this term is now applied to the entire disease regardless of the site of onset.

Extraocular motor nuclei are often said to be unaffected in ALS but lower motor neuron degeneration involving the oculomotor, trochlear, and abducens nuclei has been described [11, 12]. As stated by Hirano et al (this volume) further confirmatory studies of this occurrence in classical sporadic ALS are needed. However, mild spasticity of the extraocular muscles in patients with upper motor neuron degeneration [13, 14, 15] is not uncommon. ALS, as noted earlier, can be accompanied by dementia or parkinsonism although overt changes of this kind are infrequent.

It has been widely held also that sensory symptoms and signs are not present in classical ALS. However, sensory complaints and signs, such as paresthesia and diminished vibration sense, are not infrequent (25% of cases). The altered vibration thresholds are found with careful sensory testing and have been interpreted by Mulder et al [16] as due to increased cutaneous myelinated nerve fibre degeneration. Radtke et al [17] in a study of sensory-evoked potentials in ALS, found evidence of sensory dysfunction in almost half of the cases. Muscular pain is not uncommon. Probably muscle cramps or the persisting ache in muscle that follows severe cramps is the most frequent cause. Muscle or joint injury due to weakened muscles is also a cause.

Of interest are findings of histological, histochemical, and/or ultrastructural abnormalities reported in organs other than the nervous system, such as liver and skin, of ALS patients [18, 19, 20]. Liver biopsies of ALS patients have been reported as showing abnormal liver enzymes, and on electron microscopy alterations of mitochondria have been seen in hepatic cells [18]. The copper content of hepatocytes may be elevated. Pathological findings in sporadic ALS are described by Hirano et al (this volume).

Syndromes That Are Clinically Indistinguishable from Classical Sporadic ALS

FAMILIAL ALS

Familial ALS is clinically identical to classical sporadic ALS. It is estimated that about 5% of cases of ALS have a family history of the disease [2, 20, 21, 22]. Mulder et al [3] reviewed 72 families with 2 or more affected members and almost 90% had ALS in more than one generation. Familial ALS in only a single sibship suggests recessive inheritance but actual numbers of affected members are difficult to determine because of the usually late onset of the disease. Family members who might eventually develop ALS may die earlier from other disease [21, 22].

The presence of ALS and other neurological disease in the same family or in the same patient has been reported. Roe [23] described a mother with two daughters who were all diagnosed as having ALS and two other daughters who were diagnosed with multiple sclerosis. Mackay

[24] mentions the occurrence of ALS in a sister and brother and multiple sclerosis in another sister. Autopsy-proven ALS and multiple sclerosis in the same patient have been described [25].

Clinical Features

The sex ratio in familial ALS ranges from (male/female) 1:1 to 1.3:1 [1, 3, 4, 26, 27] and in sporadic ALS from 1.2:1 to 1.6:1 [2, 6, 28, 29, 30]. Familial ALS occurs at an earlier age than the sporadic disease. In the Mayo clinic studies the mean age of onset of familial ALS was 48 years and of sporadic ALS 66 years [3, 6].

The clinical features of lower and upper motor neuron signs in familial and sporadic cases are indistinguishable. Minor sensory findings such as paresthesias and vibratory sensory diminution occur in familial disease in about the same proportion (20%) as in sporadic ALS. Similarly, dementia occasionally occurs and may be slightly more frequent in familial (7%) than sporadic (3.5%) cases [2, 3].

Subtypes of Familial ALS Based on Duration of Disease

The average duration of illness in familial ALS, overall, is similar to that for sporadic ALS at approximately 2.5 years. However, it is possible to identify two subgroups based on the duration of the disease. ALS can be of very short duration if the diaphragm is affected early or in bulbar ALS with severe upper airway obstruction and aspiration, but the short-duration disease as described here advances with extraordinary rapidity regardless of the site of onset. Horton et al [22] have described both short- and long-duration cases of familial ALS but their short-duration type had an average survival of 2 years, ranging up to 5 years, which corresponds to the mean survival for both sporadic and familial ALS There are, however, families with ALS that progresses very rapidly.

Short-duration ALS Data for five families with apparently dominantly inherited ALS and a mean duration of illness of one year or less are shown in Table 2. The disease in the five families extended over two to four generations with a mean age of onset of 47 years (compared to about 60 years in sporadic ALS) and a mean duration of 9.5 months (a third of the mean duration for the sporadic disease). In family A of Engel et al [30] the duration of ALS was more variable than in the other families, ranging between 6 months and 2 years, but the average duration was about one year. In the family that we studied with four affected members over four generations ALS ranged in duration between 9 and 12 months.

TABLE 2
Short-duration familial amyotrophic lateral sclerosis

Author [reference]	Generations	Mean age of onset (range) yr	Cases (male:female)	Site of onset	Muscle wasting	Upper motor neuron signs (cases)	Duration (range) mo
Boudin and Barbizet (fam. Bl) [34]	2	49 (42–63)	3:1	Limbs, shoulder girdle	+	+ (1)	10 (9–12)
Engel et al (fam. A) [30]	4	39 (30–56)	4:7	Usually limbs	+	Autopsy evidence in some	approx 12
Hawkes et al [31]	3	53 (39–63)	2:4	Legs and arms	+	+ (4)	4.7 (3–6)
Horton et al (fam. 1) [22]	2	49 (39–56)	2:1	Limbs, bulbar*	+	+ (1)†	11 (6–16)
Present author	4	43 (41–45)	1:3	Bulbar, arms, legs	+	+ (2)	10 (9–12)

* Site of onset not specified.
† Autopsy evidence of pyramidal tract involvement.

Long-Duration ALS Data for eight families with long-duration ALS, averaging 13 years, are shown in Table 3. The disease in the eight families extended over one to four generations with a mean age of onset of 38 years, approximately 22 years or so less than the mean for sporadic ALS. Survival in some family members was only 2 to 3 years but the mean duration for these families was 7 or more years. In families 13 and 14 of Horten et al [22] the only two affected members in each family were still alive at the time of their report; in the present author's study also, two of the three cases with ALS were still alive after 7 years.

Pathology of familial ALS differs from that of sporadic and Western Pacific ALS. This is described by Hirano et al (this volume).

Conjugal ALS Conjugal ALS has been described by MacKay [24] and Paolino et al [33]. The significance of conjugal ALS is not clear but a coincidental occurrence in spouses or a common environmental cause are the most likely possibilities.

WESTERN PACIFIC ALS

There are a number of well-known high-incidence regions of ALS in the Western Pacific. These are the regions occupied by the Chamorros on Guam, Rota, and Tinian Islands; the Hobara and Kozagawa regions of the Kii Peninsula on Honshu Island in Japan; the Auyu and Jakai villages of West Irian; and, most recently, Groote Eylandt in Australia. These high-incidence areas have implicated environmental factors, especially the mineral content of soil and water [38] and a formerly important dietary constituent, the cycad seed, in the pathogenesis of ALS [39]. The westernization of the diet of the native Chamorro population of Guam and nearby islands appears to have produced a drop in incidence. There may still be other high-incidence foci in the Western Pacific and Asia [40]. Gajdusek [41] has proposed that injury to the 10-mm neurofilament from a variety of environmental causes could be responsible for neuronal breakdown in ALS and a number of other disorders.

Epidemiology

ALS in the geographically restricted foci of the Western Pacific is associated with parkinsonism and dementia (PD). The decline in the incidence and mortality rates of ALS and PD on Guam has been dramatic. The annual incidence about 30 years ago was 50 per 100,000 population whereas now it is less than 5 per 100,000, close to the mean incidence of about 1.5 per 100,000 population in Europe and North America [42,

TABLE 3
Long-duration familial amyotrophic lateral sclerosis

Author [reference]	Generations	Mean age of onset (range) yr	Cases (male:female)	Site of onset	Muscle wasting	Upper motor neuron signs (cases)	Duration (range) years
Espinosa et al [35]	2	39 (32–51)	2:6	Limbs	+	+ (3)	14 (2–33)
Metcalf* and Hirano [32]	4	40 (31–50)	8:8	Limbs, data incomplete	+	+ (5)	12 (5–21)
Giménez-Roldán and Estaban [36]	3	50 (33–61)	2:3	1 bulbar 4 distal	+	+ (1)	7 (2–13)
Albercat† et al [37]	3	30 (24–38)	8:5	Limbs	+	+ (4)	18 (5–36)
Horton et al [22]							
Fam 12	3	38 (28–52)	10:8	Limbs, bulbar‡	+	+ (4)	14 (6–27)
Fam 13	1	45 (44–45)	2:0	Limbs, bulbar‡	+	+ (2)	6§
Fam 14	1	35 (33–37)	2:0	Limbs, bulbar‡	+	+ (1)	14"
Present author	2	30 (29–30)	1:2	Limbs	+	+ (1)	18 (2 alive after 7 years)

* 6 cases had sensory symptoms; 2 had glove and stocking sensory signs.
† Information available on only 5 family members.
‡ Site of onset not specified.
§ Both cases alive after 3 years' and 9 years' duration.
" Both cases alive after 10 years' and 18 years' duration.

43]. The incidence in New Guinea and the Kii Peninsula is said to have declined but detailed studies have not been reported [42].

Rodgers-Johnson et al [42] evaluated the clinical and pathological course of Guamanian ALS and found a progressive increase in the age of clinical onset in both sexes. The mean age is now approximately 52 years as compared to 45 years three decades ago. Moreover, as occurs with classical sporadic ALS with later onset, the duration of the disease has become shorter. The mean duration is now less than 4 years, 30% to 50% less than three decades ago. The male to female ratio was approximately 2:1 and has now attained 1:1 [43]. ALS among the Chamorro migrants from Guam to the United States (mainly California), Japan, Germany, and Korea has shown a much higher incidence than normally encountered in these countries but less than on Guam [44]. Garruto et al [44] claim that the minimum exposure on Guam for contracting the disease is 18 years.

Clinical Features

ALS of the Guamanian type Guamanian ALS has a pattern and distribution of skeletal muscle weakness and wasting, beginning focally but eventually involving the skeletal musculature generally including bulbar muscles, that are indistinguishable from those of the classical form of the disease. Very few patients with ALS of the Guamanian type show intellectual loss despite close association of the disease with the Parkinson-dementia complex. All Guamanian ALS patients have lower motor neuron signs consisting of atrophy and fasciculation and about 85% to 90% have upper motor neuron signs consisting of hyperreflexia and/or the Babinski sign, the same as in classical ALS (85%) [3]. Minor sensory symptoms and signs, notably paresthesias and loss of vibration sense, are found in 30% of the Guamanian cases, which is similar to their occurrence in the classical and familial forms of ALS.

Kii Peninsula and New Guinea ALS The clinical features of Kii Peninsula and New Guinea ALS are the same as of Guamanian ALS and are identical to those of the classical disease. Gajdusek [40] has summarized the key epidemiological features in western New Guinea and Kii Peninsula cases, respectively, as follows: sex ratio 1.5:1 and 1.8:1; onset 33 and 50 years; mean duration 3.5 and 2.6 years.

Groote Eylandt motor neuron disease This disorder was recently described by Kiloh et al [45] and affects Australian aborigines who live on Groote Eylandt and the nearby Arnheim Land area of Northern Australia [46]. It is a complex disorder similar to ALS/PD inasmuch as there are at least two syndromes. One of these resembles ALS but occurs in childhood, and the other is of later onset with a clinical picture of cerebellar and upper motor neuron signs and, sometimes, supranuclear ophthalmoplegia. Because the same family can have different members affected by either of the two disorders they appear to be variations of the same condition.

Pathology

The pathological changes in Guamanian ALS, which apply for the most part to other Western Pacific forms of the disease, have been well described by Hirano and his associates (see this volume). Loss of anterior horn cells and corticobulbar and corticospinal tract degeneration are the same as in classical ALS. Posterior column degeneration is rare. However, the feature that distinguishes the Western Pacific from classical ALS is an abundance of neurofibrillary tangles (NFT) in neurons in the former. Recently, Rodgers-Johnson et al [42] have reported on the neuropathological features in Guamanian ALS patients over a 30-year period. They found cortical atrophy in 28% of cases. NFTs were found scattered diffusely throughout the cerebrum and brain-stem in 96% of cases, with a predilection for the hippocampus, and were observed in the spinal cord in 22% of cases. They also were present in the cranial nerve nuclei and anterior horn cells. Some degree of NFT formation is present in the normal Chamorro nervous system.

Pathogenesis

The explanation offered by some investigators for the high incidence of ALS/PD in these regions is the deposition of toxic metals and essential minerals in the neurons of the central nervous system. This process is said to begin with an indigenous lack of calcium and magnesium in soil and water [47], and deficiency of these minerals in the diet produces secondary hyperparathyroidism. This is followed by the deposition of calcium (mobilized from bone) and toxic elements such as aluminum, manganese, and silicon (absorbed from the diet) into neurons. Accumulation of calcium, aluminum, and silicon in neurons bearing neurofibrillary tangles has been found in these cases [47]. Garruto et al [47] suggest that these elements may interfere with slow axonal transport.

Spencer et al [39] have revived the notion that the consumption of the seed from the false sago palm (*Cycas circinalis*) is the source of the neurological disorders on Guam. The toxic component β-N-methylamino-L-alanine (L-BMAA) is viewed by Spencer and his associates as the cause of ALS/PD. Their evidence lies in the effects of L-BMAA after its oral administration to cynomolgus monkeys. The animals developed features of motor neuron disease within 8 weeks. As suggested by Yanagihara [48] there may be combinations of hormone (parathyroid, etc.), mineral dietary and metabolic factors, toxins, etc. that cause ALS-PD rather than any one of these alone. The decline in ALS/PD on Guam supports this view inasmuch as the deficient minerals, calcium and magnesium, have been made available and the cycad seed abandoned through acculturation and westernization of the Chamorro diet. If, as seems likely, ALS does not vanish but plateaus at a low incidence corresponding to the remainder of the world, then this hypothesis would be proved to be at least partially correct.

POST-ENCEPHALITIC ALS

Following the epidemics of encephalitis lethargica that peaked in 1920 and 1924 there were many reports of patients who developed ALS months or years after an attack of encephalitis [1]. The average age of onset of encephalitis was 28 years and the interval between the encephalitis and onset of ALS averaged less then 10 years. Half of the reported cases developed ALS within 5 years. While association of ALS with encephalitis could have been a coincidence, it seems improbable because two-thirds of these cases also had parkinsonism, a condition that is a well-recognized sequel of encephalitis lethargica. Moreover, the mean age of onset of ALS was less than 40 years, which is unusually young for the classical disease. A pathological feature common to both the Western Pacific and post-encephalitic types of ALS was the presence of intraneuronal neurofibrillary tangles.

PRESUMABLY INFECTIVE MOTOR NEURON DISEASE

It has long been debated whether virus infection can produce motor neuron disease resembling ALS in man. A syndrome that was clinically indistinguishable from ALS occurred in a patient who was bitten on an ankle by a cat [49]. The injury was accompanied by severe local infection requiring debridement, and within 6 months of the bite paralysis appeared at the ankle and advanced proximally causing death from pulmonary failure within a year. At autopsy there was both severe lower motor neuron loss and corticospinal degeneration but, in addition, perivascular inflammation was present in the meninges and spinal cord, suggesting an infectious cause. A careful search for virus was made but none was found. There was oligoclonal banding in the cerebrospinal fluid and marked elevation of the ANA titre in serum, both of which are very unusual findings in ALS. There were no signs of autoimmune disease. This case appears to be the only report of an ALS-like syndrome with central nervous system inflammatory changes involving a possible animal source.

JUVENILE NEURONAL INCLUSION-BODY ALS

There are a number of reports of a sporadic syndrome in young adolescents that is clinically and pathologically indistinguishable from ALS except for the unusually young age of the patient and the pathological finding of neuronal intracytoplasmic inclusions [1, 50]. Onset is between 12 and 16 years of age and the duration of the disease ranges from 12 to 18 months. There is lower motor neuron and pyramidal tract degeneration but no other long-tract changes. Neuronal degeneration and/or intracytoplasmic basophilic inclusions are found in the cortex, subcortical and brain-stem nuclei, and spinal motor neurons.

Distinct But Clinically Similar Disease States That May Be Confused with Classical ALS

POST-POLIOMYELITIS PROGRESSIVE AMYOTROPHY

The 'post-polio' syndrome is a disorder in which progressive muscular weakness and wasting develops some years after an acute attack of poliomyelitis from which there has been, as a rule, considerable recovery (see Dalakas, this volume). The recurrence of muscular weakness in the post-polio syndrome involves both previously partially or fully affected muscles and also formerly clinically normal muscles. As in poliomyelitis the new weakness and wasting is asymmetrical and appears after an interval of 1 to 6 decades following an attack of acute poliomyelitis [51]. The loss of muscle strength is very slow and can periodically plateau. Fasciculation may be present in both the clinically affected and unaffected muscles. Fibrillation potentials and positive sharp waves may also be present but, as a rule, they are sparse or moderate, suggesting very scattered slow denervation. Oligoclonal bands (IgG) in the cerebrospinal fluid are found in half of the post-polio patients with no evidence of elevated antibodies to poliovirus [51]. Muscle biopsy shows no evidence of group atrophy but rather isolated, atrophic angulated fibres in the intercises between large fibres. This suggests a loss of the individual nerve terminals of surviving motor neurons. Motor neurons that have survived poliomyelitis take over the muscle fibre territory of the destroyed motor neurons by means of axonal sprouting. Dalakas et al [51] have proposed that the enlarged motor units constitute a burden to the cell, which must be metabolically hyperactive if it is to maintain the metabolic demands of its enlarged axonal territory. It is believed that if these demands cannot be met, as presumed in the post-polio syndrome, then individual nerve terminals from the formerly expanded population of axonal sprouts will be progressively lost. This could explain a clinical picture of slowly progressive muscular weakness emerging. An alternative interpretation of weakening of muscles is a further dropping out of an already polio-depleted population of anterior horn cells (rather than axonal sprouts) as the individual ages. However, the normal loss of anterior horn cells is generally not significant before the age of 60 years and many post-polio cases are under this age [52].

LIPID DISORDER AND MOTOR NEURON DISEASE

Lipid Abnormalities in ALS

The possiblity that lipids are in some manner involved in the pathogenesis of ALS has been supported by two recent observations. First, Dawson and Stefansson [53] described a difference from the normal in ganglioside content of the spinal cord of ALS patients (see also Dawson et al. this volume). They observed sialosyl-(2→3)-globotetraosylceramide (SPG) in 9 ALS spinal cords, which with one exception, was not found in normal cords. This ganglioside, which was also found by Kundu et al [54] in ALS skeletal muscle, was not present in normal or facioscapulo-humeral muscular dystrophy muscle. The concentration can rise with the severity of the disease. As pointed out by Dawson and Stefansson the gangliosides influence neuronal sprouting, and the relative increase of one or more of these may reflect an attempt at recovery by the motor neuron. The second observation on lipid changes in ALS was the finding of altered ganglioside patterns in the brain of ALS patients, not only in the motor cortex but in the frontal and temporal lobes and parahippocampal gyrus cortex (see Dawson et al, this volume) [55].

Gangliosides and Motor Neuron Disease

Abnormality in lipid metabolism giving rise to an ALS-like motor neuron disease is rare but has been described in several cases of G_{M2} gangliosidosis resulting from a deficiency of a N-acetyl-β-D-hexosaminidase, a lysosomal hydrolase (called also β-Hex). An isozyme of β-Hex, hexosaminidase A or 'Hex A,' is composed of alpha and beta chains, and genetic alteration of either chain can cause impaired Hex A activity (see

TABLE 4
Motor neuron disease and hexosaminidase deficiency

Case or family [reference]	Sex, age at onset (years)	Age last examined (years)	Muscle atrophy	Fascic	UMN signs	Other signs
Navon et al [63]	F, child	43	+	−	+	Tremor
	M, child	38	+	nr	+	−
	F, child	35	+	nr	−	Psychosis
	F, child	30	weakness	nr	+	−
Rapin et al [64]	F, 2	24	nr	−	+	Ataxia
	M, 2	29	+	nr	+	Ataxia
	F, 2	16	nr	nr	+	Psychosis
Kaback et al [57]	M, 16	22	+	nr	+	nr
Willner et al [65]	F, child	27	+	nr	+	Parkinson's
	M, child	26	+	nr	+	Parkinson's
Mitsumoto et al [56]	M, 16	30	+	+	+	Ataxia, dementia
	M, child	32	+	−	+	Ataxia, dementia
	M, child	36	+	+	−	−
Cashman et al [66]	F, 7	24	+	−	+	Ataxia
Yaffe et al [67]	M, 16	22	+	+	+	Depression

ABBREVIATIONS: Fascic, fasciculation; UMN, upper motor neuron; nr, not recorded

Dawson et al, this volume) and G_{M2} gangliosidosis. This disorder consists of a spectrum of conditions that include Tay-Sachs disease, Sandhoff's disease, and various juvenile or young adult disorders. As Dawson and others point out, G_{M2} gangliosidosis is clinically heterogeneous and can be present with a large variety of clinical signs and symptoms because of involvement of virtually all parts of the nervous system to a variable degree. Among the variations are cases that resemble different motor neuron disorders, including ALS [56–62].

Clinical features Gangliosidosis resembling ALS shows wasting, fasciculation, hyperactive deep tendon reflexes, and the Babinski sign with denervation potentials on electromyography but is distinguishable from ALS for a number of reasons, as shown in Table 4. The patients are usually very young at the time of onset of disability and the duration of the disease is very long (10–30 years, much more than the 2.7 years in classical ALS) [56, 57, 63–67]. Not infrequently, there are associated features such as ataxia, dementia, parkinsonism, and psychosis. The large majority of patients with the ALS-like syndrome have had onset of symptoms and signs by mid-adolescence and have shown relatively symmetrical muscular wasting. In this respect the wasting can more closely resemble Charcot-Marie-Tooth disease or limb-girdle muscular dystrophy than ALS, which usually has a focal onset. These patients have severe Hex A deficiency while their normal parents show only partial deficiency. Membranous cytoplasmic bodies can be found in biopsied rectal ganglion cells.

MERCURY POISONING

Elemental and Inorganic Mercury Poisoning

Elemental and inorganic mercy poisoning can produce a wide variety of neurological syndromes including a disorder with close resemblance to ALS. Adams et et [68] described a patient who had undergone elemental mercury exposure over a 2 day period during which he salvaged mercury from industrial thermometers. The neurological findings consisted of weakness, muscular wasting, fasciculation, and hyperactive tendon reflexes. Urinary mercury was moderately elevated. The patient gradually and spontaneously improved with no residual signs. Barber [69] also described inorganic mercury (HgO) exposure in which the subjects had flu-like symptoms of muscular pain, tremor, burning pain in the feet and legs, and loss of appetite and weight. Fasciculation, cramps, and brisk tendon reflexes were present but there was no muscular atrophy and sensory conduction velocities were reduced; recovery was rapid and complete without treatment. Soluble inorganic mercury salts such as mercuric chloride are highly toxic to various organs, notably kidneys and gastrointestinal tract, which obscures their neurological effects.

Organic Mercury Poisoning

Methyl mercury and other forms of alkyl mercury poisoning carry widespread neurological effects and a grave prognosis (e.g. Minamata disease). There are, however, accounts of an illness accompanying organic mercury poisoning identical to ALS [70]. Determinations of mercury and pathological evidence of mercury poisoning are lacking; therefore, there is no reliable indication that the syndrome is due to mercury poisoning rather than a merely coincidental association of mercury exposure with classical ALS.

MOTOR NEUROPATHY ACCOMPANYING HODGKIN'S DISEASE

Motor neuron disease has been reported accompanying Hodgkin's disease but has clear differences from classical ALS. Rowland and Schneck [17] described two cases of combined Hodgkin's and motor neuron disease but the cases were much younger (ages 14 and 27 years) than in classical ALS. These patients showed distal weakness and wasting with absent or reduced tendon reflexes. Neither patient showed fasciculation and there were no long-tract signs – findings that tend not to favour a diagnosis of ALS. Autopsies showed widespread and marked loss of anterior horn cells and posterior column demyelination. In one case there was also perivascular round-cell infiltration and demyelination of the anterior and *posterior* roots. Walton et al [72] described a case with weakness that was predominantly proximal and left-sided but, nevertheless, generalized with muscular wasting and fasciculation. Tendon reflexes were absent and there were no corticospinal tract signs. At autopsy there was widespread degeneration of the anterior horn cells throughout the spinal cord with inflammatory cells in and around the areas of degenerated motor neurons which, the authors commented, resembled the reaction in acute anterior poliomyelitis. There was no corticospinal degeneration but some involvement of the posterior horns and dorsomedial columns. Recine et al [73] described still another case of Hodgkin's disease with diffuse muscular weakness and wasting and some fasciculation. At autopsy there was loss of anterior horn cells but, as in the previously mentioned cases, there was also demyelination in the posterior roots.

From the reported cases it appears that motor neuron disease accompanying Hodgkin's disease and showing anterior horn cell degeneration is both neuronopathic and neuropathic without corticospinal tract degeneration. Neither clinically nor pathologically does the disorder truly resemble classical ALS.

AUTOIMMUNE DISEASE AND ALS

The evidence that an autoimmune disease process is involved in ALS comes from both clinical and experimental sources. A family history of thyroid disease and other autoimmune disease has ben reported as unusually high in ALS and a significant increase in Ia antigen-positive T-cells has been observed [74]. Certain histocompatibility antigens have been identified with ALS [75–78] and immune-complex formation in renal glomeruli has been found in ALS patients, but this is most likely secondary to tissue breakdown [79, 80].

Gurney et al [81] have found an antibody in ALS patients to a protein (molecular weight 56,000 – the '56K protein') that is derived from skeletal muscle and stimulates axonal sprouting (see Antel et al, this volume). This antibody inhibited terminal axonal sprouting of neurons and the subsequent reinnervation of skeletal muscle. Whether it is etiologically important in ALS in not known but it provides evidence of trophic communication from muscle to the motor neurons.

Histocompatibility Antigens in ALS

Histocompatibility antigens have been investigated, with the disclosure of an unusually high incidence of the HLA-A2 and HLA-A28 by some investigators [76]. A high incidence of HLA-A3 has been reported but has not been confirmed. [76, 77]. A marginally increased frequency of Bw16 has been found on Guam. A group of ALS patients on Guam with diminished cellular immunity and shorter life expectancy had an increased frequency of HLA-Bw35 [78].

Monoclonal Gammopathy

Monoclonal gammopathy can be defined as an excessive and/or altered production of immunoglobulins (M-components) that are derived from single, usually neoplastic, clones of the B cell series of immunocytes (plasma cells and their precursors). The clinical conditions that have been identified with these are distinguished by the nature of the neoplasm or the M-component that is produced (e.g. multiple myeloma, amyloidosis, Waldenstrom's macroglobulinemia, heavy chain diseases). When the cause of the gammopathy is unrecognized or unclear the condition is termed a 'monoclonal gammopathy of unknown significance'. This may occur in relation to neoplasms of other than the B cell series or various non-neoplastic diseases. M-components occur in the general population without evident disease and may sometimes be due to antecedent illness, especially chronic infections. Axelsson et al [82] found that 1% of the population had M-components of low concentration and that this level rose with age, reaching almost 6% by the 9th decade of life.

According to Shy et al [83] there is a significantly higher occurrence of serum immunological abnormality in motor neuron disorder than would be expected by chance alone. These authors included essentially two groups of patients in their study: (1) those with only lower motor findings suggesting motor neuropathy and (2) others with both upper and lower motor neuron signs compatible with ALS. Patients with essentially lower motor neuron signs tended to have IgM paraproteins whereas those with both lower and upper motor neuron disease had IgG or IgM paraproteins in equal proportion. The association of motor disorders and monoclonal gammopathy on clinicopathological grounds proves, as a rule, to be either a motor neuropathy or a condition that is indistinguishable from classical ALS. These two conditions and their significance will now be discussed in more detail.

Motor Neuropathy or Radiculoneuropathy

The clinical characteristics of motor neuropathy are muscular wasting, fibrillation, and (at least in some cases) fasciculation that are characteristics of anterior horn cell degeneration but these patients, in contrast to those with classical ALS, have no upper motor neuron signs. Table 5 covers cases on which autopsy studies have been done. The anterior horn cells in these cases are present well in excess of expectation for ALS and show only chromatolysis. Pure motor disorder of this type occurring in association with monoclonal gammopathy is very rare. In a review of the literature Driedger and Pruzanski [88] found that less than 1% of patients with plasma cell neoplasia have peripheral neuropathy and in only 15% of these is the deficit purely motor. Some patients with monoclonal gammopathy are much improved by immunosuppression therapy or plasmaphoresis whereas other motor neuropathy patients have a relentless downhill course. Neuropathy accompanying *multiple* myeloma does not appear to respond to treatment of the myeloma [89] whereas excision or radiation of a *solitary* myeloma has been accompanied by recovery of the neuropathy in some cases [90]. Patients with neuropathy sometimes have reduced motor conduction velocities, in which case they usually have a demyelinating neuropathy. Others with no conduction loss probably have axonal neuropathy. Antibody activity against peripheral nerve myelin has occasionally been identified, and there also may be antibodies against the perikaryon and axons of anterior horn cells although there is little evidence for this [91, 92]. Fasciculation in neuropathy, if present at all, is ordinarily not a prominent feature. It is of interest, therefore, that some patients with monoclonal gammopathy and neuropathy have very active fasciculation – a feature not ordinarily found in neuropathies although occasional (mild) fasciculation is not uncommon. Active fasciculation gives an appearance that is indistinguishable from classical ALS. The explanation for fasciculation of this

TABLE 5
Motor neuropathy and monoclonal gammopathy – autopsy cases

Disease [reference]	Gammopathy type	Sex and age of onset (yr)	Duration	Neurological features				Neuropath features	
				UMN	LMN	Fascic		UMN	LMN
Multiple myeloma [84]	Lambda chains	M, 50	4 mo	–	+	–		–	Chromatolysis; slight cell loss
Waldenström macroglobulinemia [85]	–	M, 58	9 yr	–	+	+		–	–
Unknown significance [86]	IgM$_k$	M, 48	14 mo	–	+	+		–	Chromatolysis only
Unknown significance [87]	IgM	M, 38	< 1 yr	–	+	–		–	Chromatolysis only

ABBREVIATIONS: UMN, upper motor neuron; LMN, lower motor neuron; Fascic, fasciculation kind in motor neuropathy is that the perikaryon of the anterior horn cell, the presumed source of the fasciculation, is also affected.

ALS Syndrome

By comparison with the syndrome of motor neuropathy, the ALS syndrome with monoclonal gammopathy has both upper and lower motor neuron signs identical to those of classical ALS. A literature search revealed only four autopsy cases with pathological features that were consistent with the ALS syndrome (Table 6). The anterior horn cells in these cases were markedly diminished in number and showed the characteristic degenerative changes of ALS; there was also pyramidal tract degeneration. Patients with the classical ALS syndrome and monoclonal gammopathy have not responded to treatment, and it is our view that these are classical ALS cases with an associated (secondary or coincidental) monoclonal gammopathy.

OTHER UNCOMMON MOTOR NEURON DISEASE

While some confusion can exist between ALS and other motor neuron disorders, they are not dealt with in detail here because they are usually clinically distinguishable from ALS for a number of reasons. The most important of these disorders are referred to below.

Kugelberg-Welander disease and other spinal muscular atrophies (SMA) Kugelberg-Welander disease occurs in much younger (adolescent) individuals, as a rule, than does classical ALS, and the muscular weakness and wasting is proximal and symmetrical in distribution. The course of illness is usually very slow, lasting more than a decade. Fasciculation is usually evident but upper motor neuron signs are infrequent. There are other very rare, more complex forms of chronic adult SMA.

Primary lateral sclerosis This is a rare disorder in which patients show only upper motor neuron signs, often with extreme spasticity of the limb, trunk, and eventually bulbar muscles. It has a life expectancy that is long, usually greater than 10 years as long as the patient receives proper care. The PET scan is useful in identifying loss of the motor area in the cortex (see Garnet et al, this volume).

The muscular pain fasciculation syndrome This and other benign, nonprogressive neuropathies can cause confusion with ALS because of the presence of fasciculation [98]. The symptoms are very persistent and accompanied by some muscular fatigue but the disorder is non-progressive without, as a rule, muscular wasting.

Amyotrophic choreo-acanthocytosis Amyotrophic signs may sometimes appear before extrapyramidal features in this disease and cause confu-

TABLE 6
Amyotrophic lateral sclerosis and monoclonal gammopathy – autopsy cases

Disease [reference]	Gammopathy type	Sex and age of onset (yr)	Duration	Neurological features			Neuropath features	
				UMN	LMN	Fascic	UMN	LMN
Multiple myeloma [93]	Lambda chains	M, 61	8 yr	+	+	nr	+	+
Plasmacytosis [94]	IgG$_A$	M, 69	9 mo	–	+	+	+	+
Waldenström macroglobulinemia [95]	IgM$_k$	M, 59	3–4 yr	+	nr	nr	+	nr
Waldenström macroglobulinemia [96]	IgM$_k$	M, 75	2 yr	nr	+	+	+	+
Unknown significance [97]	IgG$_k$	M, 63	25 mo	+	+	+	+	+

nr – not recorded

sion with ALS. Acanthocytosis is a valuable but not invariable diagnostic feature [99].

Lyme disease This disease is caused by *Borrelia burgdorferi*, a spirochete, and is reported to produce occasionally a clinical picture similar to ALS. It may be treatable with ceftriaxone [100].

Tropical and epidemic spastic paraparesis These two conditions, the former associated with HTLV-1 infection and the latter with high cyanide intake from eating toxic cassava roots, present with a chronic spastic paraparesis of long duration [101].

Spinal segmental muscular atrophy This is an insidiously progressive neuronal but often self-limited muscular atrophy of one (but sometimes more than one) limb. It is of juvenile or adult onset and has been described especially in Asian countries [102].

Combined Motor Neuropathy and Corticospinal Tract Disease Resembling Classical Sporadic ALS

THYROTOXICOSIS

Thyrotoxicosis may be accompanied by an ALS-like syndrome that upon treatment of the thyroid disorder reverses or relentlessly progresses. These are pathogenetically different disorders.

Reversible syndrome This disorder can be clinically very similar to classical ALS and it is probably due to a combination of motor neuropathy and corticospinal abnormality [103, 104] The myopathy is characterized by mainly proximal muscular weakness and wasting and dysphagia. Pain and stiffness of muscles and, less frequently, fasciculation and cramps also may be present. McComas et al [105] believe that the myopathy is largely due to a motor fibre loss with decreased functioning motor units in the affected muscles. The upper motor neuron signs can occur with or without myopathy or other clinical neurological manifestations [106]. Recovery from the thyroid disorder (treated with I^{131}) usually produces remission of the myopathy and corticospinal abnormality. Bulens [107] described a patient with spastic paraplegia, dementia, and optic neuropathy who showed dramatic recovery of all functions following treatment of the hyperthyroidism.

Progressive syndrome The clinical picture of classical ALS with hyperthyroidism has been described by McMenamin and Croxson [108] and Rosati et al [109]. The failure of the ALS syndrome in these cases to reverse on treatment of the thyroid disorder has led these authors to assume that the association of the two conditions was coincidental.

Whether thyrotoxicosis can prematurely induce classical ALS that, otherwise, would occur at a later time is not known.

HYPERPARATHYROIDISM

Primary and secondary hyperparathyroidism may be accompanied by muscular weakness and wasting that, like thyrotoxic myopathy, has a characteristically proximal distribution, especially in the pelvic girdle and thigh musculature [110–112]. A distinctive feature is the presence of bone pain in most cases. The tendon reflexes are usually normal or increased and the plantar responses normal. Fasciculation and denervation potentials are usually absent. The disorder may be myopathic but also neuropathic or neuronopathic in origin since electromyography can show reduced number and size of motor units and a muscle biopsy in some cases has shown neurogenic atrophy [111, 113]. Improvement in the neurological features usually follows treatment with calcium, phosphorus, and vitamin D. Myopathy also occurs in hypophosphatemic osteomalacia and has the same clinical findings as described above for hyperparathyroidism [114].

Whereas the myopathic picture as described above is characteristic of hyperparathyroidism, Patten and Engel [115] reported another syndrome that is similar to ALS and occurs in both primary and secondary hyperparathyroidism and phosphate deficiency. In addition to mainly proximal muscular weakness and atrophy and increased tendon reflexes there were in Patten's cases such findings as fasciculation, dysphagia, spasticity, and a Babinski sign. Decreased vibration sense in the lower extremities was noticed in some patients. On electromyography there were positive sharp waves, fibrillation potentials, and decreased numbers of motor unit potential. The syndrome must be extremely rare.

OTHER METABOLIC DISORDERS

A number of metabolic disorders can produce neuropathy that, if entirely motor, might possibly be confused with ALS. For example, Thomas [116] described two cases of *uremic neuropathy* with purely motor neuropathy and distal muscular weakness and wasting. The neuropathy improves with dialysis. *Diabetic amyotrophy* comprises moderate to marked weakness and wasting of the pelvifemoral muscles of subacute onset and slow progression without sensory impairment in middle-aged (or older) diabetic patients. Recovery occurs with proper treatment of the diabetes. EMG studies suggest a proximal axonopathy. *Critical illness polyneuropathy* described by Zochodne et al [117] occurs as a complication of sepsis and multiple organ failure in critical illness. ALS might enter into the differential diagnosis in a case of sepsis with wasting and fasciculation that is due to severe metabolic derangement.

LEAD POISONING

Lead produces both a demyelinating neuropathy and/or neuronopathy and, in the latter instance, can have a clinical picture with close resemblance to that of ALS [118]. Such cases can have muscular weakness, wasting, fasciculation, and upper motor neuron signs but are responsive to chelation therapy, with improvement or, at least, stabilization of the neurological condition. There are a number of clues to the diagnosis of lead poisoning, apart from a history of exposure, that can distinguish it from classical ALS. The patient with lead poisoning often is or has been ill with features of anorexia, abdominal pain, and personality change. Porphyrin metabolism in lead poisoning is impaired, with altered conversion of delta-aminolevulinic acid to porphobilinogen. Urine analysis will identify the increase in the former product. Also, the incorporation of iron heme is reduced, causing anemia. Lead urinary excretion is enhanced by chelation therapy with 2,3-dimercaptopropanol and $CaNa_2EDTA$.

RADIATION NEUROMYELOPATHY

There is a lower motor neuron syndrome that can follow irradiation consisting of muscular atrophy, weakness, flaccidity, and absence of the tendon reflexes and normal sensation, but it depends upon the level of the neuraxis to which irradiation has been directed. These signs occur, especially, with irradiation at the *lumbosacral cord and cauda equina level*, in which case it may be accompanied by mild impairment of bladder and bowel function. The lumbosacral syndrome tends to appear months or even a few years after irradiation and may then progress over a period of several months to, sometimes, a few years from the time of onset [119]. If the radiation dose has not been intense, then the signs stabilize but do not improve. However, if the radiation dose is large over a short period of time (e.g. 8000 rads over a month), the neurological disorder can progress relentlessly. It is debatable whether the lumbosacral neuromuscular signs are due to a radiculopathy or neuronopathy.

The most common form of post-radiation myelopathy involves the *cervical and thoracic spinal cord levels* and follows the irradiation of malignant neoplasms of the nasopharynx, tongue, and paraspinal region [120]. The signs include, depending upon the level, diffuse denervation atrophy of one or both upper limbs and spasticity of the legs. Fasciculation may or may not be present but denervation potentials are found in the affected muscles. As noted by Pallis et al [120] long-tract *sensory* signs also tend to be present. The latent interval from the time of irradiation to the first neurological signs varies from 6 to 18 months.

Sadowsky et al [121] described a case with post-radiation motor neuron syndrome that began several months after cranial and spinal irradiation for medulloblastoma. The signs consisted of flaccid weakness and atrophy of the legs, absent tendon reflexes, and flexor plantar responses. Lagueny et al [122] described three patients who developed a progressive flaccid paraparesis without sensory or sphincter disturbances following radiotherapy. In these cases the course was initially progressive and then stabilized 2 to 4 years from the time of onset.

MOTOR NEUROPATHY AND UNRELATED CORTICOSPINAL
TRACT DISEASE

The combination of muscular wasting from any of a number of possible causes and compressive or unrelated degenerative spinal cord disease may produce a clinical picture that may be confused with that of ALS. In particular, benign fasciculation due to a mild neuropathy occurring (coincidentally) in combination with spasticity from cervical spondylosis and cord compression (both of which are common in older subjects) can produce a clinical picture that can initially resemble ALS. While not characteristic, multiple sclerosis, nevertheless, may occasionally have restricted lower motor neuron wasting (e.g. in a hand) because of a plaque in the motor root exit zone that in combination with corticospinal plaques producing spasticity can lead, for a time, to an erroneous diagnosis of ALS. For these reasons it is important to rule out other diseases before reaching a firm decision on a diagnosis of ALS.

Probable Coincidental Occurrence of Classical Sporadic ALS with Other Unrelated Disease

CANCER AND AMYOTROPHIC LATERAL SCLEROSIS

ALS may accompany malignant neoplastic disease. The possibility that ALS and cancer occurring together in the same patient is merely a coincidence has been stressed by a number of workers [123, 124]. ALS and cancer are age-related diseases and the observed incidence of their combination is said to be compatible, statistically, with expectation. However, the view that an ALS-like syndrome could arise from cancer is based on there being a variety of paraneoplastic syndromes of which ALS could be yet another [125, 126]. There are also reports of a remission of a motor disorder resembling ALS following eradication of the neoplasm [127–129]. The motor neuron disease in each case in which remission was reported occurred in association with bronchial carcinoma, and resolution was said to have taken place over a period of months following resection of the growth. Thus, the argument on whether an ALS syndrome occurs with carcinoma has advocates on both sides. Unfortunately, little autopsy evidence is available. Brain et al [125], and subsequently Croft and Wilkinson [129], studied a number of cases of neuromyopathy in carcinoma. They found 13 subjects in whom there was an apparent relationship between neoplasm and an ALS-like syndrome. It is of interest that in half of their cases the neoplasm preceded the neurological disorder by as much as 19 years (mean 3.5 years) and it followed the neoplasm in the remaining half by as much as 5 years (mean 2 years). Thus, the span of time was large and diminished the significance of a relationship between the neoplasm and ALS. An autopsy was available in 2 cases. One case (number 3) had a remission on treatment of the neoplasm and the autopsy following relapse showed, essentially, preservation of the anterior horn cells despite widespread muscular wasting. There was extensive metastatic spread of the carcinoma, including the meninges and brain. The other autopsy case (number 8) also showed preservation of anterior horn cells. There were also metastases but these were not observed in the nervous system. Thus, both cases on the basis of autopsy evidence were doubtfully ALS and may have been, instead, motor neuropathy due to metastatic disease.

A possible relationship between cancer and ALS has been cited by other authors [130], including some claims of remission following treatment of the neoplasm but without subsequent autopsy or other convincing evidence as to the nature of the disorder [127, 128, 131]. A coincidental association of ALS and cancer and possibly a predominantly motor neuropathy seem the most likely explanations in some other reports [132, 133].

In summary, it is probable that in most cases the association of cancer with ALS is a coincidence of two age-related diseases. It is also possible that some patients may have motor neuropathy either due to metastatic disease or as a paraneoplastic syndrome.

IRREVERSIBLE ALS AND OTHER DISEASE

As discussed above, thyrotoxicosis and hyperparathyroidism can, through coincidence, be accompanied by ALS. Similarly, monoclonal gammopathy may accompany ALS without apparent causal significance.

While there are many possible chemicals that could be incriminated as causing or inducing ALS there are some that have received particular attention. Herbicides (such as 2,4 D), petrochemicals, and insecticides have been viewed as possible causative agents. Among the insecticides parathion (an organophosphate), pyrethrin, and chlordane have been suspected of causing a motor neurone disease [134, 135]. At present the role of these or any organic industrial toxin in the pathogenesis of ALS is unknown.

Conclusions

Using classical sporadic ALS as the bench-mark there are a number of motor neuron diseases that can be distinguished from the sporadic disease. However, there are also some that are clinically indistinguishable and these include familial ALS, Western Pacific ALS, post-encephalitic ALS, and a presumably infective form of the disease. Some distinct but clinically similar diseases such as post-poliomyelitis syndrome and hexosaminidase A deficiency can be confused with classical ALS. When related or unrelated motor neuropathy and corticospinal disorder happen in combination (as can occur in thyrotoxicosis) the findings may especially resemble those of ALS. Classical ALS sometimes occurs in association with other age-related diseases, such as cancer, and it then becomes important not to assume a causal relationship where it likely does not exist.

References

1 Hudson AJ. Amyotrophic lateral sclerosis and its association with dementia, parkinsonism and other neurological disorders. Brain 1981;104:217–247

2 Hudson AJ, Davenport A, Hader WJ. The incidence of amyotrophic lateral sclerosis in southwestern Ontario, Canada. Neurology 1986;36:1524–1528

3 Mulder DW, Kurland LT, Offord KP, Beard CM. Familial adult motor neuron disease: Amyotrophic lateral sclerosis Neurology 1986;36:511–517

4 Rosen AD. Amyotrophic lateral sclerosis. Clinical features and prognosis. Arch Neurol 1978;35:638–642

5 Gubbay SS, Kahana E, Zilber N, et al. Amyotrophic lateral sclerosis, a study of its presentation and prognosis. J Neurol 1985;232:295–300

6 Juergens SM, Kurland LT, Okazaki H, Mulder DW. ALS in Rochester, Minnesota, 1925–1977. Neurology 1980;30:463–470

7 Kurtzke, JF. Epidemiology of amyotrophic lateral sclerosis. In: Rowland LP, ed. Human Motor Neuron Diseases. New York, Raven Press, 1982;281–302

8 Murray TJ, Cameron J, Heffernan LP, et al. Amyotrophic lateral sclerosis

in Nova Scotia. In: Cossi V, Kato AC, Parlette W, Pinelli W, Pollini M, eds. Amyotrophic Lateral Sclerosis. New York, Plenum, 1987;345–349

9 Kurtzke JF, Beebe GW. Epidemiology of amyotrophic lateral sclerosis: I. A case-control comparison based on ALS deaths. Neurology 1980;30:453–462

10 Gresham LS, Molgaard CA, Colbeck AL, Smith R. Amyotrophic lateral sclerosis and history of skeletal fracture: A case-control study. Neurology 1987;37:717–719

11 Harvey DG. Torack RM, Rosenbaum, HE. Amyotrophic lateral sclerosis with ophthalmoplegia. A clinicopathologic study. Arch Neurol 1979;36:615–617

12 Hughes JT. Pathology of amyotrophic lateral sclerosis. In: Rowland LP, ed. Human Motor Neuron Diseases. New York, Raven Press. 1982;61–74

13 Leveille A, Kiernan J, Goodwin JA, Antel J. Eye movements in amyotrophic lateral sclerosis. Arch Neurol 1982;39:684–686

14 Jacobs L, Bozian D, Heffner RR, Barron SA. An eye movement disorder in amyotrophic lateral sclerosis. Neurology 1981;31:1282–1287

15 McGlone J. Hudson AJ. An eye movement disorder in ALS. Neurology 1983;33:254–255

16 Mulder DW, Bushek W, Spring E, et al. Motor neuron disease (ALS): Evaluation of detection thresholds of cutaneous sensation. Neurology 1983;33:1625–1627

17 Radtke RA, Erwin A, Erwin CW. Abnormal sensory evoked potentials in amyotrophic lateral sclerosis. Neurology 1986;36:796–801

18 Masui Y, Mozai T, Kakehi K. Functional and morphometric study of the liver in motor neuron disease. J Neurol 1985;232:15–19

19 Ono S, Toyokura Y, Mannen T, Ishibashi Y. Amyotrophic lateral sclerosis: Histologic, histochemical, and ultrastructural abnormalities of skin. Neurology 1986;36:948–956

20 Nakano Y, Hirayama K, Terao K. Hepatic ultrastructural changes and liver dysfunction in amyotrophic lateral sclerosis. Arch Neurol. 1987;44:103–106

21 Mulder DW. The clinical syndrome of amyotrophic lateral sclerosis. Proc Staff Meet Mayo Clinic 1957;32:427–436

22 Horton WA, Eldridge R, Brody JA. Familial motor neuron disease: Evidence for at least three different types. Neurology 1976;26:460–465

23 Roe PF. Familial motor neurone disease. J Neurol Neurosurg Psychiat 1964;27:140–143

24 Mackay RP. Course and prognosis in amyotrophic lateral sclerosis. Arch Neurol 1963;8:117–127

25 Hader WJ, Rozdilsky B, Nair CP. The concurrence of multiple sclerosis and amyotrophic lateral sclerosis. Can J Neurol Sci 1986;13:66–69

26 Chio' A, Brignolio F, Meineri P, Schiffer D. Phenotypic and genotypic

heterogeneity of dominantly inherited amyotrophic lateral sclerosis. Acta Neurol Scand 1987;75:277–282

27 Kurland LT, Mulder DW. Epidemiologic investigations of amyotrophic lateral sclerosis. 2. Familial aggregations indicative of dominant inheritance. Neurology 1955;5:182–267

28 Jokelainen M. The epidemiology of amyotrophic lateral sclerosis in Finland: A study based on death certificates of 421 patients. J Neurol Sci 1976;29:55–63

29 Gudmundsson KR. The prevalence of some neurological diseases in Iceland. Acta Neurol Scand 1968;44:57–69

30 Engel WK, Kurland LT, Klatzo I. An inherited disease similar to amyotrophic lateral sclerosis with a pattern of posterior column involvement. An intermediate form? Brain 1959;203–220

31 Hawkes CH, Cavanaugh JB, Mowbray S, Paul EA. Familial motor neurone disease: Report of a family with five post-morten studies. In: Rose FC, ed. Progress In Motor Neurone Disease. Bath, Pitman, 1984;70–98

32 Metcalf CW, Hirano A. Amyotrophic lateral sclerosis. Clinicopathological studies of a family. Arch Neurol 1971;24:518–523

33 Paolino E, Granieri E, Tola MR, Rosati G. Conjugal amyotrophic lateral sclerosis. Ann Neurol 1983;14:699

34 Boudin G, Barbizet J. Formes familiales de sclérose latérale amyotrophique (étude de deux familles). Revue Neurologique 1956;95:229–245

35 Espinosa RE, Okihiro MM, Mulder DW, Sayre GP. Hereditary amyotrophic lateral sclerosis. A clinical and pathologic report with comments on classification. Neurology 1972;12:1–7

36 Giménez-Roldán S, Estaban A. Esclerosis lateral amiotrofica familiar. Critica de su clasificacion y analisis de 14 familias de origen espanol. Revista Clinica Espanola 1978;148:167–173

37 Alberca R, Castilla JM, Gil-Peralta A. Heredity amyotrophic lateral sclerosis. J Neurol Sci 1981;50:201–206

38 Garruto RM. Elemental insults provoking neuronal degeneration: The suspected etiology of high incidence amyotrophic lateral sclerosis and parkinsonism-dementia of Guam. In: Hutton JT, Kenny AD, eds. Senile Dementia of the Alzheimer's Type. Neurology and Neurobiology, vol 18. New York, Alan R Liss Inc. 1985;319–336

39 Spencer PS, Nunn PB, Hugon J, et al. Motorneurone disease on Guam: Possible role of a food neurotoxin. Lancet i,1986;965

40 Gajdusek DJ. Foci of motor neuron disease in high incidence in isolated populations of East Asia and the Western Pacific. In: Rowland LP. Human Motor Neuron Diseases. New York, Raven Press, 1982;363–393

41 Gajdusek DC. Hypothesis: Interference with axonal transport of neurofila-

ment as a common pathogenetic mechanism in certain diseases of the central nervous system. New Eng J Med 1985;312:714–719

42 Rodgers-Johnson P, Garruto RM, Yanagihara R, et al. Amyotrophic lateral sclerosis and parkinsonism-dementia on Guam: A 30-year evaluation of clinical and neuropathologic trends. Neurology 1986;36:7–13

43 Garruto RM, Yanagihara R, Gajdusek DC. Disappearance on high-incidence amyotrophic lateral sclerosis and parkinsonism-dementia on Guam. Neurology 1985;35:193–198

44 Garruto RM, Gajdusek DC, Chen K-M. Amyotrophic lateral sclerosis among Chamorro migrants from Guam. Ann Neurol 1980;8:612–619

45 Kiloh LG, Lethlean AK, Morgan G, et al. An endemic neurological disorder in tribal Australian aborigines. J Neurol Neurosurg Psychiat 1980;43:661–668

46 Cawte J. Emic accounts of a mystery illness: The Groote Eylandt syndrome. Aust New Zeal J Psychiat 1984;18:179–187

47 Garruto RM, Swyt C, Yanagihara R. et al. Intraneuronal co-localization of silicon with calcium and aluminum in amyotrophic lateral sclerosis and parkinsonism with dementia of Guam. New Eng J Med 1986;315:711–712

48 Yanagihara R. Heavy metals and essential minerals in motor neuron disease. In: Rowland LP. Human Motor Neuron Diseases. New York, Raven Press, 1982;233–247

49 Hudson AJ, Vinters HV, Povey RC, et al. An unusual form of motor neuron disease following a cat bite. Can J Neurol Sci 1986;13:111–116

50 Oda M, Akagawa N, Tabuchi Y, Tanabe H. A sporadic juvenile case of amyotrophic lateral sclerosis with neuronal intracytoplasmic inclusions. Acta Neuropathol (Berl) 1978;44:211–216

51 Dalakas MC, Elder G, Hallett M, et al. A long-term follow-up study of patients with post-poliomyelitis neuromuscular symptoms. New Eng J Med 1986;314:959–963

52 Tomlinson BE, Irving D. The numbers of limb motor neurons in the human lumbosacral cord throughout life. J Neurol Sci 1977;34:213–219

53 Dawson G, Stefansson K. Gangliosides of human spinal cord: Aberrant composition of cords from patients with amyotrophic lateral sclerosis. J Neurosci Res 1984;12:213–220

54 Kundu SK, Harati Y, Misra LK. Sialosylglobotetraosylceramide: A marker for amyotrophic lateral sclerosis. Biochem Biophys Res Comm 1984;118:82–89

55 Rapport MM, Donnenfeld H, Brunner W, et al. Ganglioside patterns in amyotrophic lateral sclerosis brain regions. Ann Neurol 1985;18:60–67

56 Mitsumoto H, Sliman RJ, Schafer IA, et al. Motor neuron disease and adult hexosaminidase. A deficiency in two families: Evidence for multisystem degeneration. Ann Neurol 1985;17:378–385

57 Kaback M, Miles J, Yaffe M, et al. Hexosaminidase-A (Hex-A) deficiency in early adulthood: A new type of G_{M2} gangliosidosis. Am J Human Genet 1978;30:31A

58 Dale AJD, Engel AG, Rudd NL. Familial hexosaminidase A deficiency with Kugelberg-Welander phenotype and mental change. Ann Neurol 1983;14:109

59 Jellinger K, Anzil AP, Seemann D, Bernheimer H. Adult G_{M2} gangliosidosis masquerading as slowly progressive muscular atrophy: Motor neuron disease phenotype. Clin Neuropathol 1982;1:31–44

60 Parnes S, Karpati G, Carpenter S, et al. Hexosaminidase-A deficiency presenting as atypical juvenile-onset spinal muscular atrophy. Arch Neurol 1985;42:1176–1180

61 Johnson WG, Wigger HJ, Karp HR, et al. Juvenile spinal muscular atrophy: A new hexosaminidase deficiency phenotype. Ann Neurol 1982;11:11–16

62 Sliman RJ, Mitsumoto H, Schafer IA, Horwitz SJ. A study of hexosaminidase-A deficiency in a patient with 'atypical amyotrophic lateral sclerosis'. Ann Neurol 1983;14:148

63 Navron R, Argov Z, Brand N, Sandbank U. Adult G_{M2} gangliosidosis in association with Tay-Sachs disease: A new phenotype. Neurology 1981;31:1397–1401

64 Rapin I, Suzuki K, Suzuki K, Valsamis MP. Adult (chronic) G_{M2} gangliosidosis: Atypical spinocerebellar degeneration in a Jewish sibship. Arch Neurol 1976;33:120–130

65 Willner JP, Bender AN, Strauss L, Yahr M, Desnick RJ: Total β-hexosaminidase A deficiency in two adult Ashkenazi Jewish siblings: Report of a new clinical variant. Am J Human Genet 1979;31:86A

66 Cashman NR, Antel JP, Hancock LW, et al. N-acetyl-β hexosaminidase β locus defect and juvenile motor neuron disease: A case study. Ann Neurol 1986;19:568–572

67 Yaffe MG, Kaback M, Goldberg M, et al. An amyotrophic lateral sclerosis-like syndrome with hexosaminidase-A deficiency: A new type of G_{M2} gangliosidosis. Neurology 1979;29:611

68 Adams, CR, Ziegler DK, Lin JT. Mercury intoxication simulating amyotrophic lateral sclerosis. JAMA 1983;250:642–643

69 Barber TE. Inorganic mercury poisoning reminiscent of amyotrophic lateral sclerosis. J Occup Med 1978;20:667–669

70 Kantarjiam AD. A syndrome clinically resembling amyotrophic lateral sclerosis following chronic mercurialism. Neurology 1961;11:639–644

71 Rowland LP, Schneck SA. Neuromuscular disorders associated with malignant neoplastic disease. J Chron Dis 1963;16:777–795

72 Walton JN, Tomlinson BE, Pearce GW. Subacute 'poliomyelitis' and Hodgkin's disease. J Neurol Sci 1968;6:435–445

73 Recine U, Longhi C, Pelosio A, Massini R. An unusually severe subacute motor neuronopathy in Hodgkin's disease. Acta Haemat 1984;71:135–138

74 Appel SH, Stockton-Appel V, Stewart SS, Kerman RH. Amyotrophic lateral sclerosis: Associated clinical disorders and immunological evaluations. Arch Neurol 1986;43:234–238

75 Behan PO, Dick HM, Durward WF. Histocompatibility antigens associated with motor neurone disease. J Neurol Sci 1977;32:213–217

76 Kott E, Livini E, Zamir R, Kuritzky A. Cell-mediated immunity to polio and HLA antigens in amyotrophic lateral sclerosis. Neurology 1979;29:1040–1044

77 Cashman NR, Gurney ME, Antel JP. Immunology in amyotrophic lateral sclerosis. Springer Semin Immunopathol 1985;8:141–152

78 Hoffman PM, Robbins DS, Nolte MT, et al. Cellular immunity in Guamanians with amyotrophic lateral sclerosis and parkinsonism-dementia. New Eng J Med 1978;229:680–685

79 Oldstone MBA, Wilson CB, Perrin LH, Norris FH Jr. Evidence for immune-complex formation in patients with amyotrophic lateral sclerosis. Lancet 1976;ii:169–172

80 Palo J, Rissanen A, Jokinen E, et al. Kidney and skin biopsy in amyotrophic lateral sclerosis. Lancet 1978;i:1270

81 Gurney ME, Belton AC, Cashman N, Antel JP. Inhibition of terminal axonal sprouting by serum from patients with amyotrophic lateral sclerosis. New Eng J Med 1984;311:933–939

82 Axelsson U, Bachmann R, Hallen J. Frequency of pathological proteins (M-components) in 6,995 sera from an adult population. Acta Med Scand 1966;179:235–247

83 Shy M, Rowland LP, Smith T, et al. Motor neuron disease and plasma cell dyscrasia. Neurology 1986;36:1429–1436

84 Case Records of the Massachusetts General Hospital (Case 31-1977) New Eng J Med 1977;297:266–274

85 Peters HA, Clatanoff DV. Spinal muscular atrophy secondary to macroglobulinemia. Reversal of symptoms with chlorambucil therapy. Neurology 1968;18:101–108

86 Rowland LP, Defendini R, Sherman W, et al. Macroglobulinemia with peripheral neuropathy simulating motor neuron disease. Ann Neurol 1982;11:532–536

87 Parry GJ, Holtz SJ, Ben-Zeev D, Drori JB. Gammopathy with proximal motor axonopathy simulating motor neuron disease. Neurology 1986;36:273–276

88 Driedger H, Pruzanski W. Plasma cell neoplasia with peripheral polyneuropathy: A study of five cases and a review of the literature. Medicine 1980;59:301–310

89 Kelly JJ, Kyle RA, Miles JM, et al. The spectrum of peripheral neuropathy in myeloma. Neurology 1981;31:24–31

90 Delauche MC, Clauvel JP, Hubault A, et al. Plasmocytome condensant et polyneuropathie: A propos d'une nouvelle observation. Rev Rhummalosteoartic 1981;48:575–579

91 Latov N. Plasma cell dyscrasia and motor neuron disease. In: Rowland, LP. Human Motor Neuron Diseases. New York, Raven Press, 1982;273–279

92 Patten BP. Neuropathy and motor neuron syndromes associated with plasma cell disease. Acta Neurol Scand 1984;69:47–61

93 Brownell B, Oppenheimer DR, Hughes JT. The central nervous system in motor neurone disease. J Neurol Neurosurg Psychiat 1970;33:338–357

94 Rudnicki S, Chad DA, Drachman DA, et al. Motor neuron disease and paraproteinemia. Neurology 1987;37:335–337

95 Chazot G, Berger B, Carrier H, et al. Manifestation neurologiques des gammapathies monoclonales. Formes neurologiques pures – Etudes en immunofluorescence. Rev Neurol 1976;132:195–212

96 Bauer M, Bergstrom R, Ritter B, Olsson Y. Macroglobulinemia Waldenström and motor neuron syndrome. Acta Neurol Scand 1977;55:245–250

97 Krieger C, Melmed C. Amyotrophic lateral sclerosis and paraproteinemia. Neurology 1982;32:896–898

98 Hudson AJ, Brown WF, Gilbert JJ. The muscular pain-fasciculation syndrome. Neurology 1978;28:1105–1109

99 Serra S, Xerra A, Arena A. Amyotrophic choreoacanthocytosis: A new observation in southern Europe. Acta Neurol Scand 1986;73:481–486

100 Wraisbren BA, Cashman N, Schell RF, Johnson R. Borrelia burgdorferi and amyotrophic lateral sclerosis. Lancet 1987;ii:323–333

101 Rosling H, Gessain A, deThe G, et al. Tropical and epidemic spastic parapareses are different. Lancet 1988;i:1222–1223

102 Virmani V, Mohan PK. Non-familial, spinal segmental muscular atrophy in juvenile and young subjects. Acta Neurol Scand 1985;72:336–340

103 Mottier D, Bergeret G, Perreault MF, et al. Myopathie thyroidienne chronique simulant une sclérose latérale amyotrophique. Nouv Presse Méd 1981;10:1655

104 Fisher M, Mateer JE, Ullrich I, Gutrecht J. Pyramidal tract deficits and polyneuropathy in hyperthyroidism: Combination clinically mimicking amyotrophic lateral sclerosis. Am J Med 1985;78:1041–1044

105 McComas AJ, Sica REP, McNabb AR, et al. Neuropathy in thyrotoxicosis. New Eng J Med 1973;289:219–220

106 Garcia CA, Fleming RH. Reversible corticospinal tract disease due to hyperthyroidism. Arch Neurol 1977;34:647–648

107 Bulens C. Neurologic complications of hyperthyroidism: Remission of

spastic paraplegia, dementia, and optic atrophy. Arch Neurol 1981;38:669–670

108 McMenamin J, Croxson M. Motor neurone disease and hyperthyroid Graves' disease: A chance association? J Neurol Neurosurg Psychiat 1980;43:46–49

109 Rosati G, Aielli I, Tola R, et al. Amyotrophic lateral sclerosis associated with thyrotoxicosis. Arch Neurol 1980;37:530–531

110 Cholod EJ, Haust MD, Hudson AJ, Lewis FN. Myopathy in primary familial hyperparathyroidism: Clinical and morphologic studies. Am J Med 1970;48:700–707

111 Patten BM, Bilezikian JP, Mallette LE, et al. Neuromuscular disease in primary hyperparathyroidism. Ann Int Med 1974;80:182–193

112 Mallette LE, Patten BM, Engel WK. Neuromuscular disease in secondary hyperparathyroidism. Ann Int Med 1975;82:474–483

113 Smith R, Stern G. Myopathy, osteomalacia and hyperparathyroidism. Brain 1967;90:593–602

114 Schott GD, Wills MR. Myopathy in hypophosphatemic osteomalacia presenting in adult life. J Neurol Neurosurg Psychiat 1975;38:297–304

115 Patten BM, Engel WK. Phosphate and parathyroid disorders associated with the syndrome of amyotrophic lateral sclerosis. In: Rowland LP, ed. Human Motor Neuron Diseases. New York, Raven Press, 1982;181–200

116 Thomas PK. Metabolic neuropathy. J Roy Coll Phycns Lond 1973;7:154–160

117 Zochodne DW, Bolton CF, Wells GA, et al. Critical illness polyneuropathy: A complication of sepsis and multiple organ failure. Brain 1987;110:819–842

118 Boothby JA, deJesus PV, Rowland LP. Reversible forms of motor neuron disease. Arch Neurol 1974;31:18–23

119 Horowitz SL, Stewart JD. Lower motor neuron syndrome following radiotherapy. Can J Neurol Sci 1983;10:56–58

120 Pallis CA, Louis S, Morgan RL. Radiation myelopathy. Brain 1961;84:460–479

121 Sadowsky CH, Sachs E Jr, Ochoa J. Postradiation motor neuron syndrome. Arch Neurol 1976;33:786–787

122 Lagueny A, Aupy M, Aupy P, et al. Syndrome de la corne antérieure post-radiothérapique. Rev Neurol (Paris) 1985;141:222–227

123 Shy GM, Silverstein I. A study of the effects upon the motor unit by remote malignancy. Brain 1965;88:515–528

124 Kurland LT, Kurtzke JF, Goldberg ID, Choi NW. Amyotrophic lateral sclerosis and other motor neuron disease. In: Kurland LT, Kurtzke JF, Goldberg ID, eds. Epidemiology of Neurologic and Sense Organ Disorders. Cambridge, Mass, Harvard University, 1973;108–127

125 Brain WR, Croft PB, Wilkinson M. Motor neurone disease as a manifestation of neoplasm (with a note on the course of classical motor neurone
disease). Brain 1965;88:479–500

126 Norris FH, Engel WK. Carcinomatous amyotrophic lateral sclerosis. In:
Brain WR, Norris FH, eds. The Remote Effects of Cancer on the Nervous
System. New York, Grune and Stratton, 1965;24–34

127 Mitchell DM, Olczak SA. Remission of a syndrome indistinguishable from
motor neurone disease after resection of bronchial carcinoma. Br Med J
1979;2:176–177

128 Peacock A, Dawkins K, Rushworth G. Motor neurone disease associated
with bronchial carcinoma. Br Med J 1979;2:499–500

129 Croft PB, Wilkinson M. The course and prognosis in some types of carcinomatous neuromyopathy. Brain 1969;92:1–8

130 Gritzman MCD, Fritz VU, Perkins S, Kaplan CL. Motor neuron disease
associated with carcinoma. A report of 2 cases. SA Med J 1983;63:288–291

131 Casson IF. Motor neurone disease associated with bronchial carcinoma. Br
Med J 1979;2:499

132 Boninsegna C, Lovaste MG, Ferrari G. Carcinoma of the prostate and
motor neuron disease. Ital J Neurol Sci 1985;6:101–105

133 Buchanan DS, Malamud N. Motor neuron disease with renal cell carcinoma and postoperative neurologic remission. A clinicopathologic report.
Neurology 1973;23:891–894

134 Pall HS, Williams AC, Waring R, Elias E. Motorneurone disease as a
manifestation of pesticide toxicity Lancet 1987;ii;685

135 Hudson AJ. Amyotrophic lateral sclerosis and toxic hydrocarbons. Arch
Neurol 1977;21:721

Classic and Western Pacific Amyotrophic Lateral Sclerosis: Epidemiologic Comparisons

CARMEL ARMON AND LEONARD T. KURLAND

The basic premise of epidemiology is that disease does not occur randomly but in patterns which reflect the operation of the underlying causes; ... knowledge of these patterns is not only of predictive value with respect to future disease occurrence, but also constitutes a major key to understanding causation. [1]

This presentation is largely a review of efforts aimed at delineating geographic and population patterns of motor neuron disease. Its purpose is to show how such information may help us define the different clinical forms and guide us in the consideration of specific etiologies.

General Epidemiologic Considerations

Diagnosis

A prerequisite to all epidemiologic studies is that the diagnosis and classification of the disease should be clear and unambiguous. As this relates to our topic, motor neuron disease is a group of system degeneration diseases which include amyotrophic lateral sclerosis (ALS), progressive muscular atrophy (PMA), and progressive bulbar palsy (PBP) [2–5]. As commonly used, the term ALS is reserved for patients who have involvement of upper and lower motor neurons; the terms progressive muscular atrophy and progressive bulbar palsy are used to describe patients with primary clinical involvement of lower motor neurons and bulbar innervated muscles respectively. ALS, in its early stages, may present as either PMA or PBP. In series from the Mayo Clinic, the term ALS has been used to include all of these forms of motor neuron disease [4, 5].

Ascertainment

In order for a disease to be described and counted, it must first be recognized as such. Interestingly, this depends not only on the severity of
the disease, but on the cultural expectations and awareness, both of the
population in which the disease occurs and of the observing physicians.
For example, a first step in the recognition of the dementias was the
realization that these disorders were not part of the expected process of
ageing. In diseases with a broad clinical spectrum, one needs to consider
the possibility that people might be subclinically affected with a disease.
This consideration is important, particularly in ascertaining the presence
of chronic diseases with few or no overt manifestations, which may go
unrecognized if the patient dies of something else. In such situations,
one must consider an 'iceberg phenomenon,' whereby the cases identified may be only a small portion of those afflicted by the disease. With
regard to motor neuron disease, as it is currently understood, the course
is usually short and devastating, occurring in previously healthy individuals; thus, it is unlikely to be the 'tip of an iceberg.' However, it is
pertinent to consider the sophistication and expectations of the populations in which motor neuron disease occurs and of the diagnosing
physicians when comparing historical data to current data. In addition,
the subgroup of motor neuron disease that develops in the course of a
dementing illness has posed, until recently, a special problem of recognition and classification, with the attendant possible loss to observation
of cases presenting after the onset of a dementing illness or their mis-
classification as Jakob-Creutzfeldt disease [6, 7].

On the basis of epidemiologic and genetic features, three major types
of ALS have been identified: (1) the classic and usually sporadic form;
(2) the familial and presumably hereditary form; and (3) the Western
Pacific (Mariana Islands) form, first described among the indigenous population (Chamorros) of Guam [8], often in association with another condition prevalent in this population, the parkinsonism-dementia complex
(PDC), which is believed to be a clinical variant of the Guam form of
ALS. This same form of ALS (with PDC) was subsequently discovered
in two villages on the Kii Peninsula of Japan [9, 10]. Another focus of
ALS was also described among the Auyu and Jakai people of Irian Jaya
(western New Guinea) [11].

Figure 1, modified from Mulder et al. [12], shows the cumulative percentage for age at onset of symptoms in four data groups with motor
neuron disease. It demonstrates the following points: (1) curves are similar for all four groups, but shifted compared to each other; (2) mean age
at onset is lowest for the Mariana Islands type and increases for the

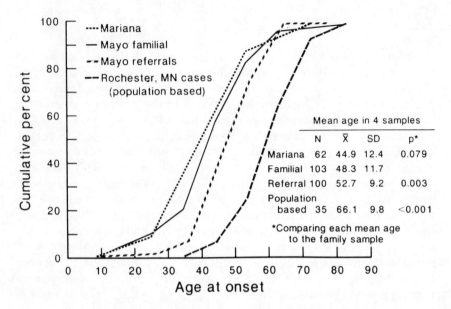

Figure 1. Cumulative per cent for age at onset of symptoms in four data groups with motor neuron disease, Mayo Clinic, Rochester, Minnesota, 1950–83 (modified from Mulder et al. Neurology 1986;36:511–517 [12])

familial, referral, and population-based groups; and (3) the referral sample has a younger mean age than the population-based group, and is the only sample to achieve a plateau (flat line after age 60 years). Both phenomena in point 3 result from referral bias, as older people are less likely to be referred to tertiary care centres. These confounding factors can be overcome by examining the population-based group before making inferences about mechanisms. The clinical and pathological features of the major types of ALS are presented in Table 1.

Classic (Sporadic) ALS

Epidemiologic Methods: Descriptive Studies

There are four major descriptive population-based parameters which can be used to describe the frequency of disease. Incidence rate refers to the number of cases starting or being diagnosed with a disease during a stated interval of time divided by the population at risk. Prevalence rate refers to the number of cases present at a given point in time divided by the population at risk. Mortality rate equals the number of deaths

TABLE 1
Clinical and pathological features of classic (sporadic), familial, and Western Pacific amyotrophic lateral sclerosis

Type	Clinical features	Pathological features
Classic (sporadic)	90% of patients Cause of death in approximately 1 of 800 men, 1 of 1200 women Male:female ratio 1.6:1 Mean age at onset 66 years (oldest group) Frequency of involvement of additional systems (sensory, autonomic, cognitive) currently a subject of investigation	Degeneration of cortical Betz cells and anterior horn cells; demyelination of corticospinal tracts
Familial	10% of patients Autosomal dominant inheritance Male:female ratio 1:1 Mean age at onset 45–50 years (intermediate age group) Three major genotypic/phenotypic variants, with variation between being greater than within families Duration generally less than in sporadic form; rarely long	Degeneration of cortical Betz cells and anterior horn cells; demyelination of corticospinal tracts Demyelination of posterior columns, involvement of spinocerebellar tracts and columns of Clarke
Western Pacific	Three foci in Western Pacific with incidence rates originally 100 times those of continental United States Linked to exposure to cycad Male:female ratio > 2:1 Mean age at onset 45 years (youngest group) Associated with parkinsonism-dementia complex	Degeneration of cortical Betz cells and anterior horn cells; demyelination of corticospinal tracts Degeneration of substantia nigra and locus ceruleus Excess neurofibrillary tangles and intracytoplasmic inclusion (granulovacuolar) bodies widespread in the central nervous system, particularly in the hippocampus, substantia nigra, locus ceruleus, and cerebellum

from the disease during a stated period of time divided by the population at risk, and the death ratio is the proportion of deaths from a specific cause divided by all deaths in the population at risk during a given period of time.

As these definitions relate to motor neuron disease, there is some evident ambiguity in the definition of incidence rate, as one to several years may elapse between the time motor neuron disease develops and the time it is diagnosed. As a corollary, estimates of prevalence rates will be underestimates to the extent that there are patients in whom the disease has begun but has not yet been diagnosed. Mortality rates and death ratios are readily available, inexpensive to obtain, and unambiguous, but depend on the methods and accuracy of reporting the disease on the death certificate. In assessing mortality rates from motor neuron disease, one has to decide whether to attribute to motor neuron disease only those deaths listed on the death certificates as specifically due to motor neuron disease, or to include all deaths in which motor neuron disease appears on the death certificate as an immediate, underlying, associated, or contributing cause of death [13].

Although there may be geographic variations of which we are not aware, it should be useful to keep in mind some 'round figures' which will provide approximate frequency values for the population of the United States and Canada. The incidence rate is about 2 per 100,000 per year and this should equal the mortality rate; however, underreporting on death certificates accounts for a lower reported rate, which in the 1980s was under 1.5 per 100,000 per year, all ages combined. Obviously, if one limited the study, the rate would increase rapidly in the older age groups. Also, the sex ratio is about 1.6 males per female, so gender should be kept in mind in providing estimates. With an average duration of nearly three years, the prevalence should be three times the incidence rate, or about 6 per 100,000 population on a given date. The death ratio incorporates the concepts of a cumulative incidence or the probability of developing the disease in a lifetime. Since all will die, the death ratio for ALS considers the proportion who can be expected to die of this cause. Again, in the United States and Canada, that ratio is 1 in 1000 deaths of those reaching adulthood, or about 1 in 800 men and about 1 in 1200 women.

Reports of annual incidence of motor neuron disease from several countries have ranged from 0.8 to 1.8 per 100,000 population. This variability may be due at least in part to different levels of ascertainment. Prevalence rates have been even more variable [14].

From 1949 to 1977, the annual crude death rate from motor neuron diseases increased from 0.7 to 1.1 per 100,000 population in the United States. Although this upward trend may reflect a true increase, it more likely is related to the ageing of the population and to better diagnosis and reporting. The principal component of the motor neuron disease group is ALS, with an annual crude death rate per 100,000 population which, from 1949 to 1977, increased from 0.5 to 1.0 [14] while that of

PMA and PBP decreased from 0.2 to 0.1. Death rates from sporadic motor neuron disease are higher in men than in women, with the male:female ratio ranging from 1.6:1 to 1.8:1. Also, the rates for whites have exceeded those for non-whites by a ratio of 1.7:1 [14].

The increasing incidence with age first noted in the population of Rochester, Minnesota [4, 5], has also been noted in the population of Israel [15], suggesting that the disease may have been severely under-diagnosed in the very elderly population in previous years. These recent population-based data, showing that the age-specific incidence of motor neuron disease increases with age (Figure 2 in Yoshida et al. [5]), are significant because they may mean that ALS is more akin to other neu-rodegenerative disorders, such as Alzheimer's disease and Parkinson's disease, than might be inferred from examining the earlier data which showed that the age-specific incidence of motor neuron disease in-creased up to age 70 years and then decreased (Figure 43 in Kurtzke's and Kurland's chapter 66 in Baker and Joynt [14]).

The increased proportion of deaths from motor neuron disease re-ported as ALS may relfect a change in physicians' diagnosing and re-porting patterns rather than a change in disease characteristics. Similarly, the purported changes in the incidence of ALS in Israel [15] may reflect better ascertainment of cases.

Analytic Comparative Studies

There is no general agreement on the cause or pathogenesis of ALS. The relatively stable death rates of the sporadic form suggest that a key etiologic factor is one that is uncommon but evenly distributed through most of the world. The uniform male majority is a clue that remains unexplained. The familial cases, with a 1:1 sex ratio, follow an autosomal dominant pattern which is responsible for some metabolic-biochemical disorder. A viral etiology for ALS seems unlikely on the basis of the persistently negative transmission experiments of Gibbs and Gajdusek [16], and also because no report has been substantiated of isolation or transmission of an infectious agent [17].

There are three major types of analytic or comparative studies which can identify potential risk factors for a disease; two of these require that the risk factor be suspected. The first is the cross-sectional study, or prevalence study, where a sample of the general population is drawn; each person in the sample is classified as to whether or not the disease is present and also as to whether or not he/she has the risk factor of interest. This aproach is not practical in ALS because of the low preva-lence of the disease.

The second type of study is the cohort (prospective or follow-up) study, where a sample from the disease-free population exposed to a factor and a second sample of people not exposed to the factor are identified; each member of each of the two samples is classified as to whether or not the disease has developed during some specified period over which all the sampled individuals are observed. Such a study, or a variation thereof, may look at exposure which occurred many years before the onset of the study itself, and select historical controls. However, two features of this type of study are, first, that the risk factor is known and, second, that the disease is not present at the time the study is initiated. These considerations make prospective cohort studies of motor neuron disease impractical, again because of its low incidence and the difficulty in identifying risk factors.

A third type of comparative or analytic study is the case-control study, where a group of persons with a particular disease and a second group of persons free of the disease are identified and each of the members of the two groups is then classified with respect to exposure to the possible risk factor(s) on the basis of an interview or, when available, from the information contained in existing medical records. Two main advantages make this type of study particularly suitable for patients with motor neuron disease. First, since the affected are selectively included, the size of the group is limited only by the clinical resources available and the perseverance of the investigator; second, it is suitable for testing multiple hypotheses with regard to possible causative agents (a 'fishing expedition'). While there are disadvantages to this method, chief of which are recall bias and the concurrent testing of multiple hypotheses, it is at the present time the only feasible epidemiologic approach for comparative or analytic studies of an uncommon disease. In other words, poor though the case-control approach may seem to be, it is the best available for the study of motor neuron disease and offers the most powerful design available when multiple exposure factors have to be evaluated simultaneously. Identification of a highly suspect risk factor, particularly if verified by several independent studies, may lead to a prospective cohort study of populations exposed and not exposed to that risk factor. However, this would still be impractical in ALS because of its low incidence.

With these considerations in mind, case-control studies that have attempted to identify possible risk factors for ALS have implicated previous mechanical, chemical, and electrical trauma, exposure to heavy metals, occupations dealing with leather, and physical (manual) labour [18–28]. In many of these studies, poor design, with leading questions by investigators trying to prove a favourite hypothesis, or recall bias by patients has often led to inconclusive and conflicting results. A notable exception is the study by Kurtzke and Beebe in which information on US military veterans obtained at the time of their enlistment was evaluated for a group who subsequently died of ALS and for a group who died of other causes. In that study, there was a slight, but significantly increased, incidence of prior trauma in the ALS group [22]. However, one must also keep in mind that when a large series of comparisons are made, by chance alone 1 in 20 can show a 'statistically significant' difference at the $P = 0.05$ level.

Familial ALS

About 5% to 10% of patients with adult onset ALS give a positive family history for the disease [14, 29]. The mode of inheritance of familial ALS is that of an autosomal dominant trait [29, 30]. The sex ratio is close to 1.0:1 in familial cases, compared to 1.6:1 in most studies of sporadic cases [31]. Between 40% and 50% of the familial cases show initial involvement of the lower extremities [12, 31, 32]. At least half of the familial cases coming to autopsy have, in addition to anterior horn cell degeneration, clinically silent involvement of spinocerebellar tracts, demyelination of the posterior columns, and involvement of the columns of Clarke [31,33, 34]. Among unselected sporadic cases of motor neuron disease, these later findings were noted in 1 out of 51 cases in the series by Lawyer and Netsky [35].

The mean age at onset for familial motor neuron disease ranges from 45.1 to 50.3 years in different series [12, 30, 31], with a standard deviation ranging from 10.5 to 12.4 years. This is 15 to 20 years earlier than the mean age at onset for the sporadic form [3, 31].

Evidence has been presented for phenotypic and genotypic variability of familial ALS [30, 36], and three major types have been identified. The first type has clinical features similar to those of the sporadic type (with the exception of age at onset and sex ratio) and a similar clinical course. The second type, perhaps comprising most of the familial cases, has involvement of the posterior columns, Clarke's columns, and the spinocerebellar tracts, and a clinical course similar to the first type and the sporadic form. The third type is similar to the second, with the exception of a survival that is much longer than the first two types, ranging from 10 to 20 years and more.

In eight families including 27 affected subjects reviewed by Chio' et al, age at onset and duration of the disease had greater variation between families than within families, consistent with the hypothesis of genetic heterogeneity of dominantly inherited ALS [30]. Thus, familial adult motor neuron disease constitutes a group of autosomal dominant disorders with high penetrance which differ on the whole from the sporadic form of the disease in that the age at onset is earlier and there is often involvement of the posterior columns, Clarke's columns, and the spinocerebellar tracts. The clinical course of the disease is comparable to that of the sporadic form, although mean duration from diagnosis to death is usually less than three years; however, a few families have been reported with an unusually long duration.

Western Pacific ALS

Epidemiologic Considerations

The Western Pacific form of ALS has aroused interest over the past 35 years, not only because of its distinctive characteristics, but because its incidence, prevalence, and mortality rates when first identified were 100 times those of the sporadic form in the continental United States. The male:female ratio approximated 2:1. Furthermore, it has occurred in three distinct geographc isolates: the Mariana Islands (primarily studied on Guam), the Kii Peninsula of Japan, and Irian Jaya (western New Guinea). Geographic isolates are important because the study of disease in a restricted population and environment may potentially demonstrate genetic or ecologic associations that otherwise might not be appreciated and may lead to recognition of a new genetic alteration, a new agent, or an unusual environmental factor that affects the host or the agent [37].

The lower and upper motor neuron degeneration in Western Pacific ALS is similar to that of sporadic ALS, with the additional and apparently specific feature of an excess of neurofibrillary tangles and intracytoplasmic inclusion (granulovacuolar) bodies, particularly in the nerve cells of the hippocampus and other subcortical areas. The neurofibrillary tangles initially described in the Guam cases may be the basic and visible neuronal degenerative process and 'common denominator' of cases in the Mariana Islands and the Kii Peninsula foci [8]. The populations of the Western Pacific foci differ so much that a simple Mendelian genetic mechanism seems unlikley; an alternative explanation has been that exposure to some exogenous factor, most likely a toxin common to these areas, accounts for their status as endemic foci. It is possible that the etiologic agents in these Western Pacific foci may be different but produce the same metabolic effect and end product in the victims of the disease. The hypothetical toxin, in smaller quantities, may also be consumed or absorbed by populations where ALS occurs sporadically and where only those excessively exposed or genetically predisposed are affected. Exposure during childhood to this or any other putative toxin may not be necessary since there appears to be an excess of ALS among Filipinos who settled in Guam as young adults. This presumes that ALS is not endemic in the Ilocos region of northwestern Luzon, the home of most Filipino immigrants to Guam [38]. An alternative etiologic hypothesis has been that low levels of calcium and magnesium in the soil and water are related to the high incidence of the disease in those foci [39, 40], though recent studies on Guam are said to disclose an adequate calcium and magnesium content in water and foods grown in the soil of areas such as Umatac where ALS and PDC are particularly prevalent [Reference 41 and McLachlan DR, personal communication]. Garruto has demonstrated deposition of aluminum in affected neurons [42], but it remains to be determined whether this is associated with cause or effect.

Cycas circinalis

As a toxic environmental or nutritional factor for Guam ALS/PDC was sought, the cycad seed (*Cycas circinalis*), which was a major food source for the Chamorros, was identified as a prime suspect in field studies by Dr Marjorie Whiting [43], and reported at the first of six international conferences held between 1962 and 1972 to explore the possible relationship between *C. circinalis* and Guam ALS/PDC (unpublished data from the first, second, fourth, and fifth and published data from the third and sixth international conferences on cycad) [44, 45]. *Cycas circinalis* is a member of the order Cycadeles, the palmlike evergreens which flourish in subtropical and tropical climates. The cycad genus dominated the vegetation of middle Mesozoic times (about 145 million years ago) and its evolution appears to have paralleled the rise and fall of the dinosaurs [46]. It is conceivable that the long survival of the plant and the demise of the dinosaurs could be related to its two toxins, cycasin and β-N-methylamino-L-alanine (BMAA). The seeds of *Cycas circinalis* have been known to be highly toxic for humans since ancient times. Some populations learned how to process the seeds for food so that acute toxicity could be avoided. Among the Chamorros of Guam, a ritual of prolonged soaking developed and, during times of famine, especially following hurricanes and in times of conflict such as World War II, cycad became an important source of carbohydrate in the diet. The husk of the nut was sometimes used as a chew and the freshly ground cycad seed was also used as a medicine, particularly in the form of a poultice applied to ulcers and other lesions of the skin.

Cycasin, a glycoside component and an exceedingly active hepatotoxic and carcinogenic agent contained in the seed of *Cycas circinalis*, was proposed for the role of the putative toxin in Guamanian ALS [47]. However, only a single animal experiment, performed in 1964, demonstrated the development of anterior horn cell disease in a young rhesus monkey fed washed cycad, with no cycasin detectable by the methods available at that time [48]. Another toxin from the cycad nut, α-amino-β-methyl-aminopropionic acid, or β-N-methylamino-L-alanine (BMAA), was isolated in the late 1960s and subsequently was found to have the lathyrogenic features Kurland had postulated at the first international cycad conference in 1962 for a candidate toxin of the Guam disease [49, 50]. Interest in and research on cycad as an etiologic agent for Western Pacific ALS reached a peak with the recent report by Spencer et al on the role of BMAA in producing an animal model of Western Pacific ALS/PDC [51].The chronology of events leading to Spencer's significant contribution is summarized here.

The Cycad Conferences: 1962–1972

By the time of the third cycad conference in 1964 [44] (i.e., within 10 years of the initiation of a stable continuing surveillance program on Guam), the following work had been completed:

1. Kurland, Mulder, and colleagues had confirmed the earlier reports of Zimmerman, Arnold et al, Koerner, and Tillema and Wynberg [52–55] that ALS, known as 'lytico' among the Chamorros of Guam, was 50 to 100 times more prevalent than in the population of the continental United States. They also found that the disease was prevalent in the Chamorros on the nearby island of Rota and among those who had moved to California in the previous 40 years [56]. It was somewhat less common among the Chamorros of Saipan and there was some uncertainty about whether ALS or some atypical form of motor neuron disease characterized by paraparesis was occurring among the Carolinians on Saipan. In the Caroline Islands to the south, neither ALS nor PDC was found [57, 58].

2. There was evidence for an increased incidence of ALS among the Chamorro population of Guam as early as 1815. Initially, the clinical and pathologic features were thought to be those of classic ALS. A genetic explanation for the observed familial aggregation was proposed initially [59], but that was soon to change. During the first surveys by Kurland and Mulder on Guam, patients were encountered with what was initially regarded as post-encephalitic parkinsonism (Japanese B encephalitis was reported on Guam in the 1940s). It soon became apparent that they had identified a new entity, which was referred to as parkinsonism-dementia complex, or PDC, but which was well recognized by the native popu-

lation as 'bodig' or 'raput,' meaning slowness or laziness. The intensive clinical, pathological, and familial studies which were carried out soon made it clear that PDC was a clinical variant of the local form of ALS [8, 60, 61].

3. It was recognized that neurofibrillary tangles and granulovacuolar bodies were present especially in the hippocampus and other subcortical areas in both ALS and PDC in the Marianas isolate, and these findings led to the realization that the ALS of Guam was a distinct form of the disease. The major pathologic difference between ALS and PDC was that cortical degeneration and loss of pigment in the substantia nigra and locus ceruleus were prominent in PDC and far less pronounced, if present at all, in the ALS cases. Among those with PDC, upper motor neuron disease was present in a large proportion of cases and in the earlier surveys about 1 in 6 had clinically obvious lower motor neuron disease as well. A small proportion also appeared to have difficulties with upward gaze but this was not regarded as a key feature of PDC at the time. Thus, it was postulated that ALS and PDC were variants of a single disease entity and that the neurofibrillary tangles were the 'common denominator' of the Guam disease. This concept was supported by later observations of Anderson et al that there was premature occurrence of neurofibrillary tangles in adult Chamorros dying of non-neurological causes, indicating that a subclinical form of the neurological disease was also present in the population [62].

4. In spite of intensive efforts to identify an infectious agent, none appeared to fit the epidemiologic pattern nor was there any such evidence from microbiological studies over the next two decades [63].

5. By 1955, familial aggregation of ALS had been described in detail in a Mayo Clinic study which reported a series of familial, and presumably hereditary, cases; such cases comprised 5% to 10% of different ALS case-series reported in the United States and Western Europe [29]. Thus, within the first 10 years, as a result of the familial studies at the Mayo Clinic and the observations of Hirano, Malamud, and the research teams on Guam, it was possible to identify at least three distinct forms of ALS: (1) the classic, sporadic form, which predominated in the West and most of Japan; (2) the familial form, which accounted for 5% to 10% of the cases in the western countries; and (3) the Western Pacific form in the Marianas and the Kii Peninsula, which was associated with PDC and characterized by neurofibrillary tangles (Table 1).

6. Changes in the collagen of the skin were observed in about half of the Chamorro patients with ALS and PDC, just as had been noted in the sporadic cases of ALS in the continental United States [64].

7. It was recognized that there was an increased incidence of diaphy-

sial aclasis (multiple exostoses) in the population, although this was not necessarily noted among the patients with ALS or PDC [65].

8. By 1962, the three features of experimental lathyrism associated with *Lathyrus odoratus* had been noted among the Chamorros, i.e., neurological disease, multiple exostoses, and collagen abnormalities, so that a search for a lathyrogenic agent was deemed an appropriate line of research even at that time.

9. Cycad had been identified by Dr Margaret Whiting, a nutritionist, and Dr F. Raymond Fosberg, a botanist, as a staple food among the Chamorros. Cycad became a prime candidate for a research effort which continued after 1964 [44, 45].

The Hiatus: 1973–1983

The long delay between the original observations on cycad and the reports by Spencer deserves explanation. It the late 1950s, Laqueur and Mickelsen et al of the National Institutes of Health showed that the glycoside cycasin, if ingested in large doses, produced acute yellow atrophy of the liver and, if ingested or applied to eroded skin in small doses, produced cancer of the liver, kidneys, and other organs after a latent period of a year or more [66, 67]. The aglycone of cycasin, methylasoxymethanol, was found to be a carcinogenic agent which biochemically was found to have a methylating mechanism similar to that of dimethylnitrosamine. However, these early efforts failed to produce, in any consistent manner, a neurological disease corresponding to ALS or PDC in animals. It was not until the third cycad conference in 1964 that Dastur, of Bombay, India, reported that one of several monkeys fed *washed* cycad (presumably free of cycasin) appeared to develop a motor neuron disease [48]. Unfortunately, this was not promptly replicated by other investigators, nor could the neurological disorder be induced in other laboratory animals, such as rodents.

A few years after the publication of the proceedings of the third cycad conference in 1964, Vega and Bell at the University of Texas described the isolation of a propionitrile from *Cycas circinalis* which had lathyrogenic features [50]. They also found that this compound (BMAA) occurred in free or bound form in other members of the cycad genus. The University of Texas group proceeded with toxicity experiments which were reported by Polsky, Nun, and Bell in the sixth cycad conference published in 1972 [49]. Only the L-isomer of BMAA was found to be toxic in the concentration tested. 'Convulsions and paralysis' were produced in mice and rats, although only with higher doses. No convulsions or paralysis were produced when the compound was injected at low concentrations over a long period of time.

With no new evidence to support Dastur's finding in a single monkey [48], interest in and support for research of the possible link between exposure to cycad and the development of neurological disease waned; nor was the report in 1975 of the induction of delayed-onset paralysis in guinea-pigs fed an extract of cycad pursued [68].

The cycad hypothesis was kept alive by Kurland and Molgaard [69]. The concept of an exogenous factor derived particular support from the reported decline in incidence of ALS in the Chamorro population of Guam [70]. There seemed to be a real reduction in the incidence and mortality rates in Guam and the Kii Peninsula which appeared most likely to be due to Westernization of life-style, particularly with regard to food sources [71]. Kurland and Mulder reiterated the cycad hypothesis in 1984 [32].

The Revival: 1983 and Beyond

The cycad hypothesis was revived by Spencer and his colleagues following their systematic study of lathyrism, a probably related motor neuron disorder induced by the neurotoxic chickling pea *Lathyrus sativus* [72]. Lathyrism is a form of irreversible non-progressive spastic paraparesis which develops in humans and in animals fed a diet containing the chickling pea. Following a limited period of exposure, lathyrism in humans presents as a non-progressive upper motor neuron degenerative disease, similar to primary lateral sclerosis in the chronic stages, and usually without involvement of other tissues. Individuals of both sexes and all ages can be affected, but the disease is more prominent among young male adults. The onset of paralysis may be acute, subacute, or insidious, and depends probably on the amount of lathyrus consumed. Neuropathologic studies conducted decades after the onset of spastic paraparesis have revealed degeneration of long ascending and descending tracts and, to a lesser extent, of spinocerebellar tracts and dorsal columns. Severe loss of Betz cells may occur, but is most noticeable in the upper part of the precentral sulcus and the paracentral lobule. Anterior horn cells display small filamentous aggregates and crystalloid inclusions [72, 73]. To the best of our knowledge, neurofibrillary tangles and granulovacuolar bodies have not been seen in cases of lathyrism. There has not been a significant problem with lathyrism in the Western Pacific nor has there been an increase in ALS and PDC in humans who have developed lathyrism or in areas where lathyrism is currently prev-

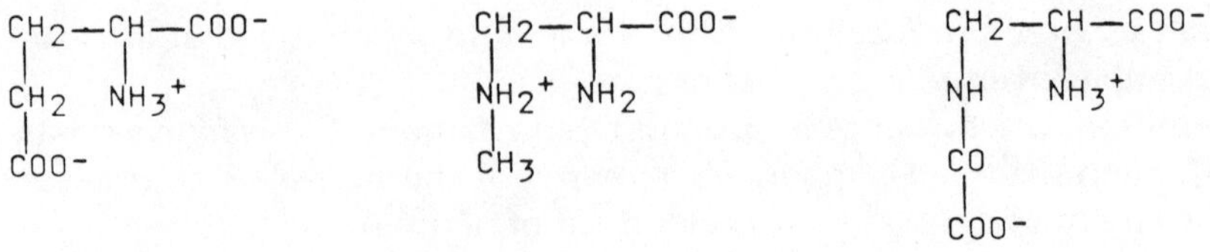

$$CH_2-CH-COO^-$$
$$CH_2 \quad NH_3^+$$
$$COO^-$$

$$CH_2-CH-COO^-$$
$$NH_2^+ \quad NH_2$$
$$CH_3$$

$$CH_2-CH-COO^-$$
$$NH \quad NH_3^+$$
$$CO$$
$$COO^-$$

Glutamic acid

β-N-methylamino-
L-alanine
(BMAA)

β-N-oxalylamino-
L-alanine
(BOAA)

Figure 2. Chemical formulae of glutamic acid, BMAA (β-N-methylamino-L-alanine), and BOAA (β-N-oxalylamino-L-alanine)

alent. It was Spencer's interest in lathyrism and the neurotoxic amino acid, β-N-oxalylamino-L-alanine (BOAA) (Fig. 2), that led him to reopen the question of a lathyrogenic mechanism in the Guam diseases [51, 73]. This time, with knowledge and experience derived from his studies of lathyrism and BOAA, he embarked on new research in an effort to understand the neurotoxic effects of BMAA, realizing that it had not been tested adequately. The application of organotypic tissue culture to compare and contrast the properties of the chemically related neurotoxic principles in *Lathyrus sativus* (BOAA) and *Cycas circinalis* (BMAA) (Fig 2) led to the development of primate models of lathyrism and of Western Pacific ALS and PDC, respectively. Using a purified L-isomer of BMAA, Spencer was able to produce in monkeys an illness with features of human ALS and possibly Parkinson's disease [73, 74]. This is described in greater detail in Spencer's chapter in this volume.

Recent field studies by Spencer also appear to have linked cycad use and motor neuron disease in both the Irian Jaya focus in western New Guinea and the Kii Peninsula focus in Japan [75, 76].

Recent reports of a decrease in the prevalence of ALS and PDC, with a shift toward a later age of onset for both conditions, and the possibility of some shift in the sex ratio [77], need to be established by careful population surveys in the Marianas. In a recent survey on Guam by Drs John Steele of Guam and Donald Calne of Vancouver, British Columbia, and others, as well as in a recent visit by one of us (L.T.K.) and Dr Steele to the nearby island of Rota, ALS appeared far less common, but PDC appeared to be as prevalent as, if not more than, had been observed 30 years earlier. Further, according to a recent survey by Dr Larry Lavine of the National Institutes of Health and Dr Steele (personal communication, February 1988), dementia alone, suggestive of Alzheimer's disease, appears more prevalent and at a much younger age (mean 65 years) than reported for the population of Rochester, Minnesota. There is also some indication from Dr Dan Perl of New York and Dr Steele that senile plaques as well as neurofibrillary tangles are present in elderly cases of the Guam disease (personal communication, October 1987).

If these findings should be borne out and if we are, indeed, seeing a decline in the incidence of ALS together with a rise in the incidence of PDC and possibly an Alzheimer's type dementia in the Western Pacific foci, one might consider the following scenario: that peak exposure to a toxic agent (BMAA) occurred during World War II when cycad was a major carbohydrate source for the Chamorros on Guam; that individuals exposed to higher doses of BMAA tended to develop ALS at a relatively early age, with or without associated PDC; that individuals exposed to a lesser dose of the toxin were less likely to develop ALS initially, but instead, at a later date, developed PDC, or possibly dementia of the Alzheimer's type. Although BMAA appears to be the most likely candidate toxin to explain these changes, one should allow that gender, genetic influences, host variability, exposure to other toxins, and other environmental factors may be potentially important in the clinical evolution of BMAA toxicity in any given individual in addition to a dose-response mechanism.

Hypothesis: Implications for Sporadic Neurodegenerative Diseases

These findings may have a bearing on the etiology of sporadic neurodegenerative diseases in view of the evidence for the presence of abnormal glutamate metabolism in sporadic ALS patients [78] and of glutamate depletion in the hippocampal perforant pathways in patients with Alzheimer's disease [79]. Glutamic acid (Fig. 2) is an excitatory neurotransmitter found primarily in the cerebellum and the spinal cord. It is also the metabolic precursor for γ-aminobutyric acid (GABA), an inhibitory neurotransmitter found in the granule cells of the olfactory bulb, in amacrine cells of the retina, in Purkinje's cells of the cerebellum, and in basket cells of both the cerebellum and the hippocampus. In the basal ganglia, there is an important inhibitory tract with endings on dopaminergic cells of the substantia nigra [80, 81]. The structural similarities between glutamic acid, BOAA, and BMAA are brought out by Figure 2, and may account for the neurotoxicity of the two latter substances in motor pathways.

In both *in vivo* and *in vitro* systems, the acute neuronotoxic action of L-BOAA is said to be mediated via quisqualate and/or kainate glutamate receptors, whereas L-BMAA action is attenuated in a dose-dependent manner by 2-amino-7-phosphonoheptanoic acid, a selective antagonist for the N-methyl-D-aspartate (NMDA) glutamate receptor [82]. In addition, BMAA may interfere with the metabolic role of glutamate in GABA synthesis or may enter into the production of a toxic analogue to GABA, accounting for the extrapyramidal changes. It may therefore be that Alzheimer's disease, Parkinson's disease, and motor neuron disease not only represent an abiotrophic interaction between agent and environment [83], but may be responses to different degrees of exposure to related ubiquitous environmental toxins affecting glutamate metabolism or glutamate neurotransmitters.

The epidemiologic similarities of the three neurodegenerative diseases ALS, PDC, and Alzheimer's dementia, namely increasing incidence with age and a 5% to 15% familial pattern, support a similar underlying environmental mechanism for all three, possibly with a single toxin playing a crucial role in what we have heretofore considered three very distinct neurological diseases. The studies underway by Spencer and others, intensively pursuing the lead provided by the epidemiologic studies of Guam 35 years ago, should soon help us know how much speculation there is in this hypothesis.

Acknowledgment

The authors are grateful to Mrs Laura Long for her invaluable editing assistance and manuscript preparation.

Supported in part by Grant NS17750 from the National Institutes of Health, Bethesda, MD.

References

1 Fox JP, Hall CE, Elveback LR. Epidemiology: Man and Disease. London, Macmillan (Collier-Macmillan), 1970;185

2 Adams RD, Victor M. Principles of Neurology, 3rd edition. New York, McGraw Hill, 1985;889

3 Kurland LT, Mulder DW. Overview of motor neuron disease. In: Poeck K, Freund HJ, Ganshirt H, eds. Neurology. Berlin/Heidelberg, Springer-Verlag, 1986;288–292

4 Juergens SM, Kurland LT, Okazaki H, Mulder DW. ALS in Rochester, Minnesota, 1925–1977. Neurology 1980;30:463–470

5 Yoshida S, Mulder DW, Kurland LT, et al. Follow-up study on amyotrophic lateral sclerosis in Rochester, Minnesota, 1925 through 1984. Neuroepidemiology 1986;5:61–70

6 Salazar AM, Master CL, Gajdusek DC, Gibbs CJ Jr. Syndromes of amyotrophic lateral sclerosis and dementia: Relation to transmissible Creutzfeldt-Jakob disease. Ann Neurol 1983;14:17–26

7 Hudson AJ. Amyotrophic lateral sclerosis and its association with dementia, parkinsonism and other neurological disorders: A review. Brain 1981;104:217–247

8 Kurland LT, Choi NW, Sayre GP. Implications of incidence and geographic patterns on the classification of amyotrophic lateral sclerosis. In: Norris FH Jr, Kurland LT, eds. Motor Neuron Diseases: Research on Amyotrophic Lateral Sclerosis and Related Disorders. New York, Grune and Stratton, 1969;28–50

9 Kimura K, Yase Y, Higashi Y, et al. Epidemiological and geomedical studies on amyotrophic lateral sclerosis. Dis Nerv Syst 1963;24:155–159

10 Shiraki H. The neuropathology of amyotrophic lateral sclerosis (ALS) in the Kii Peninsula and other areas of Japan. In: Norris FH Jr, Kurland LT, eds. Motor Neuron Diseases: Research on Amyotrophic Lateral Sclerosis and Related Disorders. New York, Grune and Stratton, 1969;80–84

11 Gajdusek DC, Salazar AM. Amyotrophic lateral sclerosis and parkinsonism syndromes in high incidence among the Auyu and Jakai people of West New Guinea. Neurology 1982;32:107–126

12 Mulder DW, Kurland LT, Offord KP, Beard CM. Familial adult motor neuron disease: Amyotrophic lateral sclerosis. Neurology 1986;36:511–517

13 Chandra V, Schoenberg BS. Motor neuron disease in the United States, 1973–1978.Neurology 1987;37:1339–1343

14 Kurtzke JF, Kurland LT. The epidemiology of neurologic disease. In: Baker AB, Joynt RJ, eds. Clinical Neurology. Philadelphia, Harper and Row, 1983; chapter 66.

15 Kahana E, Zilber N. Changes in the incidence of amyotrophic lateral sclerosis in Israel. Arch Neurol 1984;41:157–160

16 Gibbs CJ Jr, Gajdusek DC. ALS, Parkinson's disease and the ALS parkinson-dementia complex on Guam: A review and summary of attempts to demonstrate infectious etiology. J Clin Pathol 1972;25(Suppl):132–140

17 Brody JA, Hadlow WJ, Hotchin J, et al. Soviet search for viruses that cause chronic neurologic diseases in the USSR. Science 1965;147:1114–1116

18 Tandan R, Bradley WG. Amyotrophic lateral sclerosis,Part 2: Etiopathogenesis. Ann Neurol 1985;18:419–431

19 Gallagher JP, Sanders M. Trauma and amyotrophic lateral sclerosis: A report of 78 patients. Acta Neurol Scand 1987;75:145–150

20 Gawel M, Zaiwalla Z, Rose FC. Antecedent events in motor neuron disease. J Neurol Neurosurg Psychiat 1983;46:1041–1043

21 Deapen DM, Henderson BE. A case-control study of amyotrophic lateral sclerosis. Am J Epidemiol 1986;123:790–799

22 Kurtzke JF, Beebe GW. Epidemiology of amyotrophic lateral sclerosis: 1. A case-control comparison based on ALS deaths. Neurology 1980;30:453–462

23 Roelofs-Iverson RA, Mulder DW, Elveback LR, et al. ALS and heavy metals: A pilot case-control study. Neurology 1984;34:393–395

24 Plato CC, Garruto RM, Fox KM, Gajdusek DC. Amyotrophic lateral sclerosis and parkinsonism-dementia on Guam: A 25-year prospective case-control study. Am J Epidemiol 1986;124:643–656

25 Gresham LS, Molgaard CA, Golbeck AL, Smith R. Amyotrophic lateral sclerosis and occupational heavy metal exposure: A case-control study Neuroepidemiology 1986;5:29–38

26 Gunnarsson L-G, Palm R, Motor neuron disease and heavy manual labor: An epidemiologic survey of Varmland County, Sweden. Neuroepidemiology 1984;3:195–206

27 Pierce-Ruhland R, Patten BM. Repeat study of antecedent events in motor neuron disease. Ann Clin Res 1981;13:102–107

28 Campbell AMG, Williams ER, Barltrop D. Motor neurone disease and exposure to lead. J Neurol Neurosurg Psychiat 1970;33:877–885

29 Kurland LT, Mulder DW. Epidemiologic investigations of amyotrophic lateral sclerosis: 2. Familial aggregations indicative of dominant inheritance. Neurology 1955;5:182–196, 249–268

30 Chio' A, Brignolio F, Meineri P, Schiffer D. Phenotypic and genotypic heterogeneity of dominantly inherited amyotrophic lateral sclerosis. Acta Neurol Scand 1987;75:277–282

31 Emery AEH, Holloway S. Familial motor neuron diseases. In: Rowland LP, ed. Human Motor Neuron Diseases. New York, Raven Press, 1982;139–147

32 Kurland LT, Mulder DW. Overview of motor neurone disease. In: Gourie-Devi M, ed. Motor Neurone Disease: Global Clinical Patterns and International Research. New Delhi, Oxford and IBH Publishing Company, 1987;31–44

33 Engel WK, Kurland LT, Klatzo I. An inherited disease similar to amyotrophic lateral sclerosis with a pattern of posterior column involvement: An intermediate form? Brain 1959;82:203–220

34 Hirano A, Kurland LT, Sayre GP. Familial amyotrophic lateral sclerosis: A subgroup characterized by posterior and spinocerebellar tract involvement and hyaline inclusions in the anterior horn cells. Arch Neurol 1967;16:232–243

35 Lawyer T, Netsky MG. Amyotrophic lateral sclerosis: Clinicoanatomic study of 53 cases. Arch Neurol Psychiat 1953;69:171–192

36 Horton WA, Eldridge R, Brody JA. Familial motor neuron disease Neurology 1976;26:460–465

37 Kurland LT. Geographic isolates: Their role in neuroepidemiology.

In: Schoenberg BS, ed. Neurological Epidemiology: Principles and Clinical Applications. New York, Raven Pres, 1978;69–82

38 Garruto RM, Gajdusek DC, Chen K-M. Amyotrophic lateral sclerosis and parkinsonism-dementia among Filipino migrants to Guam. Ann Neurol 1981;10:341–350

39 Gajdusek DC, Garruto RM, Salazar AM. Ecology of high incidence foci of motor neuron disease in Eastern Asia and Western Pacific and the frequent occurrence of other chronic degenerative neurological diseases in these foci. Tenth International Congress on Tropical Medicine and Malaria, Manila, Philippines, 9–15 November 1980;382

40 Yase Y. The basic process of amyotrophic lateral sclerosis as reflected in Kii Peninsula and Guam. Excerp Med Int Cong Ser 1977;434:413–427

41 Zolon WJ, Ellis-Neill L. University of Guam Technical Report No, 64, 1986

42 Garruto RM. Neurotoxicity of trace and essential elements: Factors provoking the high incidence of motor neurone disease, parkinsonism and dementia in the Western Pacific. In: Gourie-Devi M, ed. Motor Neurone Disease: Global Clinical Patterns and International Research. New Delhi, Oxford and IBH Publishing Company, 1987;73–82

43 Whiting MG. Toxicity of cycads. Econ Bot 1963;17:271–302

44 Epidemiology Branch, National Institute of Neurological Diseases and Blindness, National Institutes of Health. Proceedings of the Third Conference on the Toxicity of Cycads. Fed Proc 1964;23:1337–1388

45 The American Institute of Nutrition. Sixth International Cycad Conference. Fed Proc 1972;31:1465–1546

46 Cycad. In Encyclopedia Britannica, Vol. 3. Chicago: Encyclopedia Britannica, Inc., 1974;318

47 Kurland LT. An appraisal of the neurotoxicity of cycad and the etiology of amyotrophic lateral sclerosis on Guam. Fed Proc 1972;31:1540–1542

48 Dastur DK. Cycad toxicity in monkeys: Clinical, pathological, and biochemical aspects. Fed Proc 1964;23:1368–1369

49 Polsky FI, Nunn PB, Bell EA. Distribution and toxicity of α-amino-β-methylaminopropionic acid. Fed Proc 1972;31:1473–1475

50 Vega A, Bell EA. α-amino-β-methylaminopropionic acid, a new amino acid from seeds of Cycas circinalis. Phytochemistry 1967;6:759

51 Spencer PS, Nunn PB, Hugon J, et al. Guam amyotrophic lateral sclerosis-parkinsonism-dementia linked to a plant excitant neurotoxin. Science 1987;237:517–522

52 Zimmerman HM. Monthly Report to Medical Officer in Command, U.S. Naval Medical Research Unit No. 2, 1 June 1945

53 Arnold A, Edgren DC, Palladino VS. Amyotrophic lateral sclerosis: Fifty cases observed on Guam. J Nerv Ment Dis 1953;117:135–139

54 Koerner DR. Amyotrophic lateral sclerosis on Guam. Ann Intern Med 1952;37:1204–1220

55 Tillema S, Wijnberg CJ. 'Endemic' amyotrophic lateral sclerosis on Guam: Epidemiological data, preliminary report. Doc Med Geogr Trop (Amst) 1953;5:366–370

56 Torres J, Iriarte LLG, Kurland LT. Amyotrophic lateral sclerosis among Guamanians in California. Calif Med 1957;86:385–388

57 Kurland LT, Mulder DW. Epidemiologic investigations of amyotrophic lateral sclerosis: 1. Preliminary report on geographic distribution, with special reference to the Mariana Islands, including clinical and pathologic observations. Neurology 1954;4:355–378

58 Mulder DW, Kurland LT. Amyotrophic lateral sclerosis in Micronesia. Proc Staff Meet Mayo Clin 1954;29:666–670

59 Kurland LT. Epidemiologic investigations of amyotrophic lateral sclerosis. 3. A genetic interpretation of incidence and geographic distribution. Proc Staff Meet Mayo Clin 1957;32:449–462

60 Hirano A, Kurland LT, Krooth RS, Lessell S. Parkinsonism-dementia complex, an endemic disease on the island of Guam. I. Clinical features. Brain 1961;84:642–661

61 Hirano A, Malamud N, Kurland LT. Parkinsonism-dementia complex, an endemic disease on the island of Guam. II. Pathological features. Brain 1961;84:662–679

62 Anderson FH, Richardson EP Jr, Okazaki H, Brody JA.Neurofibrillary degeneration on Guam: Frequency in Chamorros and non-Chamorros with no known neurological disease. Brain 1979;102:65–77

63 Gibbs CJ Jr, Gajdusek DC. An update on long-term *in vivo* and *in vitro* studies designed to identify a virus as the cause of amyotrophic lateral sclerosis, parkinsonism dementia and Parkinson's disease. In: Rowland LP, ed. Advances in Neurology, Vol. 36: Human Motor Neuron Diseases. New York, Raven Press, 1982;343–353

64 Fullmer HM, Siedler HD, Krooth RS, Kurland LT. A cutaneous disorder of connective tissue in amyotrophic lateral sclerosis: A histochemical study. Neurology 1960;10:717–724

65 Krooth RS, Macklin MT, Hilbish TE. Diaphysial aclasis (multiple exostoses) on Guam. Am J Human Genet 1961;13:340–347

66 Laqueur GL. Carcinogenic effects of cycad meal and cycasin, methylazoxymethanol glycoside, in rats and effects of cycasin in germfree rats. Fed Proc 1964;23:1386–1388

67 Mickelsen O, Campbell E, Yang M, et al. Studies with cycad. Fed Proc 1964;23:1363–1365

68 Louw WK, Oelofsen W. Carcinogenic and neurotoxic components in the cycad *Encephalartos altensteinii* Lehm (family Zamiaceae). Toxicon 1975;13:447–452

69 Kurland LT, Molgaard CA. Guamanian ALS: Hereditary or acquired? In: Rowland LP, ed. Human Motor Neuron Diseases. New York, Raven Press, 1982;165–171

70 Garruto RM, Yanagihara R, Gadjusek DC. Disappearance of high-incidence amyotrophic lateral sclerosis and parkinsonism-dementia on Guam. Neurology 1985;35:193–198

71 Reed DM, Brody JA. Amyotrophic lateral sclerosis and parkinsonism dementia on Guam, 1945–1972: I. Descriptive epidemiology. Am J Epidemiol 1975;101:287

72 Spencer PS, Schaumburg HH. Lathyrism: A neurotoxic disease. Neurobehav Toxicol Teratol 1983;5:625–629

73 Spencer PS. Guam ALS/parkinsonism-dementia: A long-latency neurotoxic disorder caused by 'slow toxin(s)' in food? Can J Neurol Sci 1987;14:347–357

74 Spencer PS, Nunn PB, Hugon J, et al. Motor neuron disease on Guam: Possible role of a food toxin. Lancet 1986;i:965

75 Spencer PS, Palmer VS. Herman A. Asmedi A. Cycad use and motor neurone disease in Irian Jaya. Lancet 1987;ii:1273–1274

76 Spencer PS, Ohta M, Palmer VS. Cycad use and motor neurone disease in the Kii Peninsula of Japan. Lancet 1987;ii:1462–1463

77 Rodgers-Johnson P, Garruto RM, Yanagihara R, et al. Amyotrophic lateral sclerosis and parkinsonism-dementia on Guam: A 30-year evaluation of clinical and neuropathologic trends. Neurology 1986;36:7–13

78 Plaitakis A, Caroscio JT. Abnormal glutamate metabolism in amyotrophic lateral sclerosis. Ann Neurol 1987;22:575–579

79 Hyman BT, VanHoesen GW, Damasio AR. Alzheimer's disease: Glutamate depletion in the hippocampal perforant pathway zone. Ann Neurol 1987;22:37–40

80 Schwartz JH. Chemical messengers: Small molecules and peptides. In: Kandel ER, Schwartz JH, eds. Principles of Neural Science, 2nd edition. New York, Elsevier, 1985;148–158

81 Robinson MB, Coyle JT. Glutamate and related aciclic excitatory neurotransmitters: From basic science to clinical application. FASEB J 1987;1:446–455

82 Ross SM, Seelig M, Spencer PS. Specific antagonism of excitotoxic action of 'uncommon' amino acids assayed in organotypic mouse cortical cultures. Brain Res 1987;425:120–127

83 Calne DB, Eisen A, McGeer E, Spencer P. Alzheimer's disease, Parkinson's disease, and motoneurone disease: Abiotrophic interaction between ageing and environment. Lancet 1986;ii:1067–1070

Pathological Variations and Extent of the Disease Process in Amyotrophic Lateral Sclerosis

ASAO HIRANO, MICHIO HIRANO,
AND HERBERT M. DEMBITZER

Amyotrophic lateral sclerosis (ALS) has been recognized as a distinct clinicopathological entity of unknown etiology for well over 100 years. While the major pathological component of ALS consists of a selective degeneration of the motor system, several variations in the pathology have been reported. In this chapter, we describe the three major types of ALS with which we have had the most personal experience and for each of which a number of cases have been examined pathologically. These are sporadic classic ALS, Guam ALS, and familial ALS with spinocerebellar tract and posterior column degeneration. Other types of ALS are known [1–3] but their rarity and the variations in their pathology led us to place them outside the scope of this chapter. Finally, we compare the pathology seen in several experimental animal models to the pathology of ALS.

Sporadic Classic ALS

This is the most common form, which accounts for almost all ALS cases. Descriptions of this entity are found in all textbooks of neurology and neuropathology as well as in monographs on ALS [1–4].

Topographical selectivity of the lesions is the most striking clinical and neuropathological feature in the sporadic and classic form of ALS [5]. Selective involvement of the motor system is manifested by loss of the large anterior horn cells of the spinal cord and certain motor nuclei in the lower brain-stem, such as the hypoglossal nucleus, facial motor nucleus, and the motor nucleus of the fifth cranial nerve. The striated muscles demonstrate denervation atrophy. In addition to these lower motor neurons, upper motor neurons such as the Betz cells in the motor cortex are also affected.

Involvement of the soma of these motor neurons as well as their dendrites and especially their myelinated axons gives a characteristic histological picture. Thus, myelin staining and Nissl preparations of cross-sections of the spinal cord yield pathognomonic evidence of ALS. In myelin preparations, the atrophy of the anterior horns and pallor of the antero-lateral columns, most pronounced in the crossed and uncrossed pyramidal tracts, as well as atrophy of the anterior roots are hallmarks of ALS. This selective loss in the motor system is in contrast to the preservation of the posterior columns, spinocerebellar tracts, and small myelinated axons in the antero-posterior columns. Preservation of the neurons in the posterior horns, Clarke's column, and the intermediolateral columns as well as in Onufrowicz's nucleus [6, 7] is striking in Nissl preparations. These changes are always bilateral and usually symmetric. In the brain-stem, the third, fourth, and sixth cranial nerve nuclei are spared. The involvement of the pyramidal tracts can be traced up to the Betz cells of the motor nucleus, but it is well known that involvement of the pyramidal tracts is more pronounced below the lower medulla and degeneration of the pyramidal tract appears less pronounced at upper levels of the brain-stem and internal capsule. In the involved tracts there is a loss of large-diameter axons with thick myelin and it is associated with astrocytic gliosis. Destruction of the large myelinated fibres is usually associated with the appearance of variable numbers of lipid-containing macrophages. The surviving anterior horn cells show shrinkage, and lipofuscin granules stand out. These changes are often referred to as simple atrophy or pigmentary atrophy. Astrocytic gliosis is always an associated feature but usually is not pronounced in long-standing ALS. Chromatolysis is present but is not a conspicuous feature in the usual case. Neuronophagia and perivascular lymphocytic cuffing are generally absent. Atrophy of the anterior roots is characterized by the loss of large myelinated fibres while small myelinated axons are usually spared [8–10].

According to the degree of involvement of the different levels of the neural axis, the clinicians classify ALS as either bulbar or spinal. The latter usually involves the musculature of the upper extremities more than that of the lower extremities. Pathologically, more anterior horn cells tend to survive in the lumbar cord than in the cervical cord.

Involvement of only upper motor neurons is described as 'primary lateral sclerosis.' Primary lateral sclerosis is a well-known clinical entity but actual pathological verification of this condition is rare, although it has been described recently by several investigators [11–13].

Involvement limited to the lower motor neurons is referred to as 'progressive spinal muscular atrophy.' In adults it is referred to as Aran-Duchenne disease, in infants as Werdnig-Hoffmann disease, and in juveniles as Kugelberg-Welander disease. Werdnig-Hoffmann disease, however, is actually not a pure lower motor neuron disease because involvement of other systems has been well documented [14–16]. These include certain thalamic nuclei, dorsal root ganglia, extraocular muscle nuclei, and Clarke's columns. In contrast to ALS, chromatolysis and satellitosis are conspicuous features in Werdnig-Hoffmann disease. Loss of neurons results in characteristic empty cell beds. Marked proliferation of processes of fibrillary astrocytes in the proximal portions of the spinal roots and certain cranial nerves form structures referred to as glial bundles [17]. The glial bundles are characteristic of Werdnig-Hoffmann disease but they may also appear in other conditions involving spinal roots [18, 19]. Although they were described in a single case [20], in most cases of ALS they were absent or inconspicuous. Autopsy cases of Kugelberg-Welander disease are very rare [21]. The pathology of the anterior horn cells is still not well documented in spite of the fact that it is a well-known clinical entity.

More recently, the strict selectivity of the motor system has been questioned in some sporadic classic ALS. For example, subtle involvement of the sensory system has been demonstrated by certain techniques even though the usual clinical evaluation of the sensory system indicates that it is intact [9, 22–24]. ALS characteristically spares extraocular movements except in very rare cases which were considered unusual variants of motor neuron disease [25, 26]. However, subtle disturbances of eye movement have been reported [27]. Since the extraocular nuclei themselves were not involved, they were considered to be the result of supranuclear pathomechanisms. Further pathological verification of these subtle clinical observations is needed. Alterations in widespread areas of the cerebral cortex and basal ganglia were described in positron studies [28]. Changes in ganglioside patterns were also found in non-motor as well as in motor regions of the cerebral cortex [29]. However, histological verification of these data is lacking at the present time. Involvement of the spinocerebellar tract was also reported by some investigators [30] and certain changes of Clarke's nucleus have also been documented by a few investigators [31, 32]. Systematic, well-controlled investigations are needed for clarification of these observations.

Guam ALS

ALS on Guam

In the 1950s the incidence of ALS affecting the indigenous Chamorro people on the small and isolated island of Guam was 50–100 times greater than in other parts of the world [33]. The neuropathological findings of Guam ALS were essentially similar to those of the classical sporadic ALS seen in patients in the rest of the world. In addition, however, Alzheimer's neurofibrillary tangles were present in large numbers even in relatively young patients [34]. The tangles were occasionally seen in Betz cells, but they were very rare in anterior horn cells. More interesting, in spite of widespread neurofibrillary tangles, senile plaques, characteristic of Alzheimer's disease, were usually absent.

In addition to ALS, a form of parkinsonism with dementia was also endemic among the Chamorro people [35]. This disease affected Chamorro adults in as high an incidence as ALS. It showed an insidious onset with no known previous history of encephalitis including von Economo disease. The principal neurological features were progressive parkinsonism, especially akinesia, and dementia. Tremor and rigidity may also be accompanying features but sometimes they were not conspicuous. Hyper-reflexia was very common and sometimes pyramidal signs and even signs of ALS were observed during the course of the illness. However, abnormality of eye movement was not observed except for poor convergence. Oculogyric crises were not found in any of the examined cases. There was no myoclonus or convulsive phenomena in these patients and EEGs revealed moderate voltage generalized slow activity without focal change of a paroxysmal pattern. Patients usually died after several years of a progressive course as a result of aspiration pneumonia or emaciation. This ailment has been termed 'parkinsonism-dementia complex (PD-complex) on Guam,' a descriptive clinical diagnosis.

Parkinson's disease was generally considered to be unassociated with dementia in the 1950s. The impairment of memory in some of the Chamarro patients, however, was obvious. Neuropathologically, the most conspicuous changes were severe atrophy and depigmentation of the substantia nigra and locus ceruleus in addition to cerebral atrophy, especially in Ammon's horns, the amygdaloid nucleus, and adjacent temporal cortex [36]. Microscopically, in addition to neuronal loss, many neurons exhibited Alzheimer's neurofibrillary changes. However, senile plaques were absent except in rare instances.

Ammon's horn showed not only Alzheimer's neurofibrillary changes but also abundant granulovacuolar degeneration (Simchowicz bodies) and eosinophilic rodlike structures [37], later termed Hirano bodies [38]. Interestingly, Lewy bodies, the cytological hallmark of Parkinson's disease, were not observed in most cases, and only a few of these bodies were found after an extensive survey. Neurons with Lewy bodies were present in only 10% of the cases (7 out of 70 examined cases) [39]. In these seven cases both Alzheimer's neurofibrillary changes and Lewy bodies could be identified in a single field. This observation is noteworthy because Greenfield and Bosanquet [40] described Lewy bodies only in idiopathic parkinsonism and Alzheimer's neurofibrillary tangles were limited to post-encephalitic parkinsonism in their investigation in England. It is, therefore, of interest to find the coexistence of both Lewy bodies and Alzheimer's neurofibrillary changes within the same neuron in the midbrain of a Guamanian case of PD-complex. These combinations were observed in several neurons.

Alzheimer's neurofibrillary changes are well known to affect cerebral cortical neurons as well as other areas in Alzheimer's disease. It is important to note that Alzheimer's neurofibrillary changes as observed in Guam PD-complex and in Guam ALS were similarly not only confined to the cerebral cortex but were also widely distributed in the subcortical as well as in certain brain-stem nuclei. The degree of involvement, however, varied from case to case.

The topographic distribution of neurofibrillary tangles in PD-complex and in Guam ALS was strikingly selective [41]. Pyramidal neurons of Sommer's sector and adjacent temporal cortex, the nucleus basalis of Meynert (substantia innominata), the amygdaloid nucleus, certain hypothalamic nuclei, the locus ceruleus, the dorsal raphe nucleus, and reticular neurons of the brain-stem were most susceptible. However, sensory and motor neurons were not affected or were highly resistant to these changes. In fact, it was rather exceptional to find Alzheimer's neurofibrillary tangles in the large anterior horn cells of the spinal cord, although Betz cells and the extraocular motor nuclei in the higher brain-stem sometimes exhibited these changes. It is noteworhty that, so far, Purkinje cells in the cerebellum, the mesencephalic nucleus of the trigeminal nerve, and neurons in the peripheral nervous system have failed to reveal Alzheimer's neurofibrillary tangles. It should be emphasized that the topographic distribution of Alzheimer's neurofibrillary changes seen in Guam material is also applicable to most of the other diverse conditions occurring elsewhere in the world, including Alzheimer's disease [42].

Histological study utilizing various staining and fine-structural techniques revealed that the neurofibrillary changes in the Guam material were identical to those observed in Alzheimer's disease. Hematoxylinophilic to eosinophilic as well as various argentophilic or thioflavin reactions were observed among abnormal filamentous accumulations. Electron microscopically, constricted and straight forms were also evident in both conditions [43, 44].

Discussion of Guam ALS

ALS on Guam has two specific features which were not recognized in classic sporadic ALS. The first is the relationship to PD-complex. Both diseases affected the indigenous Chamorro population of Guam and the incidences were very high. They affected only adults and were always progressively fatal neurological disorders. The second feature is that the two diseases may appear within the same family; indeed clinical symptoms and signs of both ALS and PD-complex have appeared in the same patient [39].

Some of the Chamorro population that migrated to California developed ALS and PD-complex and their neuropathological findings were identical to those of the Chamorro people on Guam [33]. In spite of these facts, however, at the present time no definite genetic factor has been discovered. Investigations of heavy metal intoxication and the toxic effects of cycasin as etiological agents are being actively pursued (see section 'Animal Models' below). There is no positive information with regard to infectious agents, trauma, or any other exogenous factors. Whether these two unusual disorders are based on a common etiology which may affect different parts of the nervous system or on different etiological factors remains to be clarified.

The precise significance of Alzheimer's tangles in ALS on Guam is unclear. We [39], as well as other investigators [45], observed a rather high incidence of Alzheimer's neurofibrillary changes in a certain proportion of Chamorro adults with no obvious clinical evidence of ALS or PD-complex. That these are patients in which the disease is insidious remains a possibility. In addition, the number of tangles present in Chamorros with no overt neurological symptoms does not approach the numbers seen in PD-complex patients.

There is a recent report that the number of ALS patients has been gradually decreasing on Guam [46]. This may be due to the fact that there has been a tremendous alteration in the environment of the island during the last quarter-century and the life-style of the Chamorro people has been altered considerably. However, there are approximately the same number of Filipino's and Caucasians as Chamorros living on the island of Guam and, except for a single case, PD-complex identical to that of the Chamorro people has not been discovered among them. The exception was a Filipino who was clinically diagnosed as having PD-complex and revealed neuropathological findings identical to those seen in Chamorros [47]. This patient emigrated from the Philippines to Guam, was married to a Chamorro woman, and spent 26 years with the Chamorros in their native environment. Even though this is a single case, it indicates that PD-complex may be due to environmental factors rather than genetic causes.

Guam-like ALS and PD-Complex in Other Areas

A high incidence of ALS is known on the Kii Peninsula in Japan [48]. PD-complex has also been described in these populations. The Kii patients also exhibited unusually high numbers of neurofibrillary tangles. The number of these patients has also recently been reported to be decreasing dramatically. A high incidence of ALS and PD-complex has been reported, too, in western New Guinea [49] but no post-mortem verification of these cases has been described.

A number of patients with parkinsonism and dementia have now been reported in the United States and elsewhere. Some of these cases were examined neuropathologically but the findings were usually different from those of the Chamorro cases. Some of them showed classical Parkinson's disease with many Lewy bodies but in addition to these changes they were marked by the neuropathological hallmarks of Alzheimer's disease [41]. Furthermore, clinical and pathological features of Parkinson's disease have been reported in a considerable number of patients with Alzheimer's disease [41, 50–56].

The unexpected observation of Alzheimer's neurofibrillary tangles in ALS on Guam led to the investigation of the occurrence of neurofibrillary changes in the anterior horn cells of ALS patients in the rest of the world. In spite of special attention, significant numbers of neurofibrillary tangles were not found in one large series of sporadic classic ALS [41]. The occurrence of small numbers of neurofibrillary tangles in Ammon's horn and in a few other areas was considered to be due to normal ageing and unrelated to ALS. The distribution and number of Alzheimer's neurofibrillary changes in sporadic classic ALS were far less than among the Chamorro patients.

In a very few cases, widely distributed, large numbers of Alzheimer's neurofibrillary changes have, however, been reported in sporadic ALS outside of Guam or Kii [57, 58]. One non-Chamorro patient in New York showed clinical symptoms of ALS, parkinsonism, and dementia (Laufer, personal communication) and showed widespread, numerous neurofibrillary tangles in the central nervous system without senile plaque formation. Thus, the Guamanian type of ALS-parkinsonism-dementia complex with widespread neurofibrillary tangles is apparently not exclusive to the Chamorro population and may even be present in the Western hemisphere. ALS associated with dementia and showing typical

Alzheimer's neurofibrillary tangles without senile plaque formation, resembling the findings in Chamorro patients, has also been reported in a German family [59].

Alzheimer's Neurofibrillary Changes

Neurofibrillary changes of the Alzheimer's type are well-known features not only in Alzheimer's disease but also in aged individuals and in Down's syndrome. They are also found in the brain-stem of patients with post-encephalitic Parkinson's disease [42]. In addition, subacute sclerosing panencephalitis, caused by measles virus, also results in Alzheimer's neurofibrillary tangles [60]. The aftermath of boxing is known to produce widespread neurofibrillary tangles, as previously described in detail by Corsellis et al [61]. Various lipidoses [62] and hydrocephalus [63, 64] may be associated with Alzheimer's neurofibrillary tangles. Certain tumours associated with vascular neoplasia exhibit typical Alzheimer's neruofibrillary tangles [65]. Neurofibrillary changes in the nucleus basalis of Meynert associated with long-standing vascular lesions on the same side were also recently observed [66]. It is worthwhile to note that most of the above-cited conditions are not associated with senile plaque formation. Apparently Alzheimer's neurofibrillary tangles may be produced by a variety of etiological factors.

In the early 1960s Schochet et al [67] reported a case of a long-standing motor neuron disease with dementia in the United States and showed extensive accumulations of 10-nm neurofilaments as well as occasional Hirano bodies within the anterior horn cells of the spinal cord. About this time, three experimental models revealed the presence of abnormal aggregates of 10-nm filaments in the large anterior horn cells of the spinal cord. These include aluminum intoxication in rabbits, β,β'-iminodipropionitrile (IDPN) intoxication in rats, and mitotic spindle inhibitors such as vinca alkaloids [68]. It must be emphasized, however, that these fibrillary accumulations are due to an increase in 10-nm neurofilaments and are not Alzheimer's neurofibrillary tangles.

Familial ALS

The observation of a number of ALS patients within certain Chamorro families on Guam stimulated further investigation of ALS within families among people outside of Guam. Kurland and Mulder [69] conducted an epidemiological survey of familial ALS based on the literature of the previous 100 years and described their own observations of six families.

A number of these cases of the familial disease were apparently inherited as an autosomal dominant trait and some of these were subsequently studied neuropathologically [70, 71]. As in all cases of ALS the anterior horns showed severe neuronal loss but, in contrast to most cases of sporadic ALS, the lumbar cord was the most severely affected. The clinical findings were consistent with this pathology in that the initial symptoms in these patients characteristically involved the lower extremities and then extended to the upper extremities–the opposite of most clinical courses of sporadic ALS.

Despite the fact that the clinical features were exclusively those of motor neuron involvement, pathological study revealed changes in certain other systems in addition to the motor system [70]. These included Clarke's columns, the spinocerebellar tracts, and the middle zones of the posterior column. The posterior column lesions appeared butterfly-shaped in cross-section and the extent and severity of the lesions were more pronounced in the lumbar cord than in the upper levels of the spinal cord. The involvement of the spinocerebellar tracts was more pronounced than that of the adjacent pyramidal tracts.

In addition to the differences in anatomical distribution, the cytological alterations of the familial type of ALS were also different from either classic sporadic ALS or Guam ALS. First, the anterior horns showed frequent swelling of the soma and loss of Nissl substance resembling chromatolytic alterations [70]. However, careful examination revealed that this was different from the usual chromatolytic changes seen after axotomy. In contrast to diffuse loss of Nissl substance seen in typical chromatolysis, formation of Lewy body–like structures was observed [71]. Hematoxylin-eosin staining showed that the cores of the inclusions were eosinophilic and were surrounded by poorly stained haloes. The inclusion bodies were either single or, more often, multiple and were strongly argentophilic.

Neuronal processes, both dendrites and axons, were often severely swollen and contained hyalin-like structures which sometimes contained an elongated core [71]. The swollen processes were also strongly argentophilic. The argentophilia and histochemical reactions of the inclusions both within the soma and in the processes suggested that they represented neurofilaments. These Lewy body–like inclusion bodies were not only observed in the large anterior horn cells, but also seen in Clarke's columns and Monakow's nucleus in the brain-stem; the latter is analogous to Clarke's column in the spinal cord.

Unlike classic or Guam ALS, perivascular lymphocytic accumulations were occasionally identified. However, Bunina bodies, which were originally described in the familial cases of ALS in the USSR [37], were searched for in vain [72]. It should be mentioned that small, 2–3 microns wide, eosinophilic Bunina bodies were sometimes observed in sporadic and Guam ALS [37].

Betz cells were relatively well preserved but showed changes. Typical neuronophagia of Betz cells was found in familial ALS [71], but was not a feature of either Guam or classical ALS.

In the electron microscope the Lewy body–like structures were seen to be made up of at least two types of fibrillary structures [73]. The component fibrils were usually randomly distributed but occasionally showed a radial arrangement in the periphery of the inclusion body. One type of fibrillary structure was morphologically identical to 10-nm neurofilaments with characteristic side arms. The other fibres were much thicker than neurofilaments and these were decorated by irregularly shaped granular structures which resembled ribosomes. These morphological features very much resembled the ribosome-associated lineal structures described in the juvenile form of ALS by Oda et al [74]. In contrast to randomly arranged fibrils in the Lewy-like bodies in the soma, uniformly swollen neuronal cell processes were characterized by compactly arranged 10-nm neurofilaments which ran parallel to the long axis [73]. They were occasionally mixed with a small number of mitochondria, fragments of endoplasmic reticulum, and other organelles. Microtubules were not identified, probably because of post-mortem changes, even though the autopsies were performed within a relatively short period of time after death.

The observation of hyalin inclusions in cases of familial ALS with short clinical courses suggests the possibility that the inclusions may represent early changes in ALS. If so, and if sporadic ALS and familial ALS are related disorders, they might also be present in sporadic cases of short clinical courses. In 1968, Carpenter studied a series of sporadic ALS cases including some with short clinical courses. Argentophilic bodies in axons in the anterior horns were described [75]. Some, larger than 20 microns, were called spheroids and they were more common in those cases with short clinical courses. Electron microscopic study revealed that the spheroids represented accumulations of 10-nm neurofilaments. Some of the spheroids were connected to normal-appearing soma of large anterior horn cells. The spheroids were regarded as focal axonal swellings due to accumulation of 10-nm neurofilaments.

Since more spheroids were present in cases with short clinical courses, it was suggested that the spheroids may be an early morphological change of ALS. This finding was later confirmed by other investigators [76–78]. In addition to the axons, accumulations of 10-nm neurofilaments were also observed in the soma of anterior horn cells in some sporadic ALS cases of short clinical course [79, 80]. The arrangement of 10-nm neurofilaments in the spheroids in sporadic ALS, however, was different from that observed in familial ALS. In sporadic ALS small bundles of 10-nm neurofilaments formed characteristic interwoven tangles [79, 80]. It should be mentioned here that spheroids are not pathognomonic for ALS since identical structures are also present in conditions other than ALS and even in aged-matched controls, although the number of spheroids is generally lower in the spinal cords of non-ALS patients.

In summary, this type of dominantly inherited familial ALS has distinct multiple system involvement. In addition, there are certain unusual histological changes which were not previously recognized in other forms of ALS. Since these earlier studies similar cases of familial ALS have been reported in the United States [72, 81, 82] and in Japan [83–85].

Whether this type of familial ALS constitutes a distinct disease, and whether it occurs sporadically, is at present uncertain [4]. So far as we are aware, only two cases of sporadic ALS have been reported to show almost the precise pathological features of this form of familial ALS [86, 87].

In addition, other sporadic cases have shown some similarities. A few reports of sporadic ALS showing hyalin-like inclusions in the soma of anterior horn cells have appeared [88–91]. A few other cases with diffusely swollen axonal processes in the anterior horn have also been described in sporadic ALS [75] and in other conditions [92–94]. Finally, some sporadic cases showing multisystem degeneration involving the spinocerebellar tract [90, 95], posterior column [95, 96], and other areas [90, 95] in addition to the motor system have been reported.

Familial ALS usually has a short and rapidly progressive clinical course after the appearance of symptoms in middle-aged patients. Indeed, some of the neuropathological findings in these cases may be related to the short duration of this illness. However, there are other families in which ALS patients have a very prolonged clinical course, such as one family in Illinois [97]. Although the severity of involvement in this Illinois family was more pronounced, the pattern of distribution was essentially the same as for the other familial cases described above, except for the additional involvement of Goll's tract.

It is important to understand that other cases of familial ALS have been studied in which the pathology differs somewhat from the type of familial ALS described here. They all, of course, show the major findings of ALS including anterior horn cell loss. In fact, a number of these familial cases are indistinguishable pathologically from classic, sporadic ALS [71].

Whether these various presentations of familial ALS represents one or multiple disease processes is not yet known. To elucidate the genetic defect or defects that cause familial ALS and the relationship of familial

ALS to other forms of the disease remains an important fundamental undertaking.

Animal Models of Motor Neuron Degeneration

Experimental approaches to the treatment of ALS would be greatly enhanced by the development of an animal model for ALS. A number of such models in which degeneration of anterior horn cells is seen have been described. In this section, some of these models are briefly introduced and their morphologic characteristics are compared to the pathology of human ALS.

Genetic Models

1. Hereditary Canine Spinal Muscular Atrophy
There are several hereditary motor neuron diseases affecting various animals [98]. One of the best documented among these is the hereditary canine spinal muscular atrophy affecting Brittany spaniels reported by Cork et al [98–100]. These dogs show a progressive neurogenic muscular atrophy and loss of large anterior horn cells. The most striking feature of this experimental model is the selective involvement of only the motor neuron system. No other systems are reported to be involved. Extraocular movement and the rectal and urinary sphincter muscles are intact as is the sensory system. Decubiti have not been observed, even in severely weak dogs. Another interesting pathological feature is the pronounced increase in 10-nm neurofilaments within the anterior horn cells in both proximal axons and the soma. Swellings of axons affect the intraspinal portions mostly, but they are also present occasionally within the proximal portions of the ventral root [98]. Degenerating neurons have been identified only very rarely in Clarke's columns and in the dorsal root ganglia [98].

This is probably the most well documented animal model for motor neuron disease. However, the mode of inheritance is reported to be different from that of human motor neuron disease [98]. The pathology differs from human ALS in that there is no involvement of the upper motor neuron system and in the extraordinary abundance of neurofilaments, far beyond that of human ALS, even in those cases with short clinical courses. Continuations of the swollen proximal portions of the axons and the soma are commonly seen whereas it is extremely difficult to demonstrate such connections in human ALS, although they have been seen [81; Sasaki S and Okamoto K, Personal communications]. Bunina bodies were not described in this canine model.

2. Hereditary Amyotrophy in Pointers

Igata et al reported progressive neurogenic atrophy in a litter of pointers [101]. The animals developed quadriplegia but eye movements, sphincter functions, and sensation were normal. Pathologically, the main abnormalities were observed in the motor peripheral nerves including the anterior roots at all spinal levels [101]. The anterior horn cells were apparently normal in number but contained numerous membranous cytoplasmic bodies or zebra bodies [102]. Accumulations of these bodies were also found in the hypoglossal and accessory nuclei. The lack of upper motor neuron involvement, the survival of the anterior horn cells, severe motor peripheral neuropathy associated with pronounced accumulation of membranous cytoplasmic bodies, and zebra bodies all distinguish this condition from human ALS.

3. Wobbler Mouse

The wobbler mouse was originally reported by Falconer in 1956 [103]. Duchen et al later described this mutant as a form of hereditary motor neuron disease with progressive neurogenic atrophy [104, 105]. Andrews and Maxwell [106] and Andrews [107] described the fine structure of vacuolar changes in the anterior horn cells. These were found to be the result of severe distension of the granular endoplasmic reticulum and Golgi apparatus. Axonal pathology of myelinated axons was also described [107]. Mitsumoto and Bradley [108] investigated this latter aspect in greater detail. They concluded that the earliest pathological changes of the disease start in the soma, followed by proximodistal axonal degeneration.

Pathological changes in the wobbler mouse are not confined to motor neurons but, unlike in human ALS, also affect other neurons including magnocellular reticular nuclei, deep cerebellar nuclei, and vestibular nuclei. Prominent vacuolar changes of anterior horn cells are also not features of ALS.

4. Mutant Syrian Hamster with Hindleg Paralysis

A mutant Syrian hamster with sex-linked hindleg paralysis was discovered by Nixon and Connelly in 1968 [109]. Progressive paralysis of the hindlegs begins in male animals 6 to 10 months after birth.

This mutant hamster was initially considered a possible model of human motor neuron disease [110]. Subsequent pathological studies, however, revealed that this animal represented a hereditary peripheral neuropathy [111]. Morphological alterations in this mutant are unique and differ from other peripheral neuropathies previously reported. The lesions are virtually confined to the heavily myelinated nerve fibres of the peripheral nervous system and are most pronounced in the spinal anterior roots of the lumbar region and proximal portion of the sciatic nerve. Among various changes involving the axon and the myelin sheath, the most prominent finding is the appearance of highly refractile, eosinophilic, rodlike structures (Hirano bodies) in the inner loops, distal portions of the Schmidt-Lanterman clefts, and the lateral loops of the myelin sheath. This is followed by disintegration and loss of myelin. The demyelinating process is accompanied by the frequent appearance of remyelination with onion bulb formation. Axonal atrophy as well as focal swelling due to accumulation of axoplasmic organelles including neurofilaments is also present. The initial morphological changes of this mutant appear to be focal accumulations of 6-nm filaments in the most distal cytoplasmic portions of the myelin sheaths. The increase of filaments results in the formation of a crystalloid pattern which presumably interferes with intracytoplasmic transport and leads to destruction of the myelin [112]. As far as we are aware, a similar neuropathy has not been described in the human.

Intoxication

1. β,β'-Iminodipropionitrile (IDPN) Intoxication
Lathyrism is a neurologic disease caused by the ingestion of the seeds of certain *Lathyrus* species [113, 114]. IDPN is a derivative of these seeds, and the administration of this material in experimental animals results in the excessive accumulation of neurofilaments in the anterior horn cells and their processes [115]. Chou and Hartman showed that the site of neurofilament accumulation is in the proximal portions of the axons, and a concept of 'axostasis' was proposed [116, 117]. Impaired axonal transport, particularly of neurofilaments, as well as further structural changes including distal axonal atrophy was documented in detail by Griffin and Price [118]. Spheroids, observed in some cases of human ALS, are similar to the filamentous accumulations seen in IDPN-treated animals. Involvement of systems other than motor neurons, such as the retina, lateral vestibular nuclei, red nuclei, reticular formation, Purkinje cells, and apparent lack of definite loss of motor neurons [118] are not features of human ALS.

2. Aluminum Intoxication
Accumulations of 10-nm neurofilaments in the perikarya of various types of neurons were induced by injection of aluminum salts into the brain

or subarachnoid space of rabbits [119–121]. Later, a chronic model of aluminum intoxication was described by Wisniewski et al [122]. In 1982, Troncoso et al reported that aluminum chloride injected into the cisterna magna of 3-to-4-week-old rabbits induced prominent neurofilament accumulation in the proximal portions of axons of affected neurons of the spinal cord and brain-stem followed by an increase of neurofilaments in the perikarya and dendrites [123]. These accumulations resemble those seen in some of the other experimental models mentioned above. The accumulation of filaments in aluminum intoxication is not limited to the motor system but affects other cells, such as cerebral cortical neurons, as well. Analysis of heavy metals in the CNS of Guam ALS patients, especially aluminum, is under intensive investigation [124, 125].

3. Retrograde Axoplasmic Transport of Adriamycin and
Ricinus communis Agglutinin (RCA)
When adriamycin, a DNA-directed RNA inhibitor, is injected into the rat sciatic nerve retrograde axoplasmic flow carries this substance into the perikarya of the anterior horn cells [126]. Chromatolysis of motor neurons appears in several days, followed by the loss of many neurons after 2 weeks. Almost all neurons within the ipsilateral motor neuron columns corresponding to the territory of the sciatic nerve efferents were reported to disappear within 3 months after the treatment. The loss of most dorsal root ganglion cells approximately 2 weeks after treatment is also seen.

This is an interesting experimental approach indicating the possibility of a neurotoxic agent entering the axon from a neuromuscular junction. A more recent report by Kondo et al [127] emphasized the greater susceptibility of primary sensory neurons, especially the small neurons in the dorsal root ganglia. This study, which utilized lower concentration of adriamycin, reported extremely mild changes in the motor neurons of the anterior horn.

Instead of adriamycin, Yamamoto et al applied *Ricinus communis* agglutinin (RCA), a potent protein synthesis inhibitor, to the same experimental model [128]. RCA was shown to be transported intra-axonally to the soma of motor neurons and dorsal root ganglia. The large motor neurons and dorsal root ganglion cells which form the sciatic nerve efferents in the lumbar spinal cord degenerated. In contrast, small and medium-sized neurons in and around the depopulated areas appeared preserved. These neurons were interpreted as internuncial. It was suggested that retrograde axoplasmic flow of neurotoxic substances and subsequent degeneration of motor neurons may be a phenonemon implicated in the pathogenesis of human motor neuron disease.

4. β-N-oxalylamino-L-alanine (BOAA) and β-N-methylamino-L-alanine (BMAA)
BOAA and BMAA are chemically related to certain excitant amino acids and are present in the seeds of *Lathyrus sativus* (BOAA) and *Cycas circinalis* (BMAA). The consumption of these seeds is believed to be linked to lathyrism and to Guam ALS respectively. The neuropathological effects of BOAA and BMAA on monkeys [129, 130] are currently under study.

Metabolic Disease: Ascorbic Acid Deficiency in Guinea-pigs

Neurogenic atrophy of the muscles, degeneration of the anterior horn cells, and demyelination of the pyramidal tract have been reported in guinea-pigs fed a diet deficient in ascorbic acid [131]. Subcutaneous hemorrhages were also observed. The absence of subacutaneous hemorrhages and the apparent lack of therapeutic value of ascorbic acid in ALS patients indicate the difference between this disease and ALS [131].

Viral Infection

1. Experimental Poliomyelitis
Cytopathological changes in motor neurons of the cervical and lumbar levels of the spinal cords of rhesus monkeys subjected to experimental poliomyelitis were reported by Bodian in 1948 [132]. Poliomyelitis infection of the central nervous system consists of a primary invasion of nerve cells which is followed by a secondary inflammatory response of variable intensity. Poliovirus has not been identified in ALS and no inflammatory reaction is present. Recurrent weakness of recovered polio patients many years later was explained by Bodian [133] and Tomlinson and Irving [134], who suggested an increased vulnerability of recovered motoneurons to cell death with increasing age as compared to the normal.

2. Spongiform Poliomyelopathy Due to Retrovirus in Mice
In 1973, Gardner and his associates described a high prevalence of a wild mouse population in certain areas of California in which both lymphoma and a progressive form of posterior limb paralysis caused by a type C RNA virus infection were found [135, 136]. The histological findings in the paralytic disease were neurogenic atrophy of posterior limb musculature and spongy changes in grey and white matter of the lumbosacral spinal cord without inflammatory changes. A C-type RNA virus was present within neurons, glia, endothelial cells, pericytes, and the extracellular space in the affected areas [137, 138]. The virus appears to spread to the nervous system via a hematogenous route [138, 139]. This

disease is also associated with a high rate of lymphoma. Later, two viruses were reported, one causing paralytic disease and the other lymphoma [138]. Spongiform changes described in these mice are not features of ALS, and viral particles have, so far, not been identified in the human disease, except in one isolated case [140].

3. Age-Dependent Polioencephalomyelitis in C 58 Mice

Age-dependent poliomyelitis, first described by Murphy et al in 1970 [141], is a progressive flaccid paralysis affecting only certain strains of mice (C 58/J, etc.). It is caused by the lactate-dehydrogenase–elevating virus in immunosuppressed, aged mice [142]. Neuropathological findings are characterized by inflammation of the anterior horns of the spinal cord followed by degeneration and loss of anterior horn cells [143]. Under prolonged immunosuppression, however, inflammatory changes are absent. Severe neuronal degeneration and loss in the anterior horns were observed along with axonal degeneration in the white matter surrounding the anterior horn as well as in the anterior roots. These changes were most severe in the lumbar cord and mildest in the cervical and sacral cords. Affected anterior horn cells showed reduction of rough endoplasmic reticulum without increase in neurofilaments. The Golgi apparatus was remarkably prominent. Neither spheroids nor Bunina bodies were identified. Structural changes observed in the affected anterior horns differ considerably from those observed in human ALS [144].

Clearly, none of the animal systems described here are precise models for ALS. However, their continued study provides important clues for our understanding of human motor neuron disease. A possible clue is also offered by the studies showing that anterior horn cell damage may be initiated in the periphery. Our search for toxic substances, initial changes due to genetic factors, or even infectious agents should perhaps be focused on areas outside the CNS. The most impressive fact is the realization that a wide variety of etiologic agents can result in apparently similar neuropathologic effects, such as destruction of anterior horn cells and the formation of neurofilament accumulations. This fact must be borne in mind when we speculate on the interrelatedness of the human motor neuron diseases.

In conclusion, ALS has been considered a distinct clinicopathological entity. In fact, however, a number of clinical as well as pathological variations occur in this motor neuron disease. The overwhelming majority of cases of ALS are of the classic sporadic type. These are characterized by a selective loss of motor neurons, especially anterior horn cells. Other forms of ALS share this feature but may include other changes as well. In the Guamanian type of ALS, Alzheimer-type neurofibrillary tangles are seen in certain areas of the CNS. In the most well known familial type of ALS, the posterior columns and spinocerebellar tracts are also involved. A number of animal models showing involvement of the anterior horn cells have been described. While interesting in themselves, none have shown themselves to be precise models of ALS. These models have, however, strongly suggested that various etiological agents may result in anterior horn cell damage or loss.

Acknowledgments

This work was supported in part by NIH Grant No. 2 P 50 NS 11605-09.

References

1 Bounduelle M. Amyotrophic lateral sclerosis. In: Vinken PJ, Bruyn GW, eds. Handbook of Clinical Neurology. Amsterdam, North Holland, 1979;22:281–338

2 Hudson AJ. Amyotrophic lateral sclerosis and its association with dementia, parkinsonism and other neurological disorders: A review. Brain 1981;104:217–247

3 Rowland LP. Human Motor Neuron Diseases: Advances in Neurology, Vol 36. New York, Raven Press, 1982

4 Oppenheimer DR. Diseases of the basal ganglia, cerebellum and motor neurons. In: Adams JH, Corsellis JAN, Duchen LW, eds. Greenfield's Neuropathology, 4th ed. New York, John Wiley & Son, 1984;699–747

5 Iwata M, Hirano A. Current problems in the pathology of amyotrophic lateral sclerosis. In: Zimmerman HM, ed. Progress in Neuropathology. New York, Raven Press, 1979;4:277–298

6 Mannen T, Iwata M, Toyokura Y, et al. The Onuf's nucleus and the external anal sphincter muscles in amyotrophic lateral sclerosis and Shy-Drager syndrome. Acta Neuropathol (Berl) 1982;58:255–260

7 Schroder HD, Reske-Nielsen E. Preservation of the nucleus X-pelvic floor motorsystem in amyotrophic lateral sclerosis. Clin Neuropathol 1984; 3:210–216

8 Sobue G, Matsuoka Y, Mukai E, et al. Spinal cord cranial motor nerve roots in amyotrophic lateral sclerosis and X-linked recessive bulbospinal muscular atrophy: Morphometric and teased-fiber study. Acta Neuropathol (Berl) 1981;55:227–235

9 Kawamura Y, Dick PJ, Shimono M, et al. Morphometric comparison to the vulnerability of peripheral motor and sensory neurons in amyotrophic lateral sclerosis. J Neuropathol Exp Neurol 1981;40:667–675

10 Kusaka H, Hirano A. Fine structural changes of anterior spinal roots in amyotrophic lateral sclerosis. Neurol Med (Tokyo) 1985;23:374–384

11 Fisher CM. Pure spastic paralysis of corticospinal origin. Can J Neurol Sci 1977;4:251–258

12 Beal MF. Richardson EP. Primary lateral sclerosis: A case report, Arch Neurol 1981;38:630–633

13 Kuzuhara S, Ohkawa Y, Toyokura Y, et al. Primary lateral sclerosis. Report of 2 autopsy cases. Abstracts, Xth International Congress of Neuropathology. Stockholm, 1986;227

14 Iwata M, Hirano A. A neuropathological study of Werdnig-Hoffmann disease. Neurol Med (Tokyo) 1978;8:40–53

15 Maya K, Inoue K, Hirano A. Pathological findings of prolonged Werdnig-Hoffmann disease. Neurol Med (Tokyo) 1981;14:243–252

16 Towfighi J, Young RSK, Ward RM. Is Werdnig-Hoffmann disease a pure lower motor neuron disorder? Acta Neuropathol (Berl) 1985;65:270–280

17 Chou S-M, Fakadej AV. Ultrastructure of chromatolytic motoneurons and anterior spinal roots in a case of Werdnig-Hoffmann disease. J Neuropathol Exp Neurol 1971;30:368–379

18 Iwata M, Hirano A. 'Glial bundles' in spinal cord late after paralytic anterior poliomyelitis. Ann Neurol 1978;4:562–563

19 Hirano A. Aspects of the ultrastructure of amyotrophic lateral sclerosis. In: Rowland LP, ed. Human Motor Neuron Diseases. New York, Raven Press, 1982;75–88

20 Ghatak NR, Nochlin D. Glial outgrowth along spinal nerve roots in amyotrophic lateral sclerosis. Ann Neurol 1982;11:203–206

21 Campbell MF, Liversedge LA. The motor neuron diseases (including the spinal muscular atrophies). In: Walton J, ed. Disorders of Voluntary Muscle. 4th ed. Edinburgh, Churchill Livingstone, 1981;725–752

22 Dick PJ, Stevens JC, Mulder DW. Frequency of nerve fiber degeneration of peripheral motor and sensory neurons in amyotrophic lateral sclerosis. Neurology 1975;25:781–785

23 Bradley WG, Good P, Rasool CG, et al. Morphometric and biochemical studies of peripheral nerve in amyotrophic lateral sclerosis. Ann Neurol 1983;14:267–277

24 Mulder DW, Bushek W, Spring E, et al. Motor neuron disease (ALS): Evaluation of detection thresholds of cutaneous sensation. Neurology 1983;33:1625–1627

25 Harvey DG, Torack RM, Rosenbaum HE. Amyotrophic lateral sclerosis with ophthalmoplegia. A clinicopathologic study, Arch Neurol 1979;36:615–617

26 Kushner M, Parrish M, Burke A, et al. Nystagmus in motor neuron disease: Clinicopathological study of two cases. Ann Neurol 1984;16:71–77

27 Leveille A, Kiernan J, Goodwin JA, et al. Eye movements in amyotrophic lateral sclerosis. Arch Neurol 1982;39:684–686

28 Dalakas MC, Hatazawa J, Brooks RA, et al. Lowered cerebral glucose utilization in amyotrophic lateral sclerosis. Ann Neurol 1987;22:580–586

29 Rapport MM, Donnenfeld H, Brunner W, et al. Ganaglioside patterns in amyotrophic lateral sclerosis brain regions. Ann Neurol 1985;18:60–67

30 Swash M, Scholtz CL, Vowles G, et al. Selective vulnerability of the corticospinal pathways in motor neuron disease. Abstracts Xth International Congress of Neuropathology, Stockholm 1986;216

31 Averback P, Crocker P. Regular involvement of Clarke's nucleus in sporadic amyotrophic lateral sclerosis. Arch Neurol 1982;39:155–156

32 Williams C, Kozlowski M, Miller CA. Spinal border cells in ALS. J Neuropathol Exp Neurol 1987;46:342 (abst)

33 Hirano A. Progress in the pathology of motor neuron diseases. In: Zimmerman HM, ed. Progress in Neuropathology. New York, Grune & Stratton, 1973;2:181–215

34 Malamud N, Hirano A, Kurland LT. Pathoanatomic changes in amyotrophic lateral sclerosis on Guam. Special reference to the occurrence of neurofibrillary changes. Arch Neurol 1961;5:401–415

35 Hirano A, Malamud N, Kurland LT, et al. Parkinsonism-dementia complex, an endemic disease on the island of Guam. I. Clinical features. Brain 1961;84:642–661

36 Hirano A, Malamud N, Kurland LT. Parkinsonism-dementia complex, an endemic disease on the island of Guam. II. Pathological features. Brain 1961;84:662–679

37 Hirano A. Pathology of amyotrophic lateral sclerosis. In: Gajdusek DC, Gibbs CJ, Jr, Alpers M, eds. Slow, Latent, and Temperate Virus Infections. NINDB Monograph No. 2. Washington, National Institutes of Health, 1965;23–26

38 Schochet SS Jr, Lampert PW, Lindenberg R. Fine structure of the Pick and Hirano bodies in a case of Pick's disease. Acta Neuropathol (Berl) 1968;11:330–337

39 Hirano A, Malamud N, Elizan TS, et al. Amyotrophic lateral sclerosis and parkinsonism-dementia complex on Guam. Arch Neurol 1966;15:35–51

40 Greenfield JG, Bosanquet FD. The brain-stem lesions in parkinsonism. J Neurol Neurosurg Psychiat 1953;16:213–226

41 Hirano A, Zimmerman HM. Alzheimer's neurofibrillary changes. A topographic study. Arch Neurol 1962;7:227–242

42 Hirano A. A Guide to Neuropathology. New York, Igaku-Shoin, 1981

43 Hirano A, Dembitzer HM, Kurland LT, et al. The fine structure of some intraganglionic alternations. Neurofibrillary tangles, granulovacuolar bod-

ies and 'rod-like' structures as seen in Guam amyotrophic lateral sclerosis and parkinsonism-dementia complex. J Neuropathol Exp Neurol 1968;27:167–182

44 Hirano A. Neuropathologic hallmarks of neuropsychiatric disorders in the elderly. In: Hirano A, Miyoshi K, eds. Neuropsychiatric Disorders in the Elderly. New York, Igaku-Shoin, 1983;3–15

45 Anderson TH, Richardson EP, Jr, Okazaki H, et al. Neurofibrillary degeneration on Guam. Frequency in Chamorros and non-Chamorros with no known neurological disease. Brain 1979;102:65–77

46 Garruto RM, Yanagihara R, Gajdusek DC. Disappearance of high-incidence amyotrophic lateral sclerosis and parkinsonism-dementia on Guam. Neurology 1985;35:193–198

47 Chen K-M, Makifuchi T, Garruto RM, et al. Parkinsonism-dementia in a Filipino migrant: Clinicopathologic case report. Neurology 1983;32:1221–1226

48 Chen KM, Yase Y. Amyotrophic Lateral Sclerosis in Asia and Oceania. Taiwan, National Taiwan University, 1984

49 Gajdusek DC, Salazar AM. Amyotrophic lateral sclerosis and parkinsonian syndromes in high incidence among the Auyu and Jakai people of West New Guinea, Neurology 1982;32:107–126

50 Lieberman A, Dziatolowski M, Kupersmith M. Dementia in Parkinson disease. Ann Neurol 1979;6:355–359

51 Hakim AM, Mathieson G. Dementia in Parkinson disease: A neuropathologic study. Neurology 1979;29:1209–1214

52 Boller F, Mitzutani T, Roessmann U, et al. Parkinson disease, dementia and Alzheimer disease. Clinicopathological correlation. Ann Neurol 1980;7:329–335

53 Gaspar P, Gray F. Dementia in idiopathic Parkinson's disease. A neuropathological study of 32 cases. Acta Neuropathol (Berl) 1984;64:43–52

54 Leverenz J, Sumi SM. Parkinson's disease in patients with Alzheimer's disease. Arch Neurol 1986;43:662–664

55 Ditler SM, Mirra SS. Neuropathologic and clinical features of Parkinson's disease in Alzheimer's disease patient. Neurology 1987;37:754–760

56 Hirano A, Llena JF. Neuropathological features of parkinsonism-dementia complex on Guam: Reappraisal and comparative study with Alzheimer's disease and Parkinson's disease. In: Zimmerman HM, ed. Progress in Neuropathology. New York, Raven Press, 1986;6:17–31

57 Meyers KR, Dorencamp DG, Suzuki K. Amyotrophic lateral sclerosis with diffuse neurofibrillary changes. Report of a case. Arch Neurol 1974;30:84–89

58 Forno LS, O'Flanagan TJ. Amyotrophic lateral sclerosis of the Guam type in a US veteran. Neurology 1973;23:876–880

59 Schmitt HP, Emser M, Heimes C. Familial occurrence of amyotrophic lateral sclerosis, parkinsonism, and dementia. Ann Neurol 1984;16:642–648

60 Malamud N, Hirano A. Atlas of Neuropathology. Second, revised edition. Berkeley, University of California Press, 1974;100–105

61 Corsellis JAN, Burton CJ, Freeman-Brown D. The aftermath of boxing. Psychol Med 1973;3:270–303

62 Horoupian DS, Yang SS. Paired helical filaments in neurovisceral lipidosis (juvenile dystonic lipidosis). Ann Neurol 1978;4:404–411

63 Fan KJ, Pezeshkpour G. Widespread neurofibrillary tangles in a retarded patient with progressive congenital hydrocephalus. J Neuropathol Exp Neurol 1986;45:367 (abst)

64 Wisniewski HM, Popovitch ER, Kaufman MA, et al. Neurofibrillary changes in advanced hydrocephalus. A clinicopathological study. J Neuropathol Exp Neurol 1987;46:26 (abst)

65 Halper J, Scheithauser BW, Okazaki H, et al. Meningoangiomatosis: A report of six cases with special reference to the occurrence of neurofibrillary tangles. J Neuropathol Exp Neurol 1986;45:426–446

66 Kato T, Hirano A. Observation of many Alzheimer neurofibrillary changes in the homolateral nucleus basalis of Meynert in a patient with an extensive old cerebral infarct. Neuropathology, in press (abst)

67 Schochet SS Jr, Hardman JM, Ladewig PP, et al. Intraneuronal conglomerates in sporadic motor neuron disease. Arch Neurol 1969;20:548–553

68 Hirano A, Iwata M. Pathology of motor neurons with special reference to amyotrophic lateral sclerosis and related diseases. In: Tsubaki T, Toyokura Y, ed. Amyotrophic Lateral Sclerosis. Baltimore, University Park Press, 1979;107–133

69 Kurland LT, Mulder DW. Epidemiologic investigations of amyotrophic lateral sclerosis. 2. Familial aggregations indicative of dominant inheritance. Neurology 1955;5:249–268

70 Engel WK, Kurland LT, Klatzo I. An inherited disease similar to amyotrophic lateral sclerosis with a pattern of posterior-column involvement. An intermediate form? Brain 1959;82:203–220

71 Hirano A, Kurland LT, Sayre GP. Familial amyotrophic lateral sclerosis. A subgroup characterized by posterior and spinocerebellar tract involvement and hyaline inclusions in the anterior horn cells. Arch Neurol 1967;16:232–243

72 Nakano I, Hirano A, Kurland LT, et al. Familial amyotrophic lateral sclerosis. Neuropathology of two brothers in American 'C' family. Neurol Med (Tokyo) 1984;20:458–471

73 Hirano A, Nakano I, Kurland LT, et al. Fine structural study of neurofibrillary changes in a family with amyotrophic lateral sclerosis. J Neuropathol Exp Neurol 1984;43:471–480

74 Oda M, Akagawa N, Tabuchi Y, et al. A sporadic juvenile case of the amyotrophic lateral sclerosis with neuronal intracytoplasmic inclusions. Acta Neuropathol (Berl) 1978;44:211–216

75 Carpenter S. Promimal axonal enlargement in motor neuron disease. Neurology 1968;18:842–851

76 Inoue K, Hirano A. Early pathological changes of amyotrophic lateral sclerosis. Autopsy findings of a case of 10 months' duration. Neurol Med (Tokyo) 1979;11:448–455

77 Nakano I, Donnenfeld H, Hirano A. A neuropathological study of amyotrophic lateral sclerosis: With special reference to central chromatolysis and spheroids in the spinal ventral horn and some pathological changes of motor cortex. Neurol Med (Tokyo) 1983;18:134–144

78 Delisle MB, Carpenter S. Neurofibrillary axonal swellings and amyotrophic lateral sclerosis. J Neurol Sci 1984;63:241–250

79 Hirano A, Inoue K. Early pathological changes of amyotrophic lateral sclerosis. Electron microscopic study of chromatolysis, spheroids and Bunina bodies. Neurol Med (Tokyo) 1980;13:148–160

80 Hirano A, Donnenfeld H, Sasaki S. Fine structural observations of neurofilamentous changes in amyotrophic lateral sclerosis. J Neuropathol Exp Neurol 1984;43:461–470

81 Power JM, Horoupian DS, Schaumberg HH, et al. Documentation of a neurological disease in a Vermont family 90 years later. Can J Neurol Sci 1974;1:139–140

82 Kato T, Hirano A, Kurland LT. Asymmetric involvement of the spinal cord involving both large and small anterior horn cells in a case of familial amyotrophic lateral sclerosis. Clin Neuropathol 1987;6:67–70

83 Kubo H, Ikuta F, Tsubaki T. An autopsy case with a history of familial amyotrophic lateral sclerosis and posterior column involvement. Clin Neurol 1967;7:45–50

84 Takahashi K, Nakamura H, Okada E. Hereditary amyotrophic lateral sclerosis–histochemical and electron microscopic study of hyaline inclusions in motor neurons. Arch Neurol 1972;27:292–299

85 Tanaka J, Nakamura H, Tabuchi Y, et al. Familial amyotrophic lateral sclerosis: Features of multisystem degeneration. Acta Neuropathol (Berl) 1984;64:22–29

86 Brownell B, Oppenheimer DR, Hughes JT. The central nervous system in motor neurone disease. J Neurol Neurosurg Psychiat 1970;33:338–357

87 Hughes JT, Jerome D. Ultrastructure of anterior horn motor neurons in the Hirano-Kurland-Sayre type of combined neurological system degeneration. J Neurol Sci 1971;13:389–399

88 Mizusawa H, Hirano A. Lower motor neuron disease associated with focal

onion bulb formation in an anterior spinal root. Neurol Med (Tokyo) 1987;26:309–311

89 Kato T, Katagiri T, Hirano A, et al. Sporadic lower neuron disease with Lewy body-like inclusions: A new subgroup? Acta Neuropathol (Berl) submitted

90 Kuroda S, Kuyama K, Morioka E, et al. Sporadic amyotrophic lateral sclerosis with intracytoplasmic eosinophilic inclusions. A case closely akin to familial ALS. Neurol Med (Tokyo) 1986;24:31–37

91 Kusaka H, Imai T, Hashimoto S, et al. Ultrastructural study of chromatolytic neurons in an adult-onset sporadic amyotrophic lateral sclerosis. Acta Neuropathol (Berl) in press

92 Kato T, Hirano A, Weinberg ML, et al. Spinal cord lesions in progressive supranuclear palsy: Some new observations. Acta Neuropathol (Berl) 1986;71:11–14

93 Kretzchmar HA, Berg BO, Davis RL. Giant axonal neuropathy. A neuropathological study. Acta Neuropathol (Berl) 1987;73:138–144

94 Shintaku M, Hirano A, Llena JF. Increased diameter of demyelinated axons in chronic multiple sclerosis of the spinal cord. J Neuropathol Exp Neurol 1987;46:367 (abst)

95 Moss TH, Campbell MJ. Atypical motor neuron disease with features of a multisystem degeneration: A non-familial case with prominent sensory involvement. Clin Neuropathol 1987;6:55–60

96 Kusaka H, Nakano I, Hirano A, et al. A case of amyotrophic lateral sclerosis with posterior column involvement. Neurol Med (Tokyo) 1985;22:220–225

97 Metcalf CW, Hirano A. Amyotrophic lateral sclerosis. Clinicopathological studies of a family. Arch Neurol 1971;24:518–523

98 Griffin JW, Cork LC, Hoffman PN, et al. Experimental models of motor neuron degeneration. In: Dyck PJ, Thomas PK, Lambert EH, Bunge R, ed. Peripheral Neuropathology. Philadelphia, WB Saunders Company, 1984;1:621–635

99 Cork LC, Griffin JW, Munnell JF, et al. Hereditary canine spinal muscular atrophy. J Neuropathol Exp Neurol 1979;38:209–221

100 Cork LC, Griffith JW, Padula CA, et al. The pathology of motor neurons in accelerated hereditary canine spinal muscular atrophy. Lab Invest 1982;46:89–99

101 Igata A, Osame M, Inada S. Hereditary amyotrophic dogs. In: Tsubaki T, Toyokura Y, eds. Amyotrophic Lateral Sclerosis. Baltimore, University Park Press, 1979;351–362

102 Uzumo S, Ikuta F, Igata A, et al. Morphological study on the hereditary neurogenic amyotrophic dogs: Accumulation of lipid compound-

like structures in lower motor neurons. Acta Neuropathol (Berl) 1983;61:270–274

103 Falconer DS. Wobbler (wr) mouse. Mouse Newsletter 1956;15:23

104 Duchen LW, Falconer DS, Strich SJ. Hereditary progressive neurogenic muscular atrophy in mouse. J Physiol (Lond) 1965;783:53–55

105 Duchen LW, Strich SJ. An hereditary motor neurone disease with progressive denervation of muscle in the mouse: The mutant 'wobbler' (with an appendix by Falconer DS). J Neurol Neurosurg Psychiat 1968;31:535–542

106 Andrews JM, Maxwell DS. Motor neuron diseases in animals. In: Norris FH, Kurland LT, eds. Motor Neuron Diseases: Research on Amyotrophic Lateral Sclerosis and Related Disorders. New York, Grune & Stratton, 1969;369–385

107 Andrews JM. The fine structure of the cervical spinal cord, ventral root and brachial nerves in the wobbler (wr) mouse. J Neuropathol Exp Neurol 1975;34:12–27

108 Mitsumoto H, Bradley WG. Axonal pathology of myelinated fibers in murine motor neuron disease (Wobbler mouse). In: Adachi M, Hirano A, Aronson SM, eds. The Pathology of the Myelinated Axon. New York, Igaku-Shoin, 1985;126–149

109 Nixon CW, Connelly ME. Hind-leg paralysis: A new sex-linked mutation in the Syrian hamster. J Heredity 1968;59:276–278

110 Homburger F, Bajusz E. New models of human disease in Syrian hamsters. JAMA 1970;212:604–610

111 Hirano A. Fine structural changes in the mutant hamster with hind leg paralysis. Acta Neuropathol (Berl) 1977;39:225–230

112 Hirano A. A possible mechanism of demyelination in the Syrian hamster with hindleg paralysis. Lab Invest 1978;38:115–121

113 Striefler M, Cohn DF, Hirano A, et al. The central nervous system in a case of neurolathyrism. Neurology 1977;27:1176–1178

114 Hirano A, Llena JF, Striefler M, et al. Anterior horn cell changes in a case of neurolathyrism. Acta Neuropathol (Berl) 1976;35:277–283

115 Ule G. Experimentellen Neurolathrysmus. Verh dtsch Ges Path 1961;45:333–338

116 Chou SM, Hartman HA. Neuroaxonal lesions produced by β,β'-iminodi-propionitrile, with a concept of 'axostasis.' Acta Neuropathol (Berl) 1964;3:428–450

117 Chou SM, Hartman HA. Electron microscopy of focal neuroaxonal lesions produced by β,β'-iminodipropionitrile (IDPN) in rats. I. The advanced lesions. Acta Neuropathol (Berl) 1965;4:590–603

118 Griffin JW, Price DL. Proximal axonopathies induced by toxic chemicals.

In: Spencer PS, Schaumburg HH, eds. Experimental and Clinical Neurotoxicology. Baltimore, Williams & Wilkins, 1980;161–178

119 Klatzo I, Wisniewski H. Streicher E. Experimental production of neurofibrillary degeneration. J Neuropathol Exp Neurol 1965;24:187–199

120 Terry RD, Pena C. Experimental production of neurofibrillary degeneration. 2. Electron microscopy, phosphatase histochemistry and electron
probe analysis. J Neuropathol Exp Neurol 1965;24:200–210

121 Wisniewski H, Narkiewicz O, Wisniewski K. Topography and dynamics of
neurofibrillary degeneration in aluminum encephalopathy. Acta Neuropathol (Berl) 1967;9:127–133

122 Wisniewski HM, Sturman JA, Shek JW. Aluminum chloride induced
neurofibrillary changes in the developing rabbit: A chronic animal model.
Ann Neurol 1980;8:479–490

123 Troncoso JC, Price DL, Griffin JW, et al. Neurofibrillary axonal pathology
in aluminum intoxication. Ann Neurol 1982;12:278–283

124 Yoshimasu F. Aluminum neurotoxicity with special reference to its relation to the degenerative CNS diseases. Neurol Med (Tokyo) 1980;13:26–33

125 Yase Y. The role of trace metals in the pathogenesis of motor neuron
disease. In: Gourie-Devi M, ed. Motor Neurone Disease. New Delhi,
Oxford & IBH Publishing Co PVT Ltd, 1987;61–71

126 Yamamoto T, Iwasaki Y, Konno H. Retrograde axoplasmic transport of
adriamycin: An experimental form of motor neuron disease? Neurology
1984;34:1299–1304

127 Kondo A, Ohnishi A, Nagara H, et al. Neurotoxicity in primary sensory
neurons of adriamycin administered through retrograde axoplasmic transport in rat. Neuropathol Appl Neurobiol 1987;13:177–192

128 Yamamoto T, Iwasaki Y, Konno H, et al. Primary degeneration of motor
neurons by toxic lectins conveyed from peripheral nerve. J Neurol Sci
1985;70:327–337

129 Spencer PS, Ross SM, Hugon J, et al. Acute and chronic cytotoxicity of
beta-N-amino-L-alanine derivatives linked to human motor neuron diseases. Abstracts Xth International Congress of Neuropathology. Stockholm,
1986;164

130 Spencer PS, Nunn PB, Hugon J, et al. Guam amyotrophic lateral sclerosis–
parkinsonism-dementia linked to a plant excitant neurotoxin. Science
1987;237:517–521

131 den Hartog Jager WA. Experimental amyotrophic lateral sclerosis in the
guinea pig. J Neurol Sci 1985;67:133–142

132 Bodian D. The virus, the nerve cell and paralysis. Bull Johns Hopkins
Hosp 1948;83:1–107

133 Bodian D. Motoneuron disease and recovery in experimental poliomyeli-

tis. In: Halstead LS, Wiechers DO, eds. Late Effects of Poliomyelitis. Miami, Symposia Foundation, 1985;45–55

134 Tomlinson BE, Irving D. Changes in spinal cord motor neurons of possible relevance to the late effect of poliomyelitis. In: Halstead LS, Wiechers PO, eds. Late Effects of Poliomyelitis. Miami, Symposia Foundation, 1985;57–70

135 Gardner MB, Henderson BE, Estes JD, et al. Unusually high incidence of spontaneous lymphomas in wild house mice. J Natl Cancer Inst 1973;50:1571–1579

136 Gardner MB, Henderson BE, Officer E, et al. A spontaneous lower motor neuron disease apparently caused by indigenous type C RNA virus in wild mice. J Natl Cancer Inst 1973;51:1243–1254

137 Andrews JM, Gardner MB. Lower motor neuron degeneration associated with type C RNA virus infection in mice: Neuropathological features. J Neuropathol Exp Neurol 1974;33:185–307

138 Johnson RT. Viral Infection of the Nervous System. New York, Raven Press, 1982

139 Brooks BR, Schwarz JR, Johnson RJ. Spongiform polioencephalomyelopathy caused by a murine retrovirus. I. Pathogenesis of infection in newborn mice. Lab Invest 1980;43:480–486

140 Pena CE. Viruslike particles in amyotrophic lateral sclerosis: Electron microscopical study of a case. Ann Neurol 1977;1:290–297

141 Murphy WH, Tom MR, Lanzi RL, et al. Age dependence of immunologically induced central nervous system disease in C 58 mice. Cancer Res 1970;30:1612–1622

142 Kascsak RJ, Carp RI, Donnenfeld H. et al. Kinetics of replication of lactate dehydrogenous-elevating virus on age dependent polioencephalomyelitis. Intervirology 1983;19:6–15

143 Kusaka H, Hirano A, Kascsak RJ, et al. Effect of prolonged immunosupression on age-dependent polioencephalomyelitis in C 58 mice. Neuropathological study. Neurol Med (Tokyo) 1984;21:171–82

144 Kusaka H, Hirano A, Kascsak RJ, et al. Effect of prolonged immunosupression on age-dependent polioencephalomyelitis in C 58 mice. Neuropathological study of chronic phase. Neurol Med (Tokyo) 1984;21:588–595

Nutritional Factors in Amyotrophic Lateral Sclerosis on Guam: Observations from Umatac

JOHN C. STEELE, TOMASA Q. GUZMAN,
MARJORIE G. DRIVER, WILLIAM ZOLAN,
LEROY F. HEITZ, FRANK H. KILMER,
CAROLYN M. PARKER, BLUEBELL R. STANDAL,
ANN M. POBUTSKY, AND DONALD R. CRAPPER
McLACHLAN

A History of the Mariana Islands and the Indigenous Chamorros

'Micronesia' is the name Europeans gave to a vast geographic region in the Western Pacific ocean of more than two thousand small islands, some high and volcanic, others low-lying coral atolls. All are tropical and humid. Almost all have dense forests and foliage, heavy rainfall, and some accretion of coral reef. The islands of Micronesia are the peaks of mountain ranges; the clusters they form are called archipelagos. The Mariana Islands is one of these achipelagos, a chain of 15 small islands in the far Western Pacific which spread northward from Guam toward Japan (Map 1).

About four thousand years ago, in a remarkable navigational feat involving open ocean voyages of thousands of miles, the Micronesian islands were settled by migrants from the Indo-Malay peninsula [1]. The first circumnavigation of the world took place in the 16th century when Ferdinand Magellan led a Spanish expedition around the globe. In 1521, having entered the Pacific from the east and sailing with the equatorial current before the trade winds, Magellan reached islands near 14 degrees north latitude. At first, he called them Las Velas (the sails) after the sails on native canoes but he renamed them Los Ladrones (the thieves) when island inhabitants stole one of his boats. Magellan's historic arrival marked the entry of Europeans into the Northwestern Pacific and provided the first contact between Europeans and Pacific Islanders. The expedition is believed to have landed at the village of Umatac in Guam, southernmost of the islands. At the time of Magellan's arrival, the indigenous people, the Chamorros, were healthy. Their population was large and their life-style and culture were adapted to the smallness of the

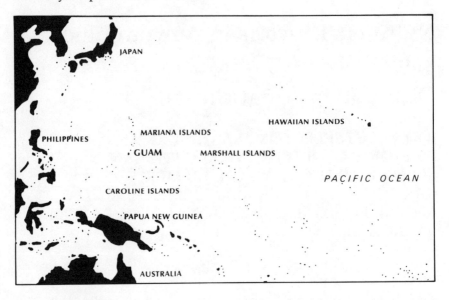

Map 1. Micronesia

islands and in harmony with their habitat's fragile ecology. They were skilled in fishing, horticulture, and navigation. They had an abundance of food for trade [2].

For 150 years after discovery, the Chamorros were mostly undisturbed by the West. Occasionally Spanish galleons sailing between Mexico and Manila stopped to provision. In 1601 and 1638 shipwrecks deposited large numbers of Mexican and Spanish sailors who scattered through the islands. In 1668, Western religion arrived on Guam when Father Diego Luis de San Vitores led a Jesuit mission to the Ladrones. He re-named them the Mariana Islands in honour of his patroness, Mariana de Austria, the Queen Regent of Spain [3]. Late in the 17th century, the Spanish sought to colonize the Mariana Islands. The Chamorros resisted and violent wars ensued. By 1710 the native population was reduced from more than 70,000 to only 1,600. The few Chamorros who survived were resettled by the Spanish in villages throughout Guam. A few hid out on the adjacent island of Rota. The depopulation and severe dis-ruption of the native society caused the remaining Chamorros to modify their traditional practices and to adopt Spain's life-styles. Chamorro women married Mexicans, Filipinos, and Spanish soldiers sent to tend the islands. It was many years, however, before the native population began to increase again [4].

During the 18th century, Jesuit missionaries guided the economic and social lives of the Chamorros. The missionaries taught the islanders European customs and encouraged agricultural production. But the lot of the islanders was a miserable one. Many fell prey to foreign diseases such as leprosy and tuberculosis brought by the Spaniards. Large numbers of Chamorros died in frequent epidemics of smallpox and measles. In 1769 the Order of Augustinian Recollects took the place of the Jesuits. The native condition deteriorated further. By the early 19th century, poverty was widespread among the indigenous people. Agriculture foundered. Many Chamorros were forced to scavenge in the forests for food [5]. As Spain's world influence waned during the 1800s, the plight of people of these distant islands grew even worse. Neglect became abandonment. In 1815, Mexico declared its independence, the Manila galleon trade ended, and the Spanish presence on Guam was reduced to a token. Although whaling ships stopped in Guam to refurbish and provision during the height of that industry from 1820 to 1840, after 1850 the whalers moved northward. During the rest of the century the Marianas were all but forsaken by outsiders.

In 1898, Guam was seized by the United States during the Spanish-American War. By terms of settlement, the island became an American territory and it has remained so to this day, except for a brief period, from 1941 to 1944, when it was occupied by the Japanese. The Northern Mariana Islands, however, were sold by Spain to Germany, which administered them until 1914. With the onset of World War I, they were occupied by Japan, who administered and developed all the islands of Micronesia except Guam, until its defeat by the United States in 1944.

Prior to World War II, Guam had been a remote US naval outpost. As such it had received little attention from the United States. There was no encouragement of economic development and the Chamorros maintained their subsistence life-style, as they had during Spanish times. In the post-war era, the United States extended its western frontier across the Pacific and promoted the rapid development and modernization of Guam and the other Micronesian islands. American military and Public Health Service physicians began to describe diseases of the region and to develop health services to address them.

Observations about ALS/PD, a Neurological Disease Occurring in Chamorros from the Mariana Islands

In 1945, a pathologist at the Guam Naval Hospital, Dr Harry Zimmerman, reported that he had seen seven Chamorro patients with amyotrophic lateral sclerosis (ALS) in only one month. In two cases, he confirmed that diagnosis by necropsy [6]. Zimmerman was not alone in his observations. Subsequent clinical studies by physicians assigned to Guam also reported remarkably high rates of ALS among Chamorros [7–9].

These reports came to the attention of Dr Leonard Kurland, who was then with the National Institute of Neurological Diseases and Blindness (NINDB). In 1953 he went to Guam to investigate the unusual phenomena detailed in the reports. He was joined by Dr Donald Mulder, a neurologist from the Mayo Clinic. Together, they made a number of important observations. They confirmed that the illness that the Chamorros suffered from was indistinguishable from classical ALS. They noted a striking familial aggregation of ALS patients; more than one-third of the affected individuals were found to have other family members who suffered from the disease [10, 11]. In addition, Kurland and Mulder found that ALS was 100 times more common on Guam than elsewhere in the world. In certain villages of southern Guam and on the adjacent island of Rota, the incidence of the disease was even higher. However, ALS was uncommon among the Chamorros and long-term residents of the other Mariana Islands. It was not found in the Caroline Islands at all [12, 13].

In 1961, Dr Asao Hirano characterized a second neurological syndrome endemic among the Chamorros of Guam and Rota. Hirano and Kurland termed it the 'parkinsonism-dementia complex' (PD) because of its clinical features. They considered ALS and PD different manifestations of a single disease process [14]. In a companion report about PD, Hirano, Nathan Malamud, and Kurland described widespread nerve cell loss, and neurofibrillary and granulovacuolar degeneration of nerve cells in cortical, subcortical, and brain-stem regions. The distribution of these changes correlated with the clinical features of dementia and parkinsonism [15]. Neurofibrillary degeneration was also present in Chamorro patients with ALS, an observation which has caused many authorities to regard the ALS suffered by Chamorros as a distinct (and separate) form of motor neuron disease.

Subsequent clinicopathological studies by Hirano et al in 1966 [16], Frank Anderson et al in 1979 [17], Leung Chen in 1981 [18], and Daniel Perl et al in 1982 [19] confirmed that neurofibrillary degeneration is very common among Chamorros, even though they have no symptoms. Some Chamorros in their 30s suffer neurofibrillary degeneration. The degeneration is similar to that which occurs in Alzheimer's disease and with ageing of the nervous system. It becomes more widespread and severe with age; by late middle life it is present in all Chamorros. Yet, despite the prevalence of severe and widespread nerve cell degeneration, senile plaques rarely occur among the Chamorros. Hundreds of careful neuropathological studies have been performed on Chamorros during the past 30 years [20]. They show that, although Chamorros suffer unusually high rates of neurofibrillary-associated neurodegenerative disease (ALS/PD), they have remarkably low rates of Alzheimer's disease and normal ageing by histological criteria. Indeed, these two conditions, Alzheimer's and ageing, so common elsewhere in the world, are distinctly uncommon in this ethnic population. This is an observation that is quite as remarkable as the observation of very high rates of incidence of ALS/PD.

In 1957, Kurland and his associates noted that Chamorros who had left Guam suffered the same high incidence of ALS as did residents of the island, even though they had lived away from Guam for many years [21]. In 1980 Dr Ralph Garruto et al [22] reviewed the occurrence of ALS among 28 Chamorros migrants from Guam. One individual had left Guam in 1935, and did not develop symptoms of ALS until 34 years later. Dr Roswell Eldridge et al discovered an elderly Chamorro in California who developed his first symptoms of parkinsonism-dementia at the age of 70 years, 46 years after leaving Guam [23, 24]. A few Filipinos who immigrated to Guam as young adults in the 1940s have been found to have histologically verified ALS/PD. However, none of them developed symptoms until at least 17 years after reaching Guam [25, 26].

These important observations about migrants show that in some, and perhaps all, ALS/PD patients there is a long interval between exposure to Guam's environment and the onset of symptoms.

In recent years, the incidence of ALS/PD on Guam has decreased. Garruto et al [27] have analysed the incidence rates of ALS in Guam since 1945 and of PD since 1955. They have noted a progressive decline in both forms of the disease and also a change in sex ratio. They note that 'the disease has disappeared in both men and women younger than 40 and ALS is now rare among those between 40 and 50, a situation strikingly different from one and two decades ago.' In addition, they note 'a greater age in onset has also occurred for PD in both sexes. Presently there are only a few cases of PD with onset before age 65 years. In the early 1960's, however, PD was occasionally observed in individuals as young as 35 years and was routinely recognized in high incidence among those in their 40's and 50's'[27].

A recent epidemiological study by Reed et al [28] confirmed the observation of Garruto et al that ALS on Guam is disappearing and that its decline began in the mid-1960s, about 20 years after World War II. Reed recently analysed the occurrence of ALS/PD in a group of Chamorros he has followed since 1968. None of the individuals he studied developed ALS during the five years between 1979 and 1983, although the annual incidence of PD was still high (i.e. 25 per 100,000 on Guam and 39 per 100,000 on Rota) during that same time [28].

Studies of Lytico (ALS) and Bodig (PD) in Umatac

From folklore accounts, the illness which the Chamorros call Lytico-Bodig has occurred among residents of Umatac for more than 150 years. Since the turn of the century, medical records indicate that village residents have suffered disproportionately higher rates of ALS/PD than those of other villages on Guam. This has been confirmed by epidemiological studies since the 1950s [10, 29]. Many patients have lived all their lives in this small village and its vicinity. The village, its people, and the surrounding countryside are a living laboratory. As such, Umatac provides a unique opportunity to study this enigmatic disease which has puzzled so many for so long.

History of Umatac

Before European contact, the Chamorros of Guam lived in 180 villages. The largest and most important were Fuuna and Agana, along the western coast. Fuuna was situated on the edge of La Fouha Bay, which is just above Umatac Bay and within the boundaries of the present-day municipality of Umatac. There were 13 other ancient settlements in this small district of only 6 square miles; 9 were along the shoreline and 4 were inland in La Fouha and Umatac valleys. By early missionary accounts 'they [the Chamorros] believe they were born from La Fouha rock – whence they all go each year for a fiesta ... They say that a woman gave birth to the land, and to the sea, and to all that is visible.' Sasalaguon, a mountain peak which dominates the southern prospect, was the Chamorro's equivalent of Hell. The spirits of those who had died violently dwelt there [30].

Magellan is believed to have anchored in Umatac Bay in 1521 and visited the village. Pigafetta, writing about this first contact with the islanders, observed 'Those people [the Chamorros] live in freedom for they have no lord or superior, and they go quite naked and some of them wear a beard ... Those people are as tall as we, and well built ... They worship nothing ... [the women] are handsome and delicate and darker than the men ... Their houses are made of wood covered with planks and fig leaves ... They are poor but ingenious and great thieves. And on this account we called those [three] islands the Islands of Thieves

[Islas de los Ladrones] ... Those thieves thought [by signs which they made] that there were no other men in the world but themselves'[2].

In 1602, Friar Juan Pobre de Zamora, one of the first Europeans to live among the Chamorros, observed: 'The men and women are hard workers, not lazy, and [they] have little regard for those who do not work ... They are naturally kind to one another ... They are so peace loving that during all the time I have spent with them, as an eyewitness, I have never seen the people of any village quarrel among themselves.'

Accounts by other early missionaries confirm the nobility, industry, and good health of the Chamorros before the era of Spanish oppression. In 1683, Father Garcia wrote about the Chamorros: 'the color of the Mariana natives is brown, a bit lighter than Filipinos. They are taller, and are more corpulent and more robust than Europeans, well featured and so stout they seem to be bloated ... They live long, and it is common for them to reach ninety or one hundred years of age ... Their principal employment is fishing, boat making, planting and decorating their homes ... These islanders obtain their ordinary food from the sea, and fish they prize more than chicken meat. For bread, they have a certain kind of fruit [i.e. breadfruit] so tasty that even newcomers from Spain do not esteem it less than wheat bread, and when this fruit is scarce they use for bread tubers similar to those found in the Philippines, like the gabe [taro], ubi [tapioca] and tugui [yam]. They also harvest enough rice to add to their enjoyment on feastdays. Their fiestas where one might expect excesses, are confined to singing their histories, and mock battles with the lance. During these entertainments, they pass around rice, cakes, tamales, fish, coconuts, bananas, sugar cane and a beverage made from rice and shredded coconut which they drink without any reprehensible excess' [31].

In 1668, Father San Vitores chose the village of Agana in central Guam as his principal residence and the headquarters for Jesuit activities. In the late 1600s the presidio (main garrison) was also established there. Though Agana thereby became the main religious and military centre in the Marianas, the early Spanish governors chose Umatac village as their main administrative centre; in part to be away from the missionaries, and in part because of Umatac's fine anchorage. In the 1690s, a palacio (governor's residence) was built by the Bay's edge and a contingent of soldiers was stationed there.

During the late 17th and 18th centuries, the native population was severely reduced by war, disease, and famine. The survivors were Christianized. Missionaries sought to change traditional Chamorro customs and practices to those of Catholicism. By 1710, the 1600 surviving Chamorros had been relocated into nine parishes (pueblos) throughout Guam, each with a church that was served by a priest [4].

Umatac was a satellite settlement and a dependency of the pueblo of Inarajan. After colonization there are accounts which tell of its poverty and neglect, and of the degradation of the Chamorro inhabitants resulting from their cultural disruption and Spanish oppression. For example, in 1819, the draftsman of a visiting French expedition described Umatac as 'about 30 hovels built on piles and constructed of the ribs of palm leaves ... The people by whom they are inhabited exhibit, outwardly, the frightful appearance of the most disgusting wretchedness. A piece of dirty, stinking cloth covers the women from the loins to the knees. The men are dressed in a sort of wide trouser ... Both are covered with a disgusting and active leprosy, that leaves on the body black and livid marks even when it disappears, and is a continual subject of dread to the Europeans who have to deal with them. Here everything is hideous; both the houses and the spectres that inhabit them.' As the expedition travelled from Umatac to Agana he observed 'When we traversed the country the mind revolts with indignation at the aspect of a soil so fertile from which nothing is obtained. Hills shadowed by vigorous and useless trees surround smiling vales, where weeds grow by thousands among a few blades of rice and Indian corn, attesting equally the goodness of the soil, the idleness of the inhabitants, and the inattention of the governors. How do these robust and almost savage men employ themselves? They live, they die ... with a few grains of Indian corn, a couple of breadfruits, half a score of segars [cigars] and a cake of the pith of the tacca pinnatifida or of the sago tree [*Cycas circinalis*] they pass the day; and I do not think they can imagine anything better in their situation, if to these productions, which the earth furnishes in abundance, they be enabled to add a bit of dried fish, or a shred of half putrid venison ... The appearance of so much wretchedness, no doubt the result of degradation into which the inhabitants of this useless archipelago have been plunged by fanatic conquerors, rends my heart, and rouses my indignation against those vain and guilty men, who fancied that the introduction of Christianity exempted them from conferring any new benefits'[32].

In 1839, an observer with the D'Urville exploration recorded the following observations: 'The village [of Umatac] is composed of badly constructed houses, open to all winds and with a repulsive dirtiness, [which] seems to clash with the fresh and gracious nature which surrounds them ... the indifference of the indigenes stops a great part of these efforts towards the good ... [and] in our travels in the countryside, we have not seen the cultivation of land respond to the idea that one must have some work from these men. Hardly have we seen any fields where potatoes are grown. Behind Umatac, and following the course of the stream, one enters into a valley where everything appears united to offer the best show of land. However, everything here is still fallow or in a near state of being abandoned ... However, in the midst of this poverty, pleasure and joy prevail. The guitar – this instrument from all Spanish countries – rings from the threshold of some houses and accompanies the soft and slow songs. Unconcern and indolence are a particular character of the Spanish nation. It is the same everywhere ... Here we see the Chamorros of Guam who would rather submit to a thousand privations and to sing in the most precarious situation on human existence ... than to devote themselves to work which would give them more comfortable circumstances' [33].

The miserable condition of Umatac and the other southern Chamorro settlements continued throughout the 19th century.

In 1870 Governor Don Felipe de la Corte observed: 'Umatac is a little hamlet which ekes out a wretched existence with the help of ships [whalers] which have to go there for water. It lies at the foot of a mountain range which leaves no room for fields; nor can it be reached by any road' [34].

In the early 1950s, 80 years later and after 50 years of American administration, Mulder confirmed the continuing poverty, isolation, and neglect of the Chamorros when he wrote: 'Conditions in Umatac have changed little [since 1870]. A road has been completed into the village but it is often impassable ... Sanitary and health conditions are poorer than in any other village on the island' [11].

Today, Umatac's residents enjoy a much more satisfactory quality of life. The population is less than 1000 and the majority of the inhabitants originate from five extended families.

Occurrence of Lytico (ALS) and Bodig (PD) in Umatac

The first folklore account of paralysis among Chamorros is from Umatac village. According to local legend, sometime after 1769 an Augustinian priest picked mangoes from a garden adjacent to his church without asking permission of the owner. The owners' anger with the priest caused the cleric to curse the man and his family with a fatal paralysis which no one could cure. The curse has continued for more than 150 years, and succeeding generations of this Umatac family have been particularly prone to this malady. Most people of Umatac believe this story.

The mango tree from which the fruits were reputedly taken still grows in a garden close to the ruins of St Dionicio's Church in the centre of the village.

Aided by the Umatac commissioner and access to National Institutes of Communicable Diseases and Stroke (NINCDS) records, we recently compiled a list of the people of Umatac who have suffered ALS/PD during the past 40 years; 108 patients have been so diagnosed and therefore more than 10% of all patients with ALS/PD on Guam have been from this small village.

At present, we identify 14 patients with ALS/PD from Umatac. Only 2 of these patients suffer from ALS and the others have the PD form of illness. Twelve of the patients have developed symptoms since 1980.

Nutritional Observations on Farms with High ALS/PD Incidence in the Three Valleys of the Umatac District

Most Umatac people live in the village, which is located by the Bay's edge. Many families also have an inland farm (ranch) in one of the three valleys where they raise their own foods. Since we believed that the environmental cause of the disease could be found on these farms and in these valleys, we began our search by targeting five farms of different families with high rates of ALS/PD in each of Cetti (2), LaFouha (1), and Umatac (2) valleys (Map 2).

Interviews which we conducted with these families indicated that the staples of their pre-World War II diets had been grown or produced on their individual farms and that those crops and products were the main source of food for each family. None of the families had depended on supplemental foods purchased from stores or provided by neighbours. The principal root crops on all farms were yams, several varieties of taro, and tapioca. These tuberous plants, important constituents of the Chamorro diet, are also carbohydrate staples in other Pacific islands. All the five families we studied also cultivated breadfruit, coconut, varieties of bananas, citruses, mango, and papaya. They raised chickens and pigs and most had several cows and carabaos which were a source of milk and meat.

The diets of the five families living in the three Umatac valleys were similar to those of families living in other villages of Guam and on other Micronesian islands. As on other Pacific islands, most Umatac children were breast-fed and not weaned until they were older than two years. Many farms had a carabao or a cow and it was usual for the children to drink its milk. Fish caught from the Bay were a main staple of the diet for young and old. Fish was eaten raw or cooked. People chewed on

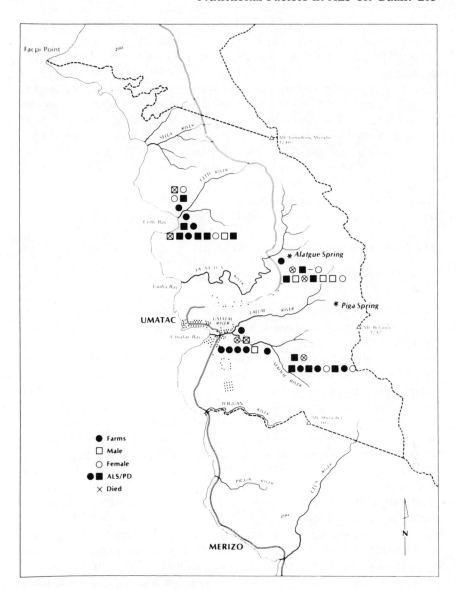

Map 2. Umatac farms with high incidence of ALS/PD

fish skeletons and also sucked on the heads. Small fish were considered a delicacy and were eaten raw.

After World War II, Guam's cultural and socioeconomic status changed profoundly. The economy altered from subsistence to wage labour, an American educational system began, and Chamorros were required to speak in English. Many became employed in government jobs and received salaries. The Chamorros began to eat processed and packaged foods imported from the United States and Japan. Although most Chamorro families continued to grow small quantities of local foods on their farms, most no longer depended exclusively on such produce.

These post-war life-style and dietary changes also occurred in Umatac. A survey conducted in 1984 revealed that four of the five ranches selected for our study were fallow; only one was being actively farmed.

The Search for the Cause of ALS/PD

THE HYPOTHESIS OF MINERAL DYSMETABOLISM

During the 1960s and 1970s, Japanese neurologists identified two valleys in the Kii Peninsula of Honshu where the small populations of several villages suffered high rates of ALS. In the first valley, called Kozagawa, residents suffered ALS but not PD. In the second valley, Hobara, some 200 kilometres distant from Kozagawa, residents suffered a somewhat different disease similar to the ALS/PD found on Guam. Some had only ALS, some had only parkinsonism-dementia, and some had features of both. Seventy per cent of the patients had other family members who were affected, and in some families the illness had occurred since the 19th century. Neuropathological studies of patients from both valleys showed widespread neurofibrillary degeneration similar to that which occurs in the ALS/PD complex of Guam.

Investigators concluded that the neurological disease of these two widely separated geographic foci in Japan and the Mariana Islands was the same and must have a common cause [35]. This very important conclusion stimulated the search for factors which would relate the two. In 1964, Whiting lived in Mitogawa Mura and compared food practices among people of this village in Kozagawa with those of Guam. She observed that cycads were often grown in Mitogawa as ornamentals, but in several months of residence she did not locate even one resident who had knowledge of the local use of them as food. Although several described uses for cycads as medicine, none of her informants had firsthand experience with medicinal use of the plant [36].

When studies by Whiting and observations by others did not identify an obvious common food or dietary practice between the peoples of these different regions, investigators began to examine the environments of each to see if there was an unusual occurrence of various elements in the soils and waters that was present in both areas. In 1967, Dr Yoshiro Yase, who was aware that manganese is neurotoxic and had been mined on Guam during the Japanese occupation, began to study environmental concentrations of that metal. He took single water samples from three rivers and five households on Guam as well as six single soil samples from different villages. These samples showed wide variations in manganese concentrations. Water and soil samples taken in Kii showed the manganese levels of river and drinking waters were not as high as on Guam. Furthermore, soil samples in Japan showed a range of values somewhat lower than on Guam. Yase then determined tissue contents of manganese in patients from Guam by neutron activation analysis (NAA). He found the manganese content to be high in the spinal cords of two patients, one with ALS and one with PD. He found the manganese level to be 5–10 times higher in the spinal cord of the ALS patients than in any other part of the central nervous system. In that same patient, the manganese level of the spinal cord was 10–20 times higher than the levels in the brain of two control cases. These findings indicated to Yase that 'manganese may possibly be one of the environmental factors responsible for the disease.' Because calcium promotes the absorption of manganese by tobacco roots and because in Guam and in Kii there are heavy deposits of calcium, he surmised that 'A hypercalcemic condition seems to be basic to the pathological process of increased manganese absorption.' He speculated that a disturbance in the metabolism of calcium may be basic to the pathological process of C.N.S. tissue degeneration' [37].

In 1962, Gajdusek encountered patients with ALS among the Auyu and Jakai people of the Kepi and Bade areas of Western New Guinea (WNG) [38]. Because of social unrest in the area, Gajdusek was not able to return to Western New Guinea until 1974. But between 1974 and 1980, he conducted five surveys of the villages of the region. Kepi and Bade are part of a low coastal plain that is 100 to 200 kilometres by river inland from tidal swamplands. The Jakai people, who have been sedentary for 30 years, live in large hilltop villages of 200 to 500 people. In contrast, the Auyu are semi-nomadic. They have established permanent smaller riverside villages only during the past few decades.

ALS was the most common neurological condition among these different tribes. Apart from a younger mean age of onset and slightly longer mean duration, their clinical illness was indistinguishable from that of classical motor neuron disease. Parkinsonism, with or without dementia, was less common than ALS but the two seemed closely related. It was not unusual for both illnesses to occur in the same village and even in the same family. In these several respects the disease mirrored the ALS/PD that occurred on Guam and in the Kii Peninsula [39]. In one of his reports on WNG, Gajdusek mentions a native woman who emigrated from the endemic area when she was 18 years of age and developed symptoms of ALS 15 years later. He emphasizes that this long interval between migration and symptoms is similar to that which occurs in migrants from Guam, some of whom may not develop symptoms of ALS/PD for many decades after leaving the island [40].

During the 1970s, Gajdusek and his associates in the United States shared Yase's opinion that the cause of ALS/PD was a disturbance in trace element metabolism in the populations of these three Western Pacific areas (i.e. Guam, Kii Peninsula of Japan, and Western New Guinea).

To test this hypothesis, Garruto et al measured the concentrations of 64 elements in the garden soils and drinking water from each of the three regions and compared them with world-wide averages [41]. Somewhat low levels of calcium were found in soil samples from all three areas, with the lowest levels in the soils of southern Guam. However, the values from all three regions were well within the world-wide range. The concentrations of calcium in the drinking water paralleled those in the soils.

The mean value of calcium in water in southern Guam was lower than in the central and northern parts of the island but only very slightly below the mean world-wide level. Values for the north and centre were above the world-wide mean. In Kii and Western New Guinea, calcium levels in drinking water were very much lower than in Guam. They, too, were within the world-wide range.

Levels of magnesium in the drinking water in Guam were similar to world-wide averages. In Western New Guinea and Kii, they were somewhat low. Soil magnesium levels in Guam and Kii were close to world-wide levels, but were low in Western New Guinea.

Manganese concentrations in 20 soil samples from Guam varied widely, ranging from 610 to 5900 ppm. Nine samples from endemic areas in the Kii Peninsula ranged in value from 265 to 2000 ppm. Twenty-four soils from Western New Guinea were tested and found to contain very low levels of manganese, ranging from 30 to only 240 ppm. Fifteen soils from the Philippines and five from the Northern Mariana Islands were measured as controls; these had concentrations ranging from 480 to 2500 and from 1600 to 2400 ppm respectively. In 24 water samples taken in Western New Guinea, manganese levels were extremely low, from less than 0.01 to 0.22 ppm. Values for the Kii Peninsula were not provided.

These various environmental samples, then, did not confirm Yase's early postulate of high environmental manganese and calcium levels in ALS/PD endemic areas [37].

Soil aluminum was found to be high in all regions. On Guam, the levels ranged from 39,000 to 120,000 ppm, in Kii from 46,000 to 130,000, and in Western New Guinea from 2300 to 60,000. Control values in the Northern Mariana Islands ranged from 78,000 to 93,000 and in the Philippines from 46,000 to 100,000. The aluminum content of Guam's waters was found to be low except in a few rare instances where very high values of up to 2.4 ppm were recorded from river sources. The aluminum concentrations in 25 samples of Western New Guinea water varied from less than 0.07 to 0.34 ppm. In the Mariana Islands, concentrations were from less than 0.07 to 0.3. Three samples from the Philippines had concentrations of less than 0.07 ppm. Values for Kii peninsula were not provided [41].

When it became apparent that high aluminum and low calcium and magnesium levels were the only seeming abnormalities in element concentrations common to all three ALS/PD foci, Yase, Gajdusek, and their associates sought to relate this observation to the pathogenesis of the disease, and to the observed accumulation of aluminum and calcium in nerve cells undergoing neurofibrillary degeneration [19, 42, 43]. They proposed that homeostatic adjustment to deficiencies of calcium and magnesium caused alterations in the absorption and metabolism of calcium, aluminum, and other di- and trivalent cations. They further proposed that these deficiencies were the cause of the early appearance of neurofibrillary degeneration [44]. In support of this hypothesis, they cited studies which showed disturbance of calcium and vitamin D metabolism in Chamorro patients with ALS/PD [45], cortical bone loss in Guamanians [46, 47], and intraneuronal accumulation of calcium and aluminum in the brain tissue of ALS/PD patients [19, 42, 43].

The Calcium Content of Umatac's Water Sources: The Piga Spring

Recently we examined calcium content in water sources in southern Guam. The principal groundwater sources in Umatac are rivers in each valley and two springs which exit from the hillside at an elevation of 400 feet (Map 2).

In Spanish times, Umatac households obtained their drinking water from wells and by rain catchment from the roofs of individual houses. Then, in the early 1900s, the US Navy constructed a dam across the lower La Fouha River and piped water from it to the village. The La Fouha River remained Umatac's main water source until the 1950s when water began to be brought from the Piga spring, a water source whose output remains constant during the dry season (unlike the La Fouha River, which is apt to dry up).

During one year from 1984 to 1985, William Zolan and Leigh Ellis-Neill of the Water and Energy Research Institute (WERI) at the University of Guam conducted a water study which measured the concentrations of aluminum, manganese, iron, and calcium each month in four southern Guam rivers, two of which are in the Umatac district (i.e. the La Fouha and Umatac rivers) [48]. Aluminum concentrations varied widely and were most irregular during the rainy season. Mean concentrations of dissolved aluminum in these southern rivers were higher than in most American rivers but the median values were similar to the US mean of 0.07 mg/l.

Zolan and Ellis-Neill [48] found that concentrations of calcium in these same rivers were consistently high and characteristic of borderline hard waters. The mean concentrations ranged from 34 to 53 mg/l. Their observation of high calcium in these rivers led us to review evidence for low calcium in the south of Guam (as earlier investigations had reported). We have now identified the Piga spring of Umatac as the likely source of confusion in earlier environmental investigations.

The Piga spring exists where a limestone is faulted in Mount Bolanos, one mile behind the village. The water of the spring is clear and has a fine taste. Three-quarters of a mile to the northwest, at about the same elevation, is a second spring, the Alatgue. Its water is also pure and has a fine taste. The only obvious difference between the two is texture; the Piga water is slippery.

Iwata et al [49] were the first to identify low calcium and magnesium levels in the Piga spring water. In a field report of 1978, they observed: 'It astonished us that the contents [of calcium and magnesium] were very low in some parts of the island, especially in southern Guam.' The report shows that the Piga spring was the only one of 32 water sources Iwata tested on Guam which had very low values of calcium and magnesium. In 1984, Garruto et al [41] also reported very low levels from this same source and from Umatac households which are supplied by water piped from the spring. Table 1 compares the values for calcium and magnesium from the Piga and Alatgue springs in 1978 (Iwata et al), in 1984 (Garruto et al), and in 1987 (WERI). All samples from the Piga spring had very low levels of both minerals. By contrast, calcium and magnesium contents of Alatgue spring water were normal.

In their report, Garruto et al compared calcium and magnesium concentrations in water samples from three different regions of Guam [41]. In the north and central parts of the island, overall values were similar

TABLE 1
Calcium and magnesium content of Alatgue and Piga springs

	Calcium (mg/l)		Magnesium (mg/l)	
	A	P	A	P
1978	80.0	4.0	6.3	1.2
1983	83.0	1.3	5.7	0.17
1987	36.4	0.28	5.9	0.03

to those elsewhere in the world. In southern Guam, averaged values were, however, found to be somewhat low. Very low values in southern Guam were found only in the Piga spring water: if one recalculates the ranges and means for the southern region and does not include Piga samples, then the values are not much different from those of other parts of Guam and the world.

Kilmer (personal communication), a geologist who has studied the Piga spring, proposes that water issuing from the spring comes from rain on the ridge, which passes rapidly downward through void spaces developed by faulting. The water contact with the volcanic sedimentary rocks that form the walls of the fractures is limited and brief. Little calcium dissolves into it.

Calcium Contents of Foods from Umatac, Guam, Palau, and Jamaica

In 1985 Crapper McLachlan et al investigated the calcium and aluminum content of vegetables and fruits eaten on the islands of Guam, Palau, and Jamaica [50]. Many of the Guam food samples were collected from the five high-incidence farms in Umatac. Palau and Jamaica were chosen for comparison because Palau (Babelthuap) has a similar geological history to Guam and neither island has reported cases of the ALS/PD.

The results of these analyses do not support the hypothesis that the Chamorro people are or were exposed to either a low calcium intake or a marked increase in aluminum content in their foods compared to native peoples of Palau and Jamaica. Indeed ingestion of 500 grams wet weight of the tuber of taro per day (about 500 calories) provides about 700 mg of calcium, which is close to the recommended intake of 800 mg of calcium per day.

When these environmental and dietary studies did not seem to confirm a disturbance of trace element metabolism and essential minerals in Umatac and on Guam, we began to search for some other environmental factor which was unique to the Chamorros of Guam and Rota.

CYCAS CIRCINALIS TOXICITY

For 40 years, investigators have searched for the cause of ALS/PD. The chronology of this quest has recently been reviewed in detail by Spencer [51] and by Steele and Guzman [52].

Since ALS was so common among Chamorros and because the aggregation of patients in many families did not conform to the usual manner of Mendelian inheritance, Kurland in the 1950s sought an environmental factor unique to the Chamorros to explain the occurrence of the disease among them. Dr Raymond Fosberg, a botanist and authority on plants of the Pacific, told Kurland that the Chamorros used the seeds of the indigenous false-sago palm, *Cycas circinalis*, for food and medicine, despite the seed's known toxicity (see Fig. 1).

Between 1962 and 1972, Kurland organized six international conferences to investigate the botany, pharmacology, and toxicity of cycads and to explore their role in ALS/PD. The first conference about the Identification of Toxic Elements in Cycads was held at the National Institutes of Health on 28 February 1962. In Dr. Kurland's opening remarks at this historic meeting, he noted Fullmer et al's [53] discovery of changes in skin collagen in ALS/PD and Krooth et al's [54] demonstration on Guam of the world's highest incidence of diaphyseal aclasia (multiple exostoses).

Kurland observed: 'These findings led me to suggest in our conferences here at N.I.H. in 1961 that there might be an analogy between the neurological conditions in the Marianas and odoratism and lathyrism ... The basis for the intense studies now underway is the thought that lathyrism and odoratism – human and experimental – which are due to toxic compounds found in natural products, have in appropriate species at appropriate ages and with appropriate compound neurological involvement, [caused] collagen change and a form of multiple exostoses in common with the problems described above. Consequently, it was suggested that there might be a basis for intensive studies of some of the natural products and known toxic materials to which the population of the island was exposed ... In 1954 we [Mulder and Kurland in consultation with Fosberg] encouraged Dr Marjorie Whiting, who was on the island at that time, to carry out a diet study ... Following her field studies, Dr Whiting suggested a relationship between this disease and the ingestion of *Cycas circinalis*, an important indigenous source of food for this population ... Dr Whiting has been responsible for much of the pioneering work in this area' [51].

Research has demonstrated that cycad seeds contain a potent hepatotoxic and carcinogenic agent called cycasin. But cycasin exhibits low

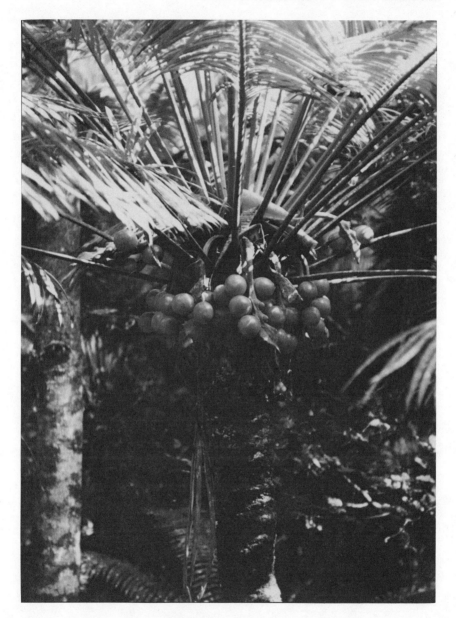

Figure 1. Cycas circinalis showing immature seeds

neurotoxicity in experimental animals. In 1961, Vega and Bell identified a second toxin, beta-N-methylamino-L-alanine (BMAA), related to the neurotoxin in the legume responsible for lathyrism, beta-N-oxalylamino-L-alanine (BOAA) [55]. However, cycad seeds were found to contain very low concentrations of free BMAA (15 mg/100 g fresh seed wt). In addition, relatively high dosages of this amino acid were required to produce convulsions in rats, chicks, and mice. These two observations led Polsky, Nunn, and Bell to conclude in 1972 'that this compound [BMAA] is unlikely to be a prime cause of neurological disease in man unless either he is more sensitive to the compound than the experimental animals, or higher concentrations of the compound occur in the plant in a bound form, or prolonged administration of low concentrations of the amino acid are as effective as a large single dose in producing neurological disorders' [56].

In 1978, Kondo concluded that the cycad hypothesis was 'unique but negative ... The search for a toxic agent has included lathyrogens because Guam ALS showed collagen changes in the skin and exostotic disease was prevalent in the population, but the effort was in vain' [57].

Although many investigators sought other explanations, the cycad hypothesis continued to be championed by Kurland and Mulder, who remained convinced that cycad was the cause of ALS/PD [58, 59, 60].

The next important observation came from Spencer et al, who reported experimental studies in primates which incriminated L-BMAA of cycad seeds as the causative agent of motor neuron disease on Guam [61]. In 1981, Spencer had proposed a relationship between lathyrism and Guam ALS and he suggested evaluating the effect of prolonged administration of BMAA (*Cycas* spp) and BOAA (*Lathyrus* spp) in a suitable animal species. During the next several years, Spencer and his colleagues investigated the clinical and neurophysiological features of lathyrism. By experimental primate studies, they confirmed the BOAA was the likely agent of (neuro)lathyrism [51]. Then, in the summer of 1985, Spencer began to study the effect of chronic BMAA administration in primates. In May 1986, he reported that this amino acid excitotoxin, a component of the cycad seed, had caused an ALS/PD-like illness in monkeys within 8 weeks of daily feedings. Furthermore, neuropathological studies showed acute degeneration of the anterior horn and Betz cells, those same cell types affected in ALS [61].

Observations Consistent with Cycad Seeds as the Cause of ALS/PD

Spencer's important report immediately led Steele and Guzman to reassess the use of cycad by the Chamorro people. By the summer of 1986, their independent field observations in the Mariana Islands convinced them that ALS/PD was most compatible with exposure to the seeds after a long interval. Their conclusions were shared with Spencer and presented at the second Canadian Conference on Neurodegenerative Diseases at Lake Louise in February 1987 [52].

Steele and Guzman's first observation regarding cycad was that ALS/PD occurs only where cycad trees grow and among people who have used their seeds for food and medicine. On Guam and Rota, there are dense cycad forests on the limestone areas. ALS/PD is most common among residents of villages in the south of Guam and Rota. Individuals in these areas depend heavily on cycad, some because of traditional practice and others because of isolation or poverty.

Folklore accounts indicate that ALS/PD has occurred among Chamorros for about 150 years. The first recorded accounts of the use of cycad for food also date from about 150 years ago [5, 54, 62, 63]. This practice was likely introduced to the Mariana Islands by Spanish-speaking migrants from Mexico, who were accustomed to preparing flour for tortillas from seeds of *Dioon edule*, the indigenous cycad of Mexico [64]. Through the course of the 19th century, cycad flour was a dietary staple for many Chamorro families, particularly those who were poor and unable to purchase or grow other foods (see Fig. 2). Its use was most widespread during times of deprivation and natural disaster. Cycad is a hardy plant; its seeds were always available when all other crops had been destroyed.

Before World War II, the use of cycad was most prevalent in the southern villages of Guam and Rota, those same villages where ALS/PD has always been most common, historically. During the Japanese occupation of Guam, from 1941 to 1944, there was severe famine. Cycad then became a staple for many families throughout Guam and Rota. Indeed, some older Chamorros today say they survived the famine only because of the cycad. In the post-war era, ALS/PD occurred in all villages of the island but was still more common in those of southern Guam. We believe the post-war geographical diversity in the incidence of the disease reflects the more widespread use of cycad during the war years.

To combat the devastation that accompanied World War II, large quantities of food were brought to the Micronesian islands. Wheat flour was one of the main imports. By the late 1940s, it had largely replaced cycad flour in the Chamorro diet, because of its greater convenience and availability. This change in food habit occurred 40 years ago. However, because of the presumed latency between exposure to cycad and the onset of neurological symptoms, a change in the annual incidence of the disease did not occur until 20 years later, in the mid-1960s. As Garruto et al and Reed and associates have shown, the decline which began then

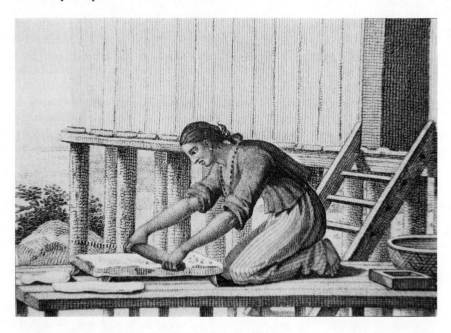

Figure 2. Preparing cycad flour in Guam in 1819

has continued in steady fashion [27, 28]. The ALS form of the disease, which is thought to have a latency ten years shorter than PD, has now almost completely disappeared. PD, because of its presumed longer latency, continues to occur at a higher rate than ALS, but it, too, is less common. It now occurs primarily among people in their sixth and seventh decades.

The first account of parkinsonism-dementia in the Mariana Islands was given by a Japanese physician in 1936. He monitored neurological illnesses among the Chamorros of Saipan between 1925 and 1939, and observed that 'progressive bulbar palsy and amyotrophic lateral sclerosis are not infrequent [among them]' [65]. Yet when NINDB neurological surveillance teams visited Saipan in the 1950s, ALS was no longer common on the island. It was very much less common than on Guam and Rota. For many years this difference in rate of disease between the Mariana islands seemed inexplicable, but interviews with elderly Saipanese and a recent historical account provide an explanation for it [66]. During Spanish and German administrations, cycad trees were abundant and the Chamorros of Saipan used cycad flour as a dietary staple in the same way people in Guam and Rota did. In 1914, the Japanese occupied Saipan and, after World War I, they began clearing the island for sugar planting. By the mid-1920s, most of the indigenous vegetation, including the cycad forests, had been cut down; local people were no longer able to prepare the flour. When the NINDB teams visited Saipan in the 1950s, cycad flour had not been used on the island for 30 years. At that time, ALS was much less common on Saipan than on Guam or Rota. All Saipanese Chamorros with the disease were either born before 1917, and could have had exposure to cycad in childhood, or had probably been exposed to cycad on Guam or Rota (where it was still being prepared) [67].

ALS/PD is particularly common among the Chamorros of Guam and Rota but it is not identified among indigenes of the Pacific islands although their life-styles and cultures are very similar to those of Chamorros [12, 13]. One notable difference between them is that other Pacific people do not use cycad although it grows on many of the islands. They therefore have had no exposure to it, at least in recent times. Even on Saipan, Carolinians who immigrated there in the early 19th century regarded cycad flour as a 'Chamorro' food and did not prepare or eat it.

Cycad flour is not regularly eaten by most of the migrant ethnic groups on Guam and the other Mariana islands, and ALS/PD has not been observed to occur among them. However, there are a few Filipinos who came to Guam in the 1940s, married Chamorro women, and adopted native life-styles and food habits. Several developed ALS/PD 17 to 26 years after their arrival on Guam. The disease has not been seen in any Filipino who arrived on Guam after 1950, when the flour ceased to be a food staple [25].

A notable feature of ALS/PD is familial occurrence: this is so prominent that at first it suggested the disease was inherited. The sharp decline in rates of ALS/PD over the past two decades, coupled with a 25-year prospective case-control study [68], now indicates that the cause of the disease must relate to environmental factors. Recent interviews by Steele and Guzman suggest that the familial aggregation of patients may relate to differences between families in the method of preparing cycad seeds. The Chamorros know that the seeds contain an acute poison (cycasin) which can be removed by soaking the seeds in water and drying them in the sun. Some families soak the seeds overnight while others wash them for three weeks. Some families change the water the seeds are soaked in every three days while others change it three times a day. Some families soak the seeds in sea water, some wash them in streams and others in vats and odd containers. Some admit to shortening the wash process so that the flour has a sharper and stronger taste. In 1964, Drs Whiting and Fosberg recognized such differences in the leaching process and suggested the possibility of a cumulative effect from small quantities of residual toxin [58]. Steele is at present collaborating with Duncan in an attempt to determine if cycad flour samples are neurotoxic in tissue culture, and if there are quantitative differences in neurotoxicity between flour samples which relate to different methods of preparation.

In publications since 1986, Spencer and his colleagues have emphasized similar epidemiological observations, many of which were first made by Whiting during her pioneering studies on Guam [69]. Taken together, they provide a plausible etiological relationship between the declining Chamorro use of cycad seed for food and medicine after World War II and the temporally associated reduction in the incidence of ALS and PD on Guam [51, 52, 70]. Furthermore, in recent articles Spencer et al report the use of cycad seeds as topical medicine in the two other Western Pacific ALS/PD foci. This practice has diminished, and rates of the disease are altering in both locales [71, 72].

At this time, we are not certain about the extent of exposure to cycad that causes ALS/PD. We wish to cite the remarkable history of a Saipanese woman and her son, both of whom began to have neurological illness in 1978, 19 years after a single feast of foods made from only four pounds of the flour, shared among six family members. The mother developed parkinsonism and her son developed ALS [67, cases 37 and 22]. This single feast was their only exposure to cycad. It occurred on the northern island of Pagan. The situation of this Chamorro family, in which ALS and PD occurred in the same year in members of different generations, is similar to that of families reported by Calne et al [73] in which members of different generations developed Parkinson's's disease within a few years of one another, observations that are in accord with their hypothesis that attributes certain neurodegenerative diseases to early, subclinical environmental damage followed by age-related attrition of neurons within the central nervous system [74].

In 1987, we obtained reliable accounts from 21 other Chamorro patients about their last known exposure to cycad. A large number of these patients indicated they had not used cycad for several decades before the onset of their symptoms. The interval was somewhat longer for those with PD than those with ALS. Few who responded had used the flour regularly since the late 1940s; no one remembered being treated with cycad medicinally [75] (Fig. 3). Two of the patients indicated that, like the Saipan family, they had had only a single exposure to cycad many years before the onset of their illness. Both are residents of Guam and could perhaps have been exposed and forgotten. In the situation of the Saipanese family, we are quite certain there was no other exposure, since cycad has been unavailable on Saipan for many years.

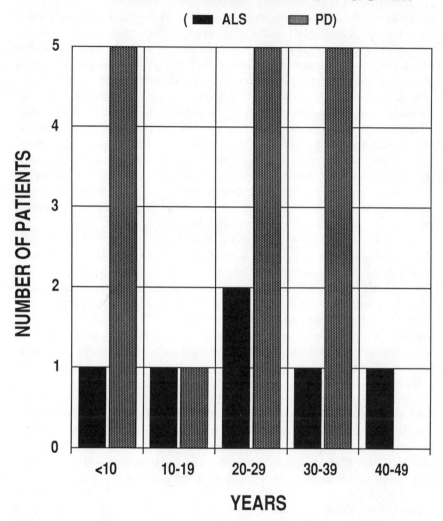

Figure 3. Interval from last cycad exposure to the onset of ALS/PD for 22 patients alive in January 1987

For more than 150 years amyotrophic lateral sclerosis (ALS) has been endemic among Chamorro indigenes of the Mariana Islands. Today it is no longer common. Incidence rates of a related disorder, the parkinsonism-dementia complex of Guam (PD), are also declining. Umatac, a small village in southern Guam with high rates of ALS/PD, is an ideal setting to search for geochemical and nutritional factors which may be the cause of this unique Pacific focus of neurodegenerative disease.

In 1985 Steele et al we studied Umatac farms where many family members suffered ALS/PD. They ate a variety of foods which provided a high daily intake of calcium. Crapper McLachlan et al measured calcium and aluminum contents of vegetables and fruits from these farms. They found that root crops were also high in calcium. We concluded that the food data did not indicate a differentially high exposure to elemental aluminum or low calcium intake in the Guamanian diet, and therefore we were unable to confirm that dietary induced dysmetabolism is the cause of this neurodegenerative disease.

In 1986 Spencer caused an ALS/PD-like illness in primates by feeding them L-BMAA, an amino acid excitotoxin in seeds of the indigenous false-sago palm, *Cycas circinalis*. Steele and Guzman reassessed the use of the seeds among Chamorros and found that ALS/PD occurs only on Micronesian islands where the trees grow and only among people who prepare them as flour or use them for medicine. The observations are in keeping with Spencer's experimental work and support his suggestion that L-BMAA and chemically related compounds deserve serious consideration as the causative agents of motor neurone disease on Guam and elsewhere.

Clarification of the etiology of ALS and parkinsonism-dementia on Guam will have widespread repercussions on the etiology of parkinsonism, the presenile dementias, and ALS elsewhere. If we can discover the cause of this disappearing disease on these distant tropical islands, we will likely be able to understand neurofibrillary-related and aluminum-associated neurodegenerative diseases in all parts of the world.

Acknowledgments

We thank Dr Arthur Hudson, chairman of the Scientific Advisory Committee, and the ALS Society of Canada and Ciba Geigy of Canada for their support of these studies by Drs McLachlan and Steele. Dr Steele thanks his daughter, Julia, Dr William Peck, and Dr Peter Spencer for their suggestions in the preparation of this manuscript.

References

1 Wenkam R, Baker BD. Micronesia: The Breadfruit Revolution. Honolulu, East-West Centre Press, University of Hawaii, 1971;1–192

2 Pigafetta A. Magellan's Voyage: A Narrative Account of the First Circum-navigation. Translated and edited by R.A. Skelton. New Haven, Yale University Press, 1969;58–61. Available at the Micronesian Area Research Centre (MARC) Library, University of Guam

3 Driver M. Guam: A Nomenclatural Chronology. Mangilao, MARC, University of Guam, 1985;1–44

4 Driver M. Cross, Sword and Silver: The Nascent Spanish Colony in the Mariana Islands. Mangilao, MARC, University of Guam, 1987;48:1–57

5 Safford W. The Mariana Islands: Notes Compiled from Documents in the Archives at Agana and from Early Voyages Found in the Libraries of San Francisco, California. Private collection. 1901;1–477. Available at the Nieves M. Flores Library, Agana, Guam

6 Zimmerman H. Monthly report to medical officer in command. USN Medical Research Unit No. 2, June 1945

7 Arnold A, Edgren D, Palladino V. Amyotrophic lateral sclerosis: Fifty cases observed on Guam. J Nerv Ment Dis 1953;117:135–139

8 Koerner D. Amyotrophic lateral sclerosis on Guam: A clinical study and review of the literature. Ann Intern Med 1952;37:1204–1220

9 Tillema S, Wijnberg C. 'Endemic' amyotrophic lateral sclerosis on Guam: Epidemiological data. Docum Med Geog Trop 1953;5:366–370

10 Kurland L, Mulder D. Epidemiological investigations of amyotrophic lateral sclerosis: 1. Preliminary report on geographic distribution with special reference to the Mariana Islands, including clinical and pathological observations. Neurology 1954;4:355–378,438–448

11 Mulder D, Kurland L, Iriarte L. Neurological diseases on the island of Guam. US Armed Forces Med J 1954;5:1724–1739

12 Elizan T, Chen K-M, Mathai K, et al. Amyotrophic lateral sclerosis and parkinsonism-dementia complex: A study in non-Chamorros of the Mariana and Caroline islands. Arch Neurol 1966;14:347–355

13 Steele J. Micronesia: Health status and neurological diseases. In: Chen KM, Yase Y, eds. Amyotrophic Lateral Sclerosis in Asia and Oceania. Taipei, National Taiwan University, 1984;173–183

14 Hirano A, Kurland L, Krooth R, et al. Parkinsonism-dementia complex, an endemic disease on the island of Guam: 1. Clinical features. Brain 1961;84:642–661

15 Hirano A, Malamud N, Kurland L. Parkinsonism-dementia, an endemic disease on the island of Guam: 11. Pathological features. Brain 1961;84:662–679

16 Hirano A, Malamud N, Elizan T. Amyotrophic lateral sclerosis and parkinsonism-dementia complex on Guam. Arch Neurol 1966;15:35–52
17 Anderson F, Richardson EP Jr, Okazaki H, et al. Neurofibrillary degeneration on Guam: Frequency in Chamorros and non-Chamorros with no known neurological disease. Brain 1979;102:65–77
18 Chen L. Neurofibrillary change on Guam. Arch Neurol 1981;38:16–18
19 Perl D, Gajdusek DC, Garruto R, et al. Intraneuronal aluminum accumulation in amyotrophic lateral sclerosis and parkinsonism-dementia of Guam. Science 1982;217:1053–1055
20 Rogers-Johnson P, Garruto R, Yanagihara R, et al. Amyotrophic lateral sclerosis and parkinsonism-dementia on Guam: a 30 year evaluation of clinical and neuropathological trends. Neurology 1986;36:7–13
21 Torres J, Iriarte L, Kurland L. Amyotrophic lateral sclerosis among Guamanians in California. Calif Med 1957;86:385–388
22 Garruto R, Gajdusek DC, Chen K-M. Amyotrophic lateral sclerosis among Chamorro migrants from Guam. Ann Neurol 1980;8:612–619
23 Eldridge R, Ryan E, Rosario J, et al. Amyotrophic lateral sclerosis and parkinsonism-dementia in a migrant population from Guam. Neurology 1969;19:1029–1037
24 Brody J, Hirano A, Scott R. Recent neuropathological observations in amyotrophic lateral sclerosis and parkinsonism-dementia of Guam. Neurology 1971;21:528–536
25 Garruto R, Gajdusek DC, Chen K-M. Amyotrophic lateral sclerosis and parkinsonism-dementia among Filipino migrants to Guam. Ann Neurol 1981;10:341–350
26 Chen K-M, Makifuchi T, Garruto R, et al. Parkinsonism-dementia in a Filipino migrant: A clinicopathological case report. Neurology 1982;32:1221–1226
27 Garruto R, Yanagihara R, Gajdusek DC. Disappearance of high-incidence amyotrophic lateral sclerosis and parkinsonism-dementia on Guam. Neurology 1985;35:193–198
28 Reed D, Labarthe D, Chen K-M, et al. A cohort study of amyotrophic lateral sclerosis and parkinsonism-dementia on Guam and Rota. Am J Epidemiol 1987;125:92–100
29 Reed DM, Brody JA. Amyotrophic lateral sclerosis and parkinsonism-dementia on Guam, 1945–1972: 1. Descriptive epidemiology. Am J Epidemiol 1975;101:287–301
30 del Valle T. Social and Cultural Change in the Community of Umatac. Mangilao, MARC, University of Guam, 1979;1–174
31 Garcia Father. The Apostle of the Marianas: The Life, Labors and Martyrdom of ven.Diego Luis De San Vitores, 1627–1672. Translated from the Spanish of Albert Risco SJ, by Juan Ledesma SJ, edited and published by

Msgr. Oscar Calvo, Diocese of Agana, Guam, 1970;106–116. Available at the Nieves Flores Library, Agana, Guam

32 Arago J. Narrative of a Voyage Around the World Commanded by Captain Freycinet. A series of letters to a friend by J. Arago, draftsman to the expedition, published by Treuttel and Wurtz, London, 1823;239–240. Available at MARC, University of Guam

33 The Guam Narrative of Cesar Degraz. Translated from the French by Robert Graig. 1984;1–57. Available at the Nieves Flores Library Agana, Guam

34 Corte y Ruano Calderon F de la. History of Mariana Islands from time of arrival of the Spaniards to 5th of May 1870. Translated by Don AT Perez. Guam Recorder 1926;3:1–70

35 Shiraki H, Yase Y. Amyotrophic lateral sclerosis in Japan. In:Vinken PJ, Bruyn GW, eds. Amsterdam, North-Holland Publishing Co. Handbook of Clinical Neurology. 1975;16:353–418

36 Whiting M. Food practices in ALS foci in Japan, the Marianas and New Guinea. Fed Proc 1964;23:1343–1345

37 Yase Y. The pathogenesis of amyotrophic lateral sclerosis. Lancet 1972;ii:292–296

38 Gajdusek DC. Motor neuron disease in natives of New Guinea. New Eng J Med 1963;268:474–476

39 Gajdusek DC, Salazar A. Amyotrophic lateral sclerosis and parkinsonian syndromes among the Auyu and Jakai people of West New Guinea. Neurology 1982;32:107–126

40 Gajdusek DC. Calcium deficiency induced secondary hyperparathyroidism and resultant CNS deposition of calcium and other metallic cations as the cause of ALS and PD in high incidence among Auyu and Jakai people in West New Guinea. In: Chen KM, Yase Y, eds. Amyotrophic Lateral Sclerosis in Asia and Oceania. Taipei, National Taiwan University, 1984; 145–171

41 Garruto R, Yanagihara R, Gajdusek DC, et al. Concentrations of heavy metals and essential minerals in garden soils and drinking water in the Western Pacific. In: Chen KM, Yase Y, eds. Amyotrophic Lateral Sclerosis in Asia and Oceania. Taipei, National Taiwan University,1984;265–329

42 Garruto R, Fukatsu R, Yanagihara R, et al. Imaging of calcium and aluminum in neurofibrillary tangle-bearing neurons in parkinsonism-dementia of Guam. Proc Natl Acad Sci (USA)1984;81:1875–1879

43 Garruto R, Swyt C, Fiori C, et al. Intraneuronal deposition of calcium and aluminum in amyotrophic lateral sclerosis of Guam. Lancet 1985;ii:1353

44 Gajdusek DC. Calcium aluminum silicon deposits in neurons lead to paired helical filaments identical to those of AD and Down's patients. Neurobiol of Aging 1986;7:555–556

45 Yanagihara R, Garruto R, Gajdusek DC, et al. Calcium and vitamin D metabolism in Guamanian Chamorros with amyotrophic lateral sclerosis and parkinsonism-dementia. Ann Neurol 1983;15:42–48

46 Plato CC, Garruto RM, Yanagihara RT, et al. Cortical bone loss and measurements of the second metacarpal bone. 1. Comparisons between adult Guamanian Chamorros and American Caucasians. Am J Phys Anthropol 1982;59:461–465

47 Plato CC, Greulich WW, Garruto RM, et al. Cortical bone loss and measurements of the second metacarpal bone: Hypodense bone in postwar Guamanian children. Am J Phys Anthropol 1984;63:57–63

48 Zolan W, Ellis-Neill L. Concentrations of Aluminum, Manganese, Iron and Calcium in Four Southern Guam Rivers. Water and Energy Research Institute (WERI), University of Guam, 1986;64:1–67

49 Iwata S, Sasajima K, Yase Y, et al. Report of investigation of the environmental factors related to occurrence of amyotrophic lateral sclerosis in Guam island. Overseas Field Research in 1976–77, financially supported by the Japanese Ministry of Education, 1978

50 Crapper McLachlan DR, McLachlan CD, Krishnan B, et al. Aluminum and calcium in Guam, Palau and Jamaica: Implications for amyotrophic lateral sclerosis and parkinsonism-dementia syndromes of Guam. Environ Geochem and Health 1989;11:45–53

51 Spencer P. Guam ALS/parkinsonism-dementia: A long-latency neurotoxic disorder caused by 'slow toxin(s)' in food? Can J Neurol Sci 1987; 14,3(suppl):347–357

52 Steele J, Guzman T. Observations about amyotrophic lateral sclerosis and the parkinsonism-dementia complex of Guam with regard to epidemiology and etiology. Can J Neurol Sci 1987;14,3(suppl):358–362

53 Fullmer H, Siedler H, Krooth R, et al. A cutaneous disorder of connective tissue in amyotrophic lateral sclerosis. Neurology 1960;10:717–724

54 Krooth R, Macklin M, Hilbish T. Diaphysial aclasia (multiple exostoses) on Guam. Am J Human Genet 1961;13:340–347

55 Vega A, Bell E. α-amino-β-methylaminopropionic acid, a new amino acid from seeds of Cycas circinalis. Phytochemistry 1967;6:759–762

56 Polsky F, Nunn P, Bell E. Distribution and toxicity of α-amino-β-methylaminopropionic acid. Fed Proc 1972;31:1473–1475

57 Kondo K. Population dynamics of motor neuron disease. In: Tsubaki T, Toyokura Y, eds. Amyotrophic Lateral Sclerosis. Baltimore, University Park Press, 1979;61–103

58 Kurland L. An appraisal of the neurotoxicity of cycad and the etiology of amyotrophic lateral sclerosis on Guam. Fed Proc 1972;31:1540–1542

59 Kurland L, Molgaard C. Guamanian ALS: Hereditary or acquired? In:

Rowland LP, ed. Human Motor Neuron Diseases. New York, Raven Press, 1982;165–171

60 Kurland L, Mulder D. Overview of motor neuron disease. Proc Int Meeting Motor Neuron Diseases, Bangalore, 1984

61 Spencer PS, Nunn PB, Hugon J, et al. Motorneurone Disease on Guam: Possible role of a food neurotoxin. Lancet 1986;i:965

62 Freycinet L de. Voyage autour du monde. Published by the Paris Imprimerie Royale, Paris, 1824. Available at MARC, University of Guam

63 Safford WE. Useful Plants of the Island of Guam. Smithsonian Institution, US National Museum, United States National Herbarium, 1905. Available at the Nieves Flores Library, Agana, Guam

64 Thieret J. Economic botany of the cycads. Econ Bot 1958;12:3–41

65 Yase Y, Brody J, Chen K-M, et al. An historical note on the parkinsonism-dementia complex of Guam. Neurol Med (Japan) 1978;8:583–589

66 Russell S. When sugar was king. Glimpses of Micronesia 1987;25/4:52–57

67 Yanagihara R, Garruto R, Gajdusek DC. Epidemiological surveillance of amyotrophic lateral sclerosis and parkinsonism-dementia in the Commonwealth of the Mariana Islands. Ann Neurol 1983;13:79–91

68 Plato C, Garruto R, Fox K, et al. Amyotrophic lateral sclerosis and parkinsonism-dementia on Guam: A 25 year prospective case-control study. Am J Epidemiol 1986;124:643–656

69 Whiting M. Toxicity of cycads. Econ Bot 1963;17:271–299

70 Spencer P, Nunn P, Hugon J, et al. Guam amyotrophic lateral sclerosis-parkinsonism-dementia linked to a plant excitotoxin. Science 1987;237:517–522

71 Spencer P, Ohta M, Palmer V. Cycad use and motor neurone disease in Kii Peninsula of Japan. Lancet 1987;ii:1462–1463

72 Spencer P, Palmer V, Herman A, et al. Cycad use and motor neurone disease in Irian Jaya. Lancet 1987;ii:1273–1274

73 Calne S, Schoenberg B, Martin W, et al. Familial Parkinson's disease: Possible role of environmental factors. Can J Neurol Sci 1987;14:303–305

74 Calne D, Eisen A. McGeer E, et al. Alzheimer's disease, Parkinson's disease and motorneurone disease: Abiotropic interaction between aging and environment. Lancet 1986;ii:1067–1070

75 Steele J, Guzman T. Amyotrophic lateral sclerosis and parkinsonism-dementia in Guam: An update. In: Fahn S, Marsden CD, Calne DB, Goldstein M, eds. Recent Developments in Parkinson's disease, Vol.11. Florham Park, NJ, Macmillan Healthcare Information, 1987;53–57

Evaluation of Environmental Factors in the Etiopathogenesis of the Amyotrophic Lateral Sclerosis / Parkinsonism-Dementia Complex of Guam

ETIENNE A. GRIMA, CATHERINE BERGERON, AND DONALD R. CRAPPER McLACHLAN

In 1869, Charcot and Joffroy first identified a slowly progressive motor neuron disease that was later named amyotrophic lateral sclerosis (ALS) [1]. The *amyotrophic* characteristics include weak atrophied muscles with decreased reflexes and fasciculations as a result of loss of lower motoneurons in the spinal cord or cranial nerve nuclei and *lateral sclerosis* refers to the degeneration of the corticospinal tracts reflected clinically by the presence of spasticity, increased tone, and hyperflexia. Most patients exhibit a combination of both features. Three varieties of ALS have been characterized: sporadic, familial, and Guamanian. All share the clinical and pathological hallmarks of ALS. The disease on Guam is associated with parkinsonism and dementia and offers important clues on the pathogenesis of ALS.

Guamanian ALS receives its name from the unprecedented high incidence of ALS among the indigenous population of modern-day Guam. Only the indigenous inhabitants, the Chamorros, and migrant Filipinos appear to be at high risk for Guamanian ALS and a second syndrome, parkinsonism-dementia complex (PDC) [2, 3].

Guamanian ALS is clinically indistinguishable from ALS occurring elsewhere in the world [3, 4]. On microscopic examination, however, the classical histopathological changes of ALS are found together with large numbers of neurons showing neurofibrillary degeneration (NFD) [5, 6, 7]. This neurofibrillary degeneration is composed of paired helical filaments (PHF) which, by light and electronmicroscopic criteria, are identical to the neurofibrillary tangles seen in Alzheimer's disease. The tangle-bearing neurons also contain high levels of aluminum [8, 9]. This type of NFD is encountered only in the Guamanian form of ALS, and predominantly affects the neocortex, hippocampus, substantia nigra, substantia innominata, hypothalamus, amygdala, locus ceruleus, nucleus raphe dorsalis, and reticular formation [6]. Neurofibrillary tangles, although reported in some ALS cases, are rare in anterior horn cells [10, 11].

In contrast to the ALS syndrome of Guam, the clinical features of the parkinsonism-dementia complex include progressive intellectual deterioration and extrapyramidal dysfunction with a mean onset of 55 years and an average duration of life of 4 years. The extrapyramidal syndrome differs from classical idiopathic parkinsonism with dementia (PD) by the frequent occurrence of isolated severe bradykinesia at onset, relatively mild rigidity until late in the disease, and mild to absent tremor. The complex is accompanied by motor neuron deficits of varying severity in over 80% of the cases [12]. Neuropathological examination reveals neuronal loss, gliosis, and widespread NFD with severe involvement of subcortical sites, especially the substantia nigra [2, 13].

Many investigations have been conducted in an effort to identify the factors responsible for a high ALS and PDC incidence in such a geographically isolated location. By the 1950s it was well established that Guam possessed the highest incidence for both ALS and PDC, the annual average being 200 per 100,000 population and over 50 per 100,000, respectively – approximately 50 times higher than the world average [3, 14]. Both syndromes are more common in males (see Table 1). During this period ALS accounted for at least 10% of all adult Chamorro deaths [15]. PDC caused a similar number [2, 16].

Initially it was thought that Guam ALS was a disorder genetically transmitted through the inheritance of a dominant gene with a 30% penetrance [17–19]. This was proposed since familial aggregates were known and members of these families could develop the disease following emigration from Guam [20]. During the Spanish occupation there was a substantial reduction of Guam's population that would have resulted in a significant reduction in the Chamorro gene pool. This, along with a subsequent introduction of Spanish/Filipino people, may have allowed for the introduction and expansion of new genetic traits that might predispose to ALS [21]. Filipinos are a more probable source of such a population susceptibility than the Spanish since (1) Mexicans have been reported to exhibit 'resistance' to ALS with a low incidence rate of 0.4/100,000 population [22]; (2) through HLA examinations it has been determined that the Spanish influence on the Chamorro gene pool has been, at best, minimal; (3) the Ilocos region of the Philippines has itself been called a high-incidence focus for ALS [23] and was the major source of the ancestral Spanish labour forces from the Philippines. It is interesting that more than 50% of all Filipinos who develop ALS or PDC were born in the Ilocos region of the Philippines [24].

Chamorro natives have had an opportunity to undergo unique genetic development. Stanhope et al [2] stated that in the southern region of Guam, an area known for its higher ALS/PDC occurrence, 'geographic isolation has resulted in a more or less closed breeding population on the island.' An underlying common gene may indeed be important. Along with the well-established male preponderance for developing Guamanian ALS/PDC there also is a high mortality rate for male offspring of ALS × ALS matings to which no single cause of death or age of death could be attributed [19].

Extensive examination of the case registry on Guam has failed to indicate a Mendelian autosomal or sex-linked pattern of inheritance for either ALS or PDC and it was concluded that a purely genetic mechanism is inadequate to account for the Guamanian disorders [2, 19]. Familial aggregates of ALS/PDC patients may relate to particular 'family' diets and habits rather than genetic links. It has been repeatedly concluded by independent investigators that environmental factors, and not genetic influences, play a direct role in ALS/PDC pathogenesis [3, 17, 25–27].

Epidemiological studies report that Chamorro and migrant Filipinos require at least an 18-year exposure to the Guamanian environment to be at high risk for ALS and PDC [28]. Those migrants who have developed ALS or PDC were found to have spent their infancy, childhood, and adolescence on Guam [23]. Individuals who then leave the island are reported to develop the Guam disorders 1 to 31 years later, regardless of country of residence [29, 30]. Migrants from Guam to the continental United States do, however, exhibit a lower probability for development of Guamanian ALS than those who remain on the island [28] although this does not prevent development of the disease [17]. United States military and construction workers who have resided on Guam for various lengths of time have not developed the Guamanian disorders. This suggests that exposure to putative agents must be more intimate than these visitors experience and/or that a genetic susceptibility is involved in the Chamorro cases [14].

Transmission studies, epidemiological evaluations, and efforts to isolate virus-related particles have provided either conflicting or negative results and do not support the view that ALS is due to a slow viral infection or bacterial pathogen [25, 31].

Environmental Factors: Looking for a Clue

The search for the environmental factor(s) involved in the development of ALS has been ongoing since the 1950s. Several characteristics of Guamanian ALS/PDC and the island itself have aided investigators in narrowing the list of possible environmental agents.

There are other geographically isolated foci of high incidence for chronic neurodegenerative diseases, including ALS. The best known are (1) isolated villages belonging to the low plains of southern West New Guinea [32]; (2) Hobara and Kozagawa of the Kii Peninsula of Japan [30, 33]; (3) Groote Eylandt and adjacent Arnhemland of Australia [34]; and (4) Ilocos on the island of Luzon in the Philippines [22, 23]. All these areas are claimed to have high environmental levels of aluminum and manganese with low levels of calcium and magnesium, as reported on Guam [23]. Cases of ALS/PDC on the Kii Peninsula are clinically and pathologically identical to those of Guamanian ALS/PDC [25]. Geographic patterns of ALS and PDC occurrence, therefore, support the hypothesis of causal environmental factors [27].

Within Guam itself there exists a distinct distribution for ALS/PDC. Four isolated villages, in the southern regions, exhibit a very high incidence of ALS/PDC, while villages in the more-developed central and western areas have the lowest rates for the island [27, 35]. One village, Umatic, on the southwest coast of Guam, demonstrates the highest risk for ALS/PDC in the world. ALS incidence for Umatic has been as high as 200 times greater than the global average and four times greater than that of Guam itself [27]. The population of Guam was redistributed after World War II, which required that surveys on the geographic distribution of ALS/PDC cases be conducted by place of birth rather than place of residence at disease onset. These surveys again indicated that southern villages possess the highest rate of incidence on Guam [15, 36]. Reed et al [27] and Stanhope et al [2] have demonstrated that population movements within this geographically isolated region have remained relatively stable since the start of World War II and emphasized that the southern region of Guam should be examined with special concern [27].

Parallel occurrences of ALS and PDC may arise, in the same villages, the same sibships, and even the same patient [15]. The similarity in neuropathological findings has led some investigators to suggest that these two disorders are different manifestations of the same disease and therefore share common etiologies [37, 38]. What is important is that in recent years the incidence of ALS is approaching global averages, while the incidence of PDC is not declining. The age-adjusted annual incidence for PDC between 1979 and 1983 was three times greater than that for Guamanian ALS [14]. This difference in incidence decline for these two diseases may indicate that they are not clinical variants of the same disease but instead represent two separate disorders of independent etiologies in a highly susceptible population. It is also important to consider that clinical PDC may be a heterogeneous group of disorders in-

TABLE 1
Comparison of Guamanian ALS and PD complex of Guam [33]

	Guamanian ALS	PD complex
Age of onset	46 years	58 years
Onset < 30 yr	12%	0%
Disease duration	4.0 years	4.4 years
Mean age at death	50 years	62 years
Male:female ratio	2:1	1.8:1
Incidence per 100,000 population	55*	35*
	15†	13†
Neurofibrillary degeneration	yes	yes

* 1982 reported values
† 1954 reported values

cluding Alzheimer's disease with extrapyramidal features, idiopathic parkinsonism with dementia, and progressive supranuclear palsy. Confusion in diagnosis may have contributed to the concept that ALS and PDC are a continuum since in its early stages Guamanian ALS can mask the presence of PDC [39]. These disorders may be difficult to distinguish on clinical grounds alone and the diagnosis must be confirmed by neuropathological examination.

Since both Chamorros and Filipinos require a minimal exposure time to the putative causal agent(s) on Guam and because both may experience a latency period of up to 30 years before clinical onset of ALS/PDC [24], the question arises whether other mammals are susceptible to the putative environmental toxins. Dogs and cats that are raised in the Guamanian environment fail to develop NFD [40 41]. This could indicate that animals are not exposed to the same toxic factors as the Chamorro natives or that the life spans of these animals are insufficient to reach a threshold for expression of a toxic response to the Guamanian environmental factor(s). Differences in diet, particularly the human utilization of natural vegetation as a food staple, may explain differential animal exposures to existing conditions. Finally, the lack of NFD in local animals may indicate that subhuman species are genetically incapable of responding to toxic agents by the formation of NFD composed of PHFs.

Neurons with neurofibrillary tangles, the hallmark of the Guamanian ALS/PDC diseases, have been repeatedly observed in clinically normal Chamorros [40, 42]. The frequency of occurrence is much higher than in non-native Guamanian controls or comparable North American controls, regardless of duration of residence on Guam. The change also occurs much earlier in the Chamorro than in the two other groups [40]. Further, the density of these lesions is known to increase with age. These observations suggest a preclinical state and may indicate that current prevalence rates for neurodegenerative disease on Guam underestimate the degree of exposure to the putative environmental agent. Neurological damage may extend over a larger proportion of this population than previously recognized [43, 44].

Mineral Metabolism and Guamanian ALS/PDC

A number of etiological mechanisms involving minerals have been postulated for ALS. For the Guamanian ALS/PDC we shall explore these, including recent studies in our laboratory, especially on the metabolism of aluminum.

Aluminum – A Neurotoxic Metal

An abundant element in our environment, aluminum (Al) accounts for approximately 8% of the earth's crust [45]. In healthy humans it is present only in very small amounts, 30–50 mg Al total body content, with 50% and 25% located in the skeleton and lungs, respectively [45]. The Al content of the respiratory system is known to increase with age and is related to continued inhalation of Al compounds which are a major aerosol contaminant [46]. Aluminum in the mammalian brain is usually very low and ranges between 1.0 and 1.9 μg Al/mg dry tissue weight [47]. Some researchers propose that one mode by which Al accumulates in the brain in some human neurodegenerative disorders is through a defect in the normally very efficient olfactory mucosa/olfactory bulb barriers [46]. The origin of Al in other body tissues is largely from the alimentary system [45], although the proportion absorbed through the skin and pulmonary epithelium has not been determined.

Aluminum has no known biological function but has been implicated, pathologically, as a toxin in several disorders which present with a variety of clinical conditions: Alzheimer's disease, Down's syndrome with Alzheimer's disease [48], atypical amyotrophic lateral sclerosis, parkinson-dementia complex [8], dialysis dementia, and dialysis-associated osteodysrophy [46, 49].

Altered Mineral Metabolism and the Guam ALS/PDC Syndromes

The unique geographic distribution of foci for ALS in the Western Pacific Ocean has led several groups of investigators to search for chemical determinants for these diseases. The volcanic soils of the regions of high incidence for ALS have been found to contain high concentrations of Al and manganese (Mn) and low concentrations of calcium (Ca) and magnesium (Mg) [9]. Trace element analysis of spinal cord from ALS victims from the Kii Peninsula of Japan and Guam, carried out by Yase [33, 38, 50, 51, 52], indicates an accumulation of Ca, Al, and Mn. They postulated that these diseases were associated with a disorder in Ca metabolism, possibly triggered by an interaction of metal ions with the Ca transport system. They further proposed that a low dietary intake of Ca and Mg might induce secondary hyperparathyroidism, resulting in increased absorption of Al and Ca. Together with other toxic metals this type of exposure may result in neuron death with Ca hydroxyapatite formation. Indeed, Yanagihara et al examined Ca and vitamin D metabolism in Chamorro peoples with ALS/PDC and found evidence in support of the altered Ca metabolism in a small percentage of cases [53].

Perl et al [8] and Garruto et al [54], by employing energy dispersive x-ray spectrometry, have detected Al in tangle-bearing neurons in brains of Guamanians affected with the parkinsonism-dementia complex. They have also found brain Ca content to be elevated but no significant differences were noted in the Mg, silicon, and iron related x-ray emission from neurofibrillary tangles (NFTs) of affected cells.

The pathophysiological significance of Al accumulation in NFTs has not been established. One possible explanation is that the accumulation of high concentrations of Al and Ca in the NFT may simply indicate that it contains ligands of high specificity for both Al and Ca and this finding is merely coincidental and of no pathophysiological significance in the disease process. There are, however, several known neurotoxic effects of Al which challenge this interpretation. Complex interactions in nervous tissues exist between the metabolism of Ca and Al and Al induces a neurofibrillary degeneration that is composed of 10-nm filament. It also alters phosphorylation of cytoskeletal proteins in some laboratory animals and produces changes which may be important in the neurofibrillary component of Guam ALS/PDC diseases. There are a large number of other neurotoxic effects of Al that affect nuclear, cytoplasmic, membrane, and neurotransmitter components. The possible role of these effects of Al in the Guam ALS/PDC diseases is unknown but certain properties of Al are discussed below.

Aluminum-Calcium Interactions

Physical and chemical considerations such as electronegativity, formal charge, and ionic radii led Nieboer and Richardson [55] to suggest that Al could be expected to bind to the same ligands as Ca. Al, however, approximates covalent bonds more than Ca and would, therefore, be expected to dissociate less readily.

Aluminum-Calcium Interactions in Gut

The metabolism of Al, including uptake from gut, transport in blood, and penetration into nervous tissue, has not been studied in the Guam ALS/PDC group of diseases. It has, however, been studied in animals. Al absorption from rat jejunum appears to involve an energy-dependent, carrier-mediated mechanism [56]. Al uptake and transport in the rat everted gut-sac preparation initially rose with increasing Al concentration in the bath and reached a plateau at high concentrations. Al transport was inhibited by the absence of glucose and a temperature of 40°C. Interestingly, in the absence of Ca, uptake of Al was maximal, while at Ca concentrations of 3.3 μmol/l, Al transport was reduced to 45% of maximum transport. This suggests the testable hypothesis that Al may bind to Ca recognition sites in the Ca transport system.

Further Al absorption studies have also suggested that Al and Ca absorption are interrelated. Yase [50] demonstrated that rats on a diet deficient in Ca and Mg exhibited a marked increase in brain Al content while Mayor and his colleagues [57] reported that in rats fed a diet containing supplemental Al, parathyroid hormone enhances gastrointestinal Al absorption and increases the deposition of Al in the brain. Chickens receiving the active metabolite of vitamin D, 1,25-(OH)2D3, also have increased brain Al content [58]. Each of these experiments supports the hypothesis that one route of absorption of Al involves the Ca transport system of the bowel. Whether Al penetrates the blood-brain barrier via Ca channels has not yet been determined.

Aluminum-Induced Calcium Alteration in Brain

Recent experimental evidence indicates that Al interferes with Ca homeostasis in the mammalian brain. Twelve days after intracranial injection of a single lethal dose of a soluble Al salt, cerebral Ca content was significantly increased to 112% of control content. By 20 days after Al injection, there was 129% rise in whole tissue content of Ca [59]. Animals in the advanced stages of the encephalopathy with motor signs had an average brain tissue Ca content which exceeded the control value by 275%.

The increase in whole brain content of Ca is associated with an alteration in the electrical property of neurons, suggesting that part of the measured increase in total brain Ca was associated with increased intracellular Ca ions. Recordings have been made from pyramidal CA_1 cells in isolated hippocampal slices maintained electrically active *in vitro*. Obtained from control animals and from animals with various stages of the Al encephalopathy, they showed a progressive loss of relationship between the compound excitatory post-synaptic potentials (EPSP) recorded from either the apical or basilar dendrites of the CA_1 cells and the amplitude of the compound action potential in CA_1 axons during the later stages of the Al encephalopathy [60]. This 'uncoupling' between EPSP and spike output was rapidly reversed when the concentration of Ca in the extracellular bathing medium was doubled. One explanation for the Ca-dependent re-establishment of excitability is that the concentration of intracellular Ca ions had increased, resulting in reduced Ca influx during EPSP-related conductance changes at the spike initiation zone. In the presence of increased extracellular Ca, the critical Ca flux required for spike initiation was re-established.

One mechanism by which Al could alter intracellular Ca concentration might involve Al binding to Ca receptor proteins, resulting in a failure in Ca extrusion. In plant cells, Siegel and Haug [61, 62] demonstrated that Al binds to calmodulin, a major intracellular messenger which regulates intracellular Ca concentration through stimulation of Ca^{2+}/Mg^{2+}ATPase. At Al to calmodulin molar ratios of 4:1, calmodulin stimulation is blocked. In the experimentally induced animal Al encephalopathy, calmodulin assayed by radioimmunoassay revealed concentrations in cerebral grey matter to be unchanged from those in control brain. However, the functional capacity of calmodulin, assayed by hydrolysis of cAMP by 3',5'-cyclic nucleotide phosphodiesterase, became progressively impaired in the later stages of the encephalopathy [59]. It may be that following an intracranial injection of Al, a major portion rapidly binds to an unidentified ligand which slowly releases Al over 14 to 21 days permitting Al to bind to cytoplasmic proteins such as calmodulin. This hypothesis would predict that many second messenger functions mediated by calcium/calmodulin would be altered as would the functional capacity of some proteins and peptides in the presence of unbuffered intracellular Ca.

Direct evidence that elevated amounts of Al alter Ca homeostasis in the human brain is not available. However, in the rabbit brain Al selectively depresses the messenger RNA pool size for calmodulin within 24 hours of application [63]. In Alzheimer's disease, a neurodegenerative disease with neurofibrillary degeneration morphologically identical to that found on Guam, Northern blots and quantitative dot blot analyses have revealed that messenger RNA pool size for calmodulin is reduced

TABLE 2
Relative yield of messenger RNA

	n	NF-L	α-Tubulin	CaM	GFA
A Guam PDC	2	4.2	5.3	4.5	19.5
Caucasion control	11	15.4 (0.85)	9.3 (0.93)	8.1 (0.9)	10.4 (3.3)
Ratio:					
Guam PDC/control		27%	57%	56%	188%
B Ratio:					
Alzheimer/control		27%	65%	68%	137%

NOTE Summary of relative yields for four specific mRNAs from temporal lobe neocortical grey matter for two cases of the Guamanian parkinsonism-dementia complex, compared to similar preparations from 11 age and post-mortem–interval matched Caucasian control and 10 Caucasian Alzheimer-affected brains. The relative yields are expressed for equal loadings of RNA in a quantitative dot-blot analysis and measured by intensity of signals generated following hybridization with nick-translated ^{32}P-labelled dCTP cDNA probes according to methods of McLachlan et al [64]. Guam, control, and Alzheimer dot-blots were prepared on the same filters. Numbers in parentheses are the standard error of the means for control. Probes: NF-L, low-molecular-weight (68 kD) moiety of neurofilaments; α-tubulin; CaM, calmodulin; GFA, glia fibrillary acidic protein. n = number of brains in each group.

to 68% of that of the age-matched controls [64] (Table 2). Moreover, calmodulin measured by radioimmunoassay or as an activator of cAMP hydrolysis by the enzyme 3′,5′-cyclic nucleotide phosphodiesterase was reduced significantly in extracts prepared from frontal, temporal, and parietal regions of the neocortex and subjacent white matter but not from neocortical grey matter from conditions unrelated to Alzheimer's dementia or from age-matched controls [65]. These observations indicate that, for Alzheimer's disease, there is a disorder in several steps involved in Ca homeostasis which resemble several of the changes induced by Al in experimental animals.

The temporal grey matter from two brains of patients who died with the Guam PD complex was analysed for messenger RNA pool size using the quantitative dot blot method outlined by McLachlan et al [64]. His-topathological examination revealed extensive and widespread neuro-fibrillary degeneration. As shown in Table 2A, the relative yield of messenger RNA coding for calmodulin, expressed as a percentage of total RNA, was only 56% of the average found in the temporal grey matter of 11 age-matched Caucasian control brains without the histopathology of Alzheimer's disease. As expected from the histopathological finding of increased numbers of reactive astrocytes in Guam PDC, the relative pool size for glial fibrillary acidic protein was 188% of that found in the control brains.

Further work is necessary to evaluate whether Al is involved in the molecular mechanisms responsible for the depression in mRNA calmodulin pool size in all cases of Guam PDC and ALS but these preliminary studies suggest a considerable similarity, at the molecular level, between these diseases and Alzheimer's disease.

Aluminum and the Cytoskeleton

The effect of Al upon the cytoskeleton was first clearly documented by Klatzo et al [66] and Terry and Pena [67]. The soluble salts of Al, applied either intracerebrally or systemically into susceptible laboratory animals, induced, in several classes of neurons including the pyramidal-shaped neurons of the neo- and pyriform cortex and anterior horn cells of the spinal cord, a marked accumulation of 10-nm single filaments which have immunochemical epitopes identical to those of neurofilaments. The neurofilaments of these Al-induced tangles have epitopes indicative of hyperphosphorylation [68]. A recent hypothesis postulates that the observed accumulation of neurofilaments in the soma and proximal process of neurons in the animal Al encephalopathy is related to a failure of anterograde movement of neurofilaments into axons [69] possibly because hyperphosphorylation has altered the mechanisms responsible for the transport of neurofilaments [70].

Johnson and Jope [71] administered 0.3% Al in the drinking water for 4–5 weeks to rats and significantly increased the *in vivo* incorporation of radioactive phosphorus in the MAP-2 microtubule-associated protein in brain-stem and cerebral cortex by 163% and 155% of control values, respectively. The phosphorylation of the neurofilament 200 Kd moiety in brain-stem and cerebral cortex of Al-treated rats was increased to 148% and 209% of control values, respectively. These results demonstrate that chronic oral Al administration in rats increases the phosphorylation of certain cytoskeletal proteins, a change which could be important in the development of the neurofibrillary component of Guamanian ALS/PDC.

The NFTs of the Alzheimer type differ morphologically from the Al-induced tangle in laboratory animals. The Alzheimer type NFT of Guam is composed of paired 10-nm filaments wound in a helix to form PHFs. The chemical composition of PHFs is uncertain at present. The most widely held model of PHFs considers them to be composed of several modified cytoskeletal proteins. A large number of immunohistochemical studies from several laboratories indicate that PHFs share epitopes with the 200 Kd moieties of neurofilaments [72, 73]. The neurofilaments are also hyperphosphorylated although the epitopes may differ from those induced by Al [70]. Epitopes from microtubule-associated proteins (MAP-2 proteins), vimentin [74], and ubiquitin [75] have also been detected in association with the Alzheimer tangle. Considerable evidence also supports the argument that the family of microtubule-associated phosphoryl proteins designated 'tau' represents a major antigenic component of PHFs [76, 77]. Indeed, structural characterization of PHFs indicates two distinctive parts, an external fuzzy region which can be removed by pronase treatment leaving a pronase resistant core [78]. The fuzzy external portion is probably composed of the C- and N-terminal fragments of the tau polypeptide and a 9.5 Kd tau fragment which is embedded in the insoluble filament core.

Among the well-characterized neuronal kinases, perhaps contributing to these hyperphosphylated proteins, are cAMP-dependent protein kinase II and Ca/calmodulin-dependent protein kinase II. Both these enzymes have been shown to phosphorylate MAP-2, neurofilament proteins, and tau proteins [79]. Al has also been reported to increase cAMP and cGMP levels [80]. Jope and co-workers are testing the hypothesis that the Al-induced changes in phosphorylation observed *in vivo* are secondary to the changes in cyclic AMP, although a cause and effect relationship has not yet been established *in vivo*. Furthermore, a disorder in dephosphorylation could also be important. The effects of Al upon this system are unknown.

Two further observations indicate that Al selectively affects the molecular mechanisms of the neuronal cytoskeletal system. Muma et al [81] report that the mRNA pool size for the low molecular moiety of neurofilaments is reduced in spinal cords of Al-intoxicated rabbits compared to controls. Our laboratory has demonstrated (Table 2B) that in the neocortex of Caucasian patients with Alzheimer neurofibrillary tangles there is a selective reduction in the mRNA pool size for second messengers in temporal grey matter in Alzheimer's disease [64]. The 5' flanking region of the gene for neurofilament 68 kD (NF-L) is masked from digestion by the enzyme micrococcal nuclease, probably by the histone H1° [82]. These two observations are consistent with the hypothesis that the reduction in mRNA pool size for NF-L is related to reduced transcription rather than messenger degradation.

Recent experimental work indicates that the increased H1° binding on dinucleosomes containing the 5' flanking region of a down-regulated NF-L gene results from Al-protein–DNA cross-linking [83]. In addition to an increase in H1° in the fraction enriched in inactive neurofilament genes in Alzheimer's disease, this dinucleosome fraction contains a fivefold increase in Al compared to age-matched controls. Furthermore, Al at concentrations found in Alzheimer's brain increases the affinity of H1 linker histones to DNA [84]. There is, therefore, a strong association between inactive genes in Alzheimer's disease, H1°, and increased Al content.

Similar investigations have only just been initiated for the Guam ALS/ PDC diseases. As shown in Table 2A, the relative abundance of messenger RNA coding for two important cytoskeletal constituents, the low-molecular-weight moiety of neurofilaments, NF-L, and α-tubulin, measured in temporal cerebral grey matter from two Guam PD cases, is reduced to 27% and 57% respectively compared to age-matched Caucasian controls. The kinetics of digestion by micrococcal nuclease, examination of the 5' flanking region for the human neurofilament NF-L gene, and measures of Al in the dinucleosome fraction are not yet available and therefore it cannot be determined whether Al is associated with the nuclear events responsible for the reduced pool size for these important cytoskeletal constituents. Nevertheless, the striking similarities between the Al encephalopathy in rabbits [81] and Alzheimer's disease strongly argue that neurotoxic effects of Al must be further investigated in relation to the Guam diseases.

It is noteworthy that Davidson [85, 86] measured total RNA in anterior horn cells in non-Guamanian ALS and reported a 42% reduction in cervical and 31% in lumbar anterior horn cells. In contrast, no difference in RNA content was observed between the ALS patients and controls in the RNA content of neurons in the nucleus dorsalis. Davidson and Hartmann [87] also reported statistically significant changes in the A/U base composition ratio in ALS anterior horn cells and argued that alterations in nucleic acid metabolism may be related to the pathogenesis of North American ALS. These observations justify a detailed examination of the molecular mechanisms involved in the regulation of the cytoskeleton in both anterior horn cells and those neurons affected in the PD complex.

Transferrin and Aluminum Transport

In addition to entry through the Ca transport system, Al may gain access to neurons when ligated to transferrin. Trapp [88] demonstrated that transferrin, a plasma protein, has a high affinity for Al and represents a major candidate for the transport of this element in blood. Experimental evidence provided by Edwardson and Candy [89] further supports this suggestion and has demonstrated that Al uptake and distribution within the brain is mediated by transferrin. The distribution of transferrin receptors appears to account for the vulnerability of certain brain cells within the hippocampus and cerebral cortex to take up Al selectively. Further study of the properties of transferrin and transferrin receptors in brain and spinal cord in the Guam diseases is required.

Ligand-Enhanced Aluminum Uptake

Ligand-enhanced Al uptake may circumvent the naturally occurring transport systems for Ca and iron (transferrin). The ability of Al to penetrate epithelium barriers is determined, in part, by lipid solubility. Employing the octenal/water partition coefficient, one finds that the most actively absorbed compounds of Al are those which are most lipid soluble. For example, when the same amount of elemental Al is given as a single oral dose to rabbits, Al bound to the naturally occurring sugar, maltol, reaches 13-fold higher concentrations in the blood than either oral Al bound to citrate or Al as the chloride salt. Furthermore, the urinary excretion of Al maltol is fivefold higher than the citrate or chloride form after 7 days. Indeed, in animals treated with Al maltol elevated amounts of Al are excreted for at least 14 days after a single oral dose. Studies evaluating Al as an environmental neurotoxic agent must consider changes in the natural barriers to Al, the ligand to which Al binds, and the bioavailability of Al.

Sources of Aluminum on Guam

Recently a study was undertaken to identify sources and amounts of Al and Ca ingested from the native diet of the Chamorro peoples [90]. In order to simulate the effect of rain upon the soils in the laboratory, soil from Guam was washed by water at neutral pH at 22°C, and the released Al measured. For comparison, samples were collected and measured from two other islands which have not reported a high incidence of ALS/PDC syndromes: Palau and Jamaica. Remarkably, for all soils collected on Guam, agricultural and non-agricultural ($n = 87$ from 48 sites), there is a 76-fold increase in bioavailable Al compared to all soils collected from Palau and Jamaica. Bioavailable Al was defined as the amount of Al eluted from 200 mg of soil exposed to 1 ml of distilled water at pH 7.0 and measured in the supernatant obtained by centrifugation for 15 minutes at 11,000 g and filtrated through a 0.45 μm MILLEX-HA filter. The average Guam value was 387 mg Al/ml with a range of 0.3–4538 μg Al/ml. Interestingly, Cocos Island, a limetone island to the southwest of Guam, contained an average of only 1.5μg Al/ml. In contrast, the elutible Al from 56 soils collected at 19 sites from the islands of Palau (Babbelthuap, Koror, Arakabesan) average 4.5 μg Al/ml with a range of 0.2–24.

Twenty-five soils collected at 10 sites from the island of Jamaica, including the bauxite mining region, had an average value of 6.5 μg Al/ml and a range between 1.4 and 15 μg Al/ml. This indicates that the soils of Guam have a particularly high elutible Al content. The organic and inorganic species of Al have not yet been measured in these elutants, but may be important determinants for human toxicity.

Aluminum was also measured in taro, a vegetable staple on these three islands. On Guam, 31 samples from 16 sites revealed that the edible core had an average Al content of 58 μg Al/g dry weight with a range of 5–335 μg Al/g. The edible leaf contained an average value of 682 μg Al/g with a range of 18–3508 μg Al/g. Whereas taro core from Palau and Jamaica averaged 33 μg Al/g and 22 μg Al/g respectively (range 3–100 μg Al/g dry weight), the edible leaf averaged 977 μg Al/g on Palau and 204 μg Al/g on Jamaica with ranges of 429–3300 μg Al/g. This indicates that taro is an Al storing plant. However, despite a much higher concentration of bioavailable Al in Guamanian soils, the taro plant must possess an ion transport system in the roots that provides a selective barrier to excess Al uptake such that leaf and root values do not significantly differ between the three geographical locations sampled. Elemental analysis for Al and Ca in 19 root vegetables and fruits from the islands has failed to reveal a differentially high exposure to elemental Al or low Ca intake in the diet of any of the populations on Guam, Palau, or Jamaica.

While the dietary survey did not indicate an excessive load of Al in the food chain of the inhabitants of Guam, the high elutible Al in the soils raises the possibility that the dust of Guam may be an important factor in the body's exposure to Al. The respiratory epithelium has long been known to contain the highest concentrations of Al in the human body [91]. Material from normal human brains also reveals that the olfactory bulb contains considerably higher concentrations of Al than other parts of the brain [47]. The Alzheimer type neurofibrillary degeneration found in the Guam diseases is often encountered in high density in regions which lie in close proximity to the projections of olfactory axons into the rhinencephalon. Roberts [92] has postulated that genetic factors may interact with ageing changes in the nasal mucosa increasing the probability that Al may enter sensory neurons of the olfactory epithelium and spread transneuronally to several olfactory-related areas of the brain to initiate pathology. Al applied to the olfactory bulb of rabbits has been demonstrated to penetrate into brain [46]. If future investigations demonstrate that transport of olfactory axons or absorption through the respiratory epithelium is a significant route of Al uptake, the dusts of Guam may represent an important source of Al to the native peoples.

Manganese and Delayed Damage to the Genetic Code

In addition to Al, the volcanic soils of southern Guam are high in manganese (Mn^{2+}) and low in Mg [9]. *In vitro* studies have shown that the fidelity of copying a polynucleotide template by the enzyme DNA polymerase is substantially reduced when Mn is substituted for Mg. For instance, at 5 mM Mg, 0.1 mM Mn increases the error rate in copying polynucleotide template by human placenta-a and -b DNA polymerase by a factor of approximately 5 [93]. These *in vitro* experiments raise the possibility that, in the presence of increased Mn and certain other metal ions, normal DNA repair might result in an increased number of randomly distributed genetic errors. If the repair error occurred in the antisense strand of DNA of a brain-specific gene, the error in the genetic code might not be expressed for many years. Only when the sense strand is damaged would the error in the antisense strand be expressed, perhaps even after the metal ion itself was no longer present within the nucleus. Errors in proteins essential to neuron survival could result in irreversible neuron damage and death or dysfunction.

Donaldson et al [94, 95, 96] have also suggested that Mn ions enhance autoxidation of dopamine and produce free radicals, particularly hydroxyl radicals and semi-quinone species. Both of these molecules possess considerable cytotoxicity.

As mentioned, the Groote Eylandt aborigines have an unusually high incidence of a unique neurological disorder, which is probably related to Mn inhalation and ingestion. Kiloh et al (34) reported seven cases who had features of motor neuron disease, two with lower motor neuron disease and five with lateral sclerosis and lower motor neuron disease. In four cases the disorder was noted soon after birth. Six additional patients also demonstrated a mixture of cerebellar and pyramidal tract involvement. Four exhibited a variety of supranuclear and internuclear ophthalmoplegias. Of 13 definite cases, one showed a mild dementia and one a possible dementia, and two patients had mild parkinsonism. This unusual neurological entity apparently first appeared in a population of about 1100 aborigines when they moved to a Mn-rich region on Groote Eylandt. Subsequent work has demonstrated that affected aborigines have elevated Mn in the blood (32.2 μg Mn/l; average of $n = 7$) compared to unaffected aborigines (18.9 μg Mn/l; $n = 5$) and Caucasians (7.3 μg Mn/l; $n = 4$) [97, 98]. Examination of native foods and soil indicates that the probable source of Mn is the native food chain. Thus, in this geographic focus, Mn appears to be a principal pathogenic factor in an ALS syndrome.

DNA Damage and ALS

Bradley and Krasin [99] presented evidence that a deficiency in DNA repair mechanisms in motor neurons may be the primary abnormality in ALS. The deficiency in normal DNA repair mechanisms would be expected to cause an accumulation of DNA damage which would result in abnormal transcription of RNA and ultimately in defective protein synthesis. Tandan and colleagues [100] have presented some evidence in support of this hypothesis. Employing agents which damage DNA, these workers examined cell survival and DNA repair capacity in cultured sporadic ALS and control skin fibroblasts. Both mean survival and mean unscheduled DNA synthesis (repair) were significantly reduced in ALS fibroblasts following treatment with the alkylating agent methyl methane sulphamate. Direct testing of the defective DNA repair hypotheses, however, in neurons affected by ALS has not yet been reported.

Traditional Foods and the Uses of Toxic Plants

Average yearly and age-specific incidences for ALS on Guam and the Kii Peninsula reflect a declining trend over the past 30 years, and an upward shift in the age of onset [23, 38, 101]. Today the occurrence of the Guamanian disorders is estimated at 5–14 per 100,000, only several times greater than the global average [30, 102]. These changes have occurred since the end of World War II, when Guam became a major military base for the United States. This recent decline in ALS incidence for Guamanians suggests that the environmental factor(s) responsible for ALS/PDC existed prior to the introduction of a Western way of life. Isolated, high-risk southern villages have been most recent to adopt a Western life-style and food supply, and exhibit the most traditional of Chamorro ways. Here the people have relied more upon subsistence than a 'wage economy,' and so have been exposed longer and more intimately to the Guamanian environment [19, 26, 36]. The Chamorro life-style has changed so much that it now resembles that of Western societies [19]. West New Guinea remains traditional and has not exhibited any drop in incidence of ALS over the same period of time [23].

The component of the traditional Guamanian life-style that has changed most significantly is the diet. In an 889-person study, covering 15 years, Reed et al conducted extensive investigations into characteristics of incidence for ALS/PDC and found that the only factor, out of a selected 23, that significantly separated affected from non-affected Chamorros was the preference for traditional foods. A general tendency for Guamanian PDC patients to be more traditional in food preference and subsistence-level occupation than were ALS patients was also observed [14].

There is recorded evidence that the people indigenous to the high-incidence foci for motor neuron disease (MND) have traditionally made use of a native plant known to possess hepato and neurotoxic properties [23, 103]. This plant is a false sago-palm belonging to the plant genus *Cycas* and its seeds have been used both as a traditional food staple and for various medicinal purposes since the late 1700s [26]. The species of this plant most used for such purposes was *Cycas circinalis*. Chamorro natives admit to the cycad seed's toxic potential and also associate ALS development with poor preparation of these seeds prior to their consumption. The uses of cycad and its toxic effects are described by other authors in this volume (see Armon and Kurland, Spencer et al, and Steele et al) and will not be detailed here. However, a brief summary will be given followed by a description of our own studies.

Cycas circinalis: A Toxic Plant

Cycas circinalis is the most common species of the family of false palm trees *Cycadaceae* found growing throughout much of the southwest Pacific where they are often, and wrongly, called 'sago palm' (*Metroxylon*) [104]. Cycad's ability to withstand adverse weather conditions has enabled it to be used as a reliable source of food while other plants and crops may be destroyed by typhoons and drought [103, 105]. Use of *Cycas circinalis* for medicinal and food purposes, by populations indigenous to the ranges of *Cycas*, has been well documented. These areas include all known geographic foci for high ALS incidence [103, 106].

α-Amino-β-methylaminopropionic Acid: A Neurotoxic Amino Acid

In 1985, new research was initiated to investigate a possible link between an incompletely examined neurotoxic amino acid from cycads and ALS/PDC of Guam. The basis for this renewed interest was the structural similarity between the amino acid α-amino-β-methylaminopropionic acid (also known as β-N-methylamino-L-alanine or BMAA) from cycad and β-N-oxalyl-L-2,3–diaminopropionic acid (also called β-N-oxalyl-amino-L-alanine or BOAA), an amino acid from the chickling pea *Lathyrus sativus* [107] (Fig. 1). The latter amino acid is a potent agonist of the excitatory neurotransmitter glutamate, and has been used in an

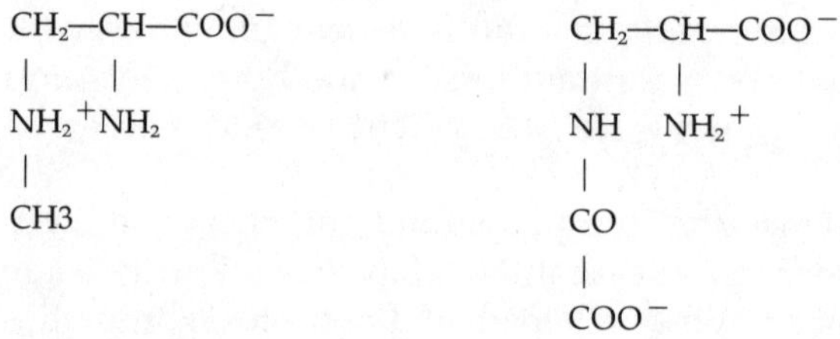

CH₂—CH—COO⁻   CH₂—CH—COO⁻

| | | |

$$\begin{array}{ll}
CH_2\text{---}CH\text{---}COO^- & CH_2\text{---}CH\text{---}COO^- \\
\quad|\quad\ \ | & \quad|\qquad\ | \\
NH_2{}^+NH_2 & NH\quad NH_2{}^+ \\
\quad| & \quad| \\
CH3 & CO \\
& \quad| \\
& COO^- \\
\textbf{BMAA} & \textbf{BOAA}
\end{array}$$

Figure 1. Structural comparison of two plant neurotoxic amino acids: α-amino-β-methylaminopropionic acid (BMAA) from *Cycas circinalis* and β-N-oxalyl-L-2,3-diaminopropionic acid (BOAA)

animal model for human neurolathyrism, which, like ALS, is a disorder of the motoneuron system in which anterior horn cells have been found to contain aggregates of 80–100 Å filaments [108].

Although BMAA was shown to be capable of causing neurological disturbances, it was not until recently, when non-human primates were orally administered the amino acid, that pathological findings suggested a possible relation between cycads and the Guamanian ALS/PDC syndromes [109]. It was reported that male *Rhesus macaques* orally administered large doses of L-BMAA developed motoneuron deficits within 8–12 weeks [110].

This was the first evidence that a systemically administered compound from seeds of *Cycas circinalis* may be involved in the unprecedented high incidence of ALS/PDC on Guam.

Variations in Cycad Toxicity: Classification and Distribution of Cycas circinalis

The Schuster classification is a taxonomic listing of which cycads may be regarded as *C. circinalis*; it contains over 40 morphological varieties. Fosberg, a botanist who wrote 'Résumé of the Cycadaceae' for the Third Conference on Toxicity of Cycads [104], emphasizes that these plant variations may indicate that the species classification of *C. circinalis* actually represents several morphologically less distinct and separate populations. Further, he states that 'it would indeed be remarkable if all these forms and local populations were identical biochemically and physiologically.'

Cycas circinalis is known to grow on the islands of Palau; however, here there have been no reports of the Guamanian ALS/PDC syndromes. Fosberg has examined the cycads growing on Palau and Guam and notes: '[*Cycas circinalis*] seems to grow better, more abundantly, and more vigorously on soils derived from limestone than from volcanic soils. However, in Guam it does grow on the northern limestone soil and also in the southern part of the island, where it seems to have become adapted to the soil of volcanic origin. The plant in the southern part of the island has slightly differently shaped seeds and perhaps other characteristics not yet observed' [104]. The cycads of Palau are found in limestone soil, like those of the northern portion of Guam. This difference in cycad habitat also occurs on New Guinea, where growing conditions are entirely different.

Similarly, Kurland [111] reports that in Kerala, South India, while *C. circinalis* was used as a food staple, there were no reports of the Guamanian disorders. Kurland remarks that although having the same botanical name the *C. circinalis* of Kerala differs morphologically from that found on Guam.

The cycad's range includes Asia, Mexico, and the southwest Pacific; however, it is not known whether plants from different localities and growing conditions all possess the same toxins. Several members of cycads have been examined: Dossaji and Herbin [112] assayed seeds from *Encephalalartos hildebrandtii* and *Cycas thuarsii* which were grown in the Coast Province of Kenya, and found that both contained the hepatotoxin cycasin, but no BMAA was detected; in a separate study, Polsky, Nunn, and Bell [113] examined all species of *Cycas*, including *C. thuarsii*, and found BMAA to be present; however, the amount varied and the source of the plants was not identified. This indicates that cycad differences are not limited to plant morphology.

Epidemiological surveillance of Guam has clearly identified the southern region of Guam as the region with the highest incidence of ALS/PDC. This, taken in concert with inter-species biochemical differences, leads to the hypothesis that cycad toxicity may be directly related to the plants' growing conditions, which may include soil nutrient composition. Whiting [103] makes reference to 'paralysis-free grazing areas' in Australia, and associates differing soil types as the factor responsible for varying toxicity. She also attributes human deaths, which followed cycad seed consumption, to unpredictable variations in this plant's toxicity. These observations may explain why other geographical areas where cycad had traditionally been utilized have not reported an increased incidence of ALS/PDC since they would have different soil compositions. One known soil characteristic which is uniquely Guamanian is a high level of bioavailable Al. These disparities between toxicity, classification, and location of *C. circinalis* require a re-evaluation of epidemiological reports on cycad consumption and ALS/PDC occurrences.

Cycad Toxicity: Processing and Consumption

Variations in ALS incidence and distribution on Guam may be due to seed selection (maturity as well as variety), cycad seed processing (duration of soaking and number of water changes), quantity of cycad flour consumed, age at which exposure occurred, and state of health at time(s) of exposure. Variations may also be suspected between processors and within different batches from the same cook. To date, the fate of BMAA in cycad seed processing has not been examined.

Diminished use of cycad has not been accompanied by a parallel decrease of disease incidence [2] owing perhaps to the long latency period reported before clinical onset. In fact, because it has been found that Chamorros continue to use native foods out of tradition, we may continue to see the Guamanian disorders persisting for quite some time.

Although previous investigations involving BMAA exposure to chickens, mice, rats, and monkeys [110, 113–118] have provided information on clinical manifestations of BMAA toxicity, they have shown non-specific general systemic toxicity(s). Data are now required on BMAA-associated histological changes to indicate a mechanism of toxic action.

Despite the large body of circumstantial evidence implicating constituents of fadang flour in the etiology of the Guamanian ALS/PDC syndromes, several difficulties accompany a hypothesis that BMAA is the responsible etiological agent: (1) although one laboratory has shown oral BMAA administration to be associated with neuron loss in subhuman primates, Alzheimer-type NFD was not induced; and (2) if it is assumed that Chamorros receive only small doses of BMAA through their fadang flour, the extremely long latency period before clinical onset makes it difficult to postulate a single mechanism for BMAA toxicity and makes the development of appropriate experimental models difficult and extremely costly to maintain.

Recent Developments in the Evaluatison of BMAA Toxicity

Based on the observations of mixed clinical effects that have been reported by other laboratories, we decided only purified BMAA should be used in our studies. Effects of the systemic route of exposure must be minimized, since it is unknown which body tissue(s) are sensitive to BMAA and therefore what the animal's response(s) would indicate. Instead, BMAA administration would be 'targeted'. Targeted exposure involves administration of varying doses of BMAA into *particular* body tissue(s), thereby reducing the number of involved tissues and organ systems.

Use of D,L-BMAA vs. L-BMAA

Cycas circinalis seeds are reported to contain approximately 15–30 mg of the L-form of BMAA per 100 grams fresh seed weight. L-BMAA extraction procedures have proven lengthy and inefficient and result in low yields, necessitating a synthetic source for toxicological evaluation. Synthetic procedures have produced three stereochemical forms of BMAA: L-BMAA, D-BMAA, and the racemic mixture D,L-BMAA.

Evaluation of the toxicity of these BMAA isomers was first conducted in 1968 when Vega, Bell, and Nunn found that natural BMAA was more toxic to chicks than their synthetic BMAA [119]. This was because the synthetic BMAA was composed of a racemic mixture (D,L-BMAA) whereas cycad BMAA occurs only in the L-form. Wistar rats, as well as 7-day post-hatch chickens (R-X-S strain), were employed in further studies which showed that the synthetic D-form of BMAA possesses no toxic properties, whereas the L-isomer does. The conclusion from this work was that one-half of the dose of the naturally occurring L-isomer of BMAA was capable of producing the same toxic response(s) as a full dose of D,L-BMAA [113, 119]. Fetal mouse spinal cord cultures have also been employed to illustrate that D-BMAA lacks neurotoxic activity [120]. This stereospecific (D,L and L) activity on neural tissue has been demonstrated with other amino acids such as D,L- and L-α-aminoadipic acid, a gliotoxic amino acid [121], and the major mammalian neurotransmitter, L-glutamate [122].

Although a method for synthesis of pure L-BMAA has been established, we have chosen to conduct our investigations with the racemic mixture of D,L-BMAA. The rationale for this decision was that D,L-BMAA is capable of reproducing L-BMAA toxicity at twice the dose and D-BMAA does not affect the toxicity of L-BMAA. Moreover, the cost of synthesizing pure L-BMAA is 100 times that for D,L-BMAA. The quality of our stock of D,L-BMAA has been verified against cycad-extracted BMAA by paper chromatography, nuclear magnetic resonance (NMR), and high-performance liquid chromatography (HPLC). By these methods the D,L-BMAA has been determined to be 99.8% pure. Steric composition analysis indicates our preparations consist of 49.8% D-BMAA and 50.2% L-BMAA. Results of initial D,L-BMAA toxicity studies have successfully reproduced BMAA-associated behavioural changes reported by other laboratories, i.e., hyperexcitability, convulsions, jumping fits, and whole body shake/ wobble (90 minutes post BMAA) [113, 117, 119].

Evaluation of Animal Models

Before administering a putative neurotoxin to animals systemically, it is prudent to first ascertain exactly how toxic the compound is when introduced directly into the mammalian central nervous system. If no toxicity is observed, then it can be assumed that the mechanism of toxicity is via the parent compound acting systemically or is via a neurotoxic metabolite that is systemically derived. It is for these reasons that intact animal models were developed involving 'targeted' stereotaxic injections of D,L-BMAA into the central nervous system.

We have developed methods for both manual and automatic microvolume intracerebral (IC) administration of D,L-BMAA test solutions for evaluation of D,L-BMAA toxicity in alert and sedated laboratory animals. Manual infusion protocols have required use of specially designed restrainers that allow for a free manipulation of the head of alert animals, thereby allowing for easy insertion of IC infusion cannulas into selected (targeted) sites through previously implanted guide cannulas. Alert animals were used so as to allow for a simple interpretation of motor response to D,L-BMAA since the presence of a circulating anesthetic could influence animal responses in an unpredictable manner.

Common cerebral consequences of immobilization-induced stress have previously been studied in non-anesthetized Wistar rats. Such evaluations have shown that a restraining technique can result in the development of an increase in whole brain metabolism [123], but an 11% to 15% decrease in regional cerebral blood flow (rCBF). These decreases were observed in all brain regions except frontal lobe and are caused by a reduction of PCO_2 from stress-induced hyperventilation. A frontal lobe increase in rCBF was associated with frontal lobe activation by pain excitation of the autonomic nervous system and/or by stimulation of primary and supplementary motor areas of the frontal cortex [123].

Although utilizing non-sedated animals in our study appears to induce changes in normal brain metabolism it is far more advantageous than using alert, paralysed, and artificially ventilated animals. Such experimental conditions are known to increase rCBF 140% to 220% above basal levels [124, 125]. The absence of an increase in rCBF in all but frontal regions of the brain in alert rats is probably due to a systemic circulatory compensation involving peripheral vasodilation. Even when heart rate was found to increase by 30%, the mean arterial blood pressure did not significantly change [123].

Cerebral consequences of long-term IC implants of inert materials in rats have also been addressed. Implants (plastic needles 2–3 mm long), inserted without damage to surrounding cortex of rats, result only in the development of an edema which completely resolves within 4 days. Following this initial period of readjustment, such implants are usually well tolerated by the cerebral cortex, and if left in place result only in deposition of a thin layer of astrocyte processes [126].

We have been very careful in the identification and classification of pathological changes at lesioned sites within targeted tissues, to ensure a complete resolution of D,L-BMAA–induced damage from those associated with mechanical disruption. Through examination of control animals' brains it has been determined that our various cannulation procedures involve minimal disruption in both rats and rabbits and that the rates (μl/min) and volumes of test solution administered do not produce any neuronal compromise.

Table 3 summarizes the general behavioural observations, doses, and surgical protocols utilized for the rat portion of our investigations.

Exposure of Neural Tissue to D,L-BMAA

Two sites were selected for the introduction of D,L-BMAA into the experimental animal brain, the cerebrospinal fluid (CSF) of the lateral ventricles and the striatum. The advantage to these two routes, intracerebroventricular (ICV) and intrastriatal (IS), is that BMAA is a very water soluble amino acid (33 mg D,L-BMAA·HCl/ml deionized distilled water) and can be expected to achieve a more even distribution, especially throughout the CSF following an ICV infusion. Once in the CSF, such a substance would have relatively free access to the brain interstitium across most of the ependyma and pial surface, therefore allowing tissue far from the site of administration to be exposed [127].

Stereotaxic infusions into the striatum (IS) have previously been used as a method for neuroanatomic characterization of lesions caused by the glutamate analogue, kainic acid [128]. Morphological changes, as well as the radius of the D,L-BMAA lesions, can then be compared to the effects of a known excitotoxin. Despite the invasive nature of this method of BMAA administration we have found that matched animal controls did not exhibit damage typical of that observed with D,L-BMAA.

Such procedures also allow for the elucidation of whether some brain regions or cell types exhibit higher sensitivity to D,L-BMAA toxicity than others. Through the characterization and mapping of induced lesions, it may be possible to gain an understanding of the existing vulnerable or protective characteristics, be they neuronal or of support cell origin, that

TABLE 3
Observed behavioural responses following single exposure to D,L-BMAA in rats (ranges expressed are in mg D,L-BMAA/g body weight for intraperitoneal injections and mg per injection for intrastriatal and intraventricular)

	Intraventricular		Intrastriatal		Intraperitoneal
	Alert	Sedated	Alert	Sedated	Alert
No abnormal behaviour	0.0 0.5 1.4	0.0 1.0 2.0	4.0	0.04–4.0	0.0
Irritability, excitability	3.6* 3.6†	3.6 S	N/O	N/O	1.5
Focal seizures	3.6	1.0	N/O	N/O	1.5
Delayed mild seizure activity	3.6	2.0 4.0	N/O	N/O	1.5*
Immediate full seizures status	(4.5)	(5.0)	N/O	N/O	N/O
Lethargic	3.6*	3.6†	N/O	N/O	1.5
Inability to lift head	3.6‡	N/A	N/O	N/O	1.5 (ataxic)
Immediate death	3.6 4.5	5.0	N/O	N/O	N/O
Delayed death	3.6‡	5.0	N/O	N/O	N/O

NOTES Alert: infusion via guide cannula, non-anesthetized. Sedated: cannulated while under anesthetic, 1–2 hours' sedation. S: additional sedation for 6–8 hours to suppress seizures. ( ): seizure preceding death. N/O: not observed. N/A: not applicable.

* 0–12 hours post-infusion
† 24 hour period post-infusion
‡ 72 hours post-infusion

will ultimately lead to an understanding of the toxic mechanism(s) of BMAA.

Intracerebral (IC) Results

D,L-BMAA is reproducibly neurotoxic to the central nervous system of mice, rats, and rabbits, in a dose-dependent and time-dependent manner, whether the animals are completely sedated or alert. The two different routes of D,L-BMAA exposure do, however, yield striking differences in relation to toxic response.

Manifestation of toxicity following single D,L-BMAA IS administration, in rats and rabbits, was limited to histopathological changes with no evidence of a drug threshold. Even at very high doses when the lesion involved the whole striatum, we observed no indications of neurological compromise (Fig. 2). In contrast, ICV infusion of D,L-BMAA were usually associated with behavioural changes, which occur promptly after animals have recovered from anesthesia. Histological changes may be present without the occurrence of behavioural changes, but only at low D,L-BMAA doses. The behavioural changes are also consistently associated with the development of a lesion. There is evidence for the existence of a drug threshold effect to ICV D,L-BMAA, since at low doses we could observe no behavioural or pathological evidence of toxicity (Fig. 2). Repeated daily and odd-day ICV administration of 0.5 mg and 1.0 mg D,L-BMAA did not precipitate behavioural changes typical of excitatory amino acids even after 57 applications.

Neuronal Lesion Characteristics

Single IC Exposures to D,L-BMAA
Three procedures were used for the single IC D,L-BMAA challenges. (1) Rats, cannulated 48 hours prior to D,L-BMAA treatment, were placed in body restrainers and infused while alert via IS and ICV routes. (2) Under surgical anesthesia, rats were stereotaxically administered D,L-BMAA via IS and ICV routes and were allowed to recover consciousness. These animals were observed for up to 10 days before histological examination. (3) The procedure was the same as number 2 except that sodium pentobarbital supplementation was used to prevent the onset of seizures following recovery from surgical anesthesia.

Histological examinations have shown the size and distribution of resultant D,L-BMAA lesions to vary according to route of administration and dose of D,L-BMAA used. However, the observed histopathological changes were consistent in all animals. At *2 hours* post-infusion, a well-demarcated lesion is identifiable, characterized by extensive vacuolation of the neuropil and myelin pallor. The cytoplasm of nerve cells is shrunken and eosinophilic, with fragmentation or clumping of the nuclear chromatin. Oligodendroglia and astrocytes also display nuclear pyknosis. All blood vessels within the lesion are filled with red blood cells, while elsewhere vessels of all sizes are well perfused and optically empty. At *18–24 hours* post-infusion, necrosis of all elements within the

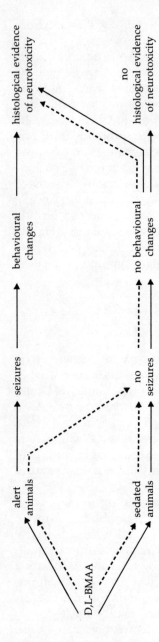

Figure 2. Behavioural *vs.* histological evidence for D,L-BMAA-mediated neurotoxicity following single intracerebroventricular (ICV) *vs.* intrastriatal (IS) routes of exposure (Route of D,L-BMAA administration: ICV ——→; IS – – – →)

lesion is evident. Necrotic blood vessels are often filled with eosinophilic granular material and surrounded by hemorrhage or fibrinoid exudates. A peripheral rim of intense edema is present and abundant polymor-phonuclear leukocytes are seen throughout the lesion. *Seven days* post-intracerebral infusion, the lesion is cavitated, filled with macrophages, and surrounded by reactive astrocytes and collections of mononuclear inflammatory cells.

Alert, guide-cannula–implanted rats, given 4.0 mg D,L-BMAA and al-lowed to develop clinical seizures, exhibited an LD_{20} by day three, the peak period of noted tissue edema. Animals that survived this critical period appear to have completely recovered motor control when ex-amined 10 days post-injection. Examination of these brains reveals an extensive lesion involving a much greater amount of tissue than was directly exposed to the amino acid injection volume. This lesion may also involve the contralateral hemisphere, but to a lesser degree.

Rats in which D,L-BMAA seizure activity was suppressed had no mor-talities. Examination of these brains indicated lesions to be similar to those of the non-sedated rats except that, in the ICV-infused rats, the lesion is smaller.

The observed D,L-BMAA–induced histological changes consist of non-selective necrosis of all elements within the lesion, including endothelial cells. These changes are very different from those observed with known excitotoxic amino acids, which produce a lesion consisting of selective neuronal necrosis without damage to other cell types, or passing axons, and no evidence of hemorrhage or inflammation [129].

Long-Term ICV Exposures to D,L-BMAA
Rats were implanted in the right lateral ventricle with guide cannulas or infusion pump cannulas 1–3 weeks prior to their first D,L-BMAA ex-posure. Suitable rats were then used to evaluate the consequences of multiple or continuous low-dose ICV infusions of D,L-BMAA. Several surgical procedures were performed in which placement of cannulas was varied to allow for estimation of surgical and cannula-related trauma. Permanent ICV implants were shown to induce the formation of con-nective tissue and reactive astrocytes in high density in the immediate vicinity of the implanted foreign bodies, but this was not unexpected [126]. However, upon examination of the whole brain of rats that re-ceived either multiple (19–57) exposures to D,L-BMAA (0.5–1.0 mg per exposure) or 1–3 days of continuous infusion via mini osmotic pumps (4–8 mg D,L-BMAA in 42 μl per day), we observed the targeted hemi-sphere to be destroyed and devoid of identifiable brain structures. Rat brains that were exposed only 4–12 times to the same daily doses exhib-

ited a less involved lesion which was clearly identifiable and radiated away from the targeted ventricle. The lesion size increased with dose and number of exposures to the toxin. These observations substantiate our initial conclusions from single ICV and IS D,L-BMAA exposures that D,L-BMAA is highly toxic to the rodent central nervous system when applied directly, but that its toxic effects are non-selective, unlike those of typical excitotoxins.

Although it is the primary lesion in human amyotrophic lateral sclerosis, we could not find evidence of neurotoxicity of anterior cells of the cervical, thoracic, or lumbar regions of the spinal cord in any of the test animals under any of our BMAA (or aluminum) exposure protocols.

Evaluation of BMAA as the Neurotoxin Involved in Guamanian ALS/PDC

Based on reported toxicological studies, quoted in the above literature, BMAA, as the naturally occurring L-isomer and the synthetic racemic mixture (D,L-BMAA), has been proposed to be an excitatory, neurotoxic amino acid. Oral L-BMAA studies, in primates, have been reported to induce specific toxicity to anterior horn cells, pyramidal cells, and extra-pyramidal systems [130]. Further investigations involving intracerebro-ventricular injections in mice and murine organotypic cultures have suggested that the toxic mechanism of BMAA involves the N-methyl-D-aspartic acid subtype of the glutamic acid receptor system. Supporting evidence includes post-synaptic swellings and attenuation of toxicity by NMDA antagonists.

We have tested this hypothesis by injecting D,L-BMAA intrastriatally in rodents. The experimental design was identical to that used in the characterization of other excitotoxins and modelled after classical kainic acid experiments. We support the hypothesis that BMAA is neurotoxic. However, our results do not support the conclusion that BMAA acts as an excitotoxic amino acid in the usual sense. Histological examination reveals a dose-dependent toxicity, resulting in non-selective tissue necrosis. These neuropathological changes are unlike those associated with known excitotoxins. Lesions resulting from excitotoxic amino acids involve degeneration of only neuronal somata and dendrites with a preservation of non-neuronal elements and axon terminals originating outside the lesion area [129].

The acute electrophysiological effects of BMAA were examined on CA_1 neurons of the *in vitro* hippocampal slice preparation [131]. Intracellular recordings made in CA_1 neurons perfused with 0.5–10 μM D,L-BMAA resulted in a 2–18 mV membrane depolarization associated with cell firing and occurred in a concentration-dependent manner. Neuron internal resistance (R_{in}) and Ca-dependent after-hyperpolarization conductance were not altered by BMAA. These findings differ from N-methyl-D-aspartate (NMDA) actions. The BMAA molecule also lacks the acidic carboxyl groups associated with excitotoxic amino acids. While our results do not support an excitatory toxic mechanism of action for this plant toxin, the mechanism of toxicity still requires further investigation, particularly the possible vasotoxic actions of this amino acid and subsequent ischemic necrosis.

Conclusion

Since D,L-BMAA animal exposures have been unable to induce the motor deficits of ALS or the histological changes to the neuronal populations involved in ALS/PDC syndromes, the relevance to the Guam diseases remains uncertain. With an absence of compromise to the anterior horn cells of the spinal cord, it does not appear that D,L-BMAA, as a parent compound or central nervous system metabolite, is directly involved in the etiopathogenesis of ALS on Guam. The possibility that a metabolite systemically derived from BMAA may be responsible should, however, be pursued.

Although BMAA may not be responsible for the unprecedented incidence of ALS/PDC on Guam, the answer to this problem may still be found in the Guamanian environment. The coexistence of elevated bio-available soil Al and heavy use of cycad seeds during the highest occurrence of these Guamanian disorders cannot be dismissed. Analysis of cycad seed endosperm composition and its variations, according to geographic location and soil types, may discover the presence of previously unrecognized toxins that, like BMAA, are toxically active on the central nervous system of mammals.

The incidence of ALS is decreasing; however, the study of this disease and Guamanian PDC remains important. If an appropriate model is developed and the environmental factors involved in the etiology and pathogenesis of ALS/PDC identified, the knowledge may be relevant to the understanding of neurodegenerative diseases outside of Guam. Such information would also be valuable in the development of preventative measures and possible treatments for neurodegenerative diseases.

(Supported by the Amyotrophic Lateral Sclerosis Society of Canada)

References

1 Mozai T. Studies on the pathogenesis of ALS with a review of the literature. Bull Osaka Med Sch 1984;14(suppl):18–35

2 Stanhope JM, Brody JA, Morris CE. Epidemiologic features of amyotrophic lateral sclerosis and parkinsonism-dementia in Guam, Mariana Islands. Int J Epidemiol 1972;1(3):199–210

3 Rodgers-Johnson P, Garruto RM, Yanagihara R, Chen K-M, Gajdusek DC, Gibbs CJ Jr. Amyotrophic lateral sclerosis and parkinsonism-dementia on Guam: A 30-year evaluation of clinical and neuropathologic trends. Neurology 1986;36:7–13

4 Iwata M, Hirano A. Current problems in the pathology of amyotrophic lateral sclerosis. In: Zimmerman M, ed. Progress in Neuropathology, Vol. 4. New York, Raven Press, 1979;277–298

5 Yanagihara RT, Garruto RM, Gajdusek DC. Epidemiological surveillance of amyotrophic lateral sclerosis and parkinsonism-dementia in the Commonwealth of the Northern Mariana Islands. Ann Neurol 1983;13:79–86

6 Hirano A, Malamud N, Elizan T, Kurland LT. Amyotrophic lateral sclerosis and parkinsonism-dementia complex on Guam. Further pathologic studies. Arch Neurol 1966;15:35–51

7 Delisle MB, Carpenter S. Neurofibrillary axonal swellings and amyotrophic lateral sclerosis. J Neurol Sci 1984;63:241–250

8 Perl DP, Gajdusek DC, Garruto RM, Yanagihara RT, Gibbs CJ Jr. Intraneuronal aluminum accumulation in amyotrophic lateral sclerosis and parkinsonism-dementia of Guam. Science 1982;217:1053–1055

9 Garruto RM, Fukatsu R, Yanagihara AR, Gajdusek DC, Hook G, Fiori, CE. Imaging of calcium and aluminum in neurofibrillary tangle-bearing neurons in parkinsonism-dementia of Guam. Proc Natl Acad Sci (USA) 1984;81:1875–1879

10 Hirano A, Donnenfeld H, Sasaki S, Nakano I. Fine structural observations of neurofilamentous changes in amyotrophic lateral sclerosis. J Neuropathol Exp Neurol 1984;43(5):461–470

11 Hirano A, Nakano I, Kurland LT, Mulder DW, Holley WP, Saccomanno G. Fine structural study of neurofibrillary changes in a family with amyotrophic lateral sclerosis. J Neuropathol Exp Neurol 1984;43(5):471–480

12 Elizan TS, Hirano A, Abrams BM, Need RL, Van Nuis C, Kurland LT. Amyotrophic lateral sclerosis and parkinsonism-dementia complex of Guam: Neurological reevaluation. Arch Neurol 1966;14:356–368

13 Deapen DM, Henderson BE. A case-control study of amyotrophic lateral sclerosis. Am J Epidemiol 1986;123(5):790–799

14 Reed D, Labarthe D, Chen KM, Stallones R. A cohort study of amyotrophic lateral sclerosis and parkinsonism-dementia on Guam and Rota. Am J Epidemiol 1987;125(1):92–100

15 Kurland LT, Mulder DW. Epidemiologic investigations of amyotrophic lateral sclerosis: 1. Preliminary report on geographic distribution, with

special reference to the Mariana Islands, including clinical and pathologic observations. Neurology 1954;4:355–378,438–448

16 Whiting MG. Toxicity of Cycads: Implications for Neurodegenerative Diseases and Cancer. Transcripts of four cycad conferences. 1st cycad conference 1962; 15. New York, Third World Medical Research Foundation, 1988

17 Torres J, Irarte LLG, Kurland LT. Amyotrophic lateral sclerosis among Guamanians in California. Calif Med 1957;86(6):385–388

18 Plato CC, Reed DM, Elizan TS, Kurland LT. Amyotrophic lateral sclerosis/ parkinsonism-dementia complex of Guam: IV. Familial and genetic investigations. Am J Human Genet 1967;19(5):617–632

19 Reed DM, Brody JA. Amyotrophic lateral sclerosis and parkinsonism-dementia on Guam, 1945–1972: I. Descriptive epidemiology. Am J Epidemiol 1975;101(4): 287–301

20 Eldridge R, Ryan E, Rosario J, Brody JA. Amyotrophic lateral sclerosis and parkinsonism-dementia in a migrant population from Guam. Neurology 1969;19(11):1029–1037

21 Plato CC, Cruz M. Blood group and haptoglobin frequencies of the Chamorros of Guam. Am J Human Genet 1967;19(6):722–731

22 Olivares L, San Esteban E, Alter M. Mexican 'resistance' to amyotrophic lateral sclerosis. Arch Neurol 1972;27:397–402

23 Gajdusek DC. Foci of motor neuron disease in high incidence in isolated populations of East Asia and the Western Pacific. In: Rowland LP, ed. Human Motor Neuron Diseases. New York, Raven Press, 1982:363–393

24 Garruto RM, Gajdusek DC, Chen L-M. Amyotrophic lateral sclerosis and parkinsonism-dementia among Filipino migrants to Guam. Ann Neurol 1981;10:341–350

25 Kurtzke JF: Epidemiology of amyotrophic lateral sclerosis. In: Rowland LP, ed. Human Motor Neuron Diseases. New York, Raven Press, 1982;281–302

26 Steele JC, Guzman T. Observations about amyotrophic lateral sclerosis and the parkinsonism-dementia complex of Guam with regard to epidemiology and etiology. Can J Neurol Sci 1987;14:358–362

27 Reed DM, Torres JM, Brody J. Amyotrophic lateral sclerosis and parkinsonism-dementia on Guam, 1945–1972: II. Familial and genetic studies. Am J Epidemiol 1975;101(4):302–310

28 Garruto RM, Gajdusek DC, Chen L-M. Amyotrophic lateral sclerosis among Chamorro migrants from Guam. Ann Neurol 1980;8:612–619

29 Hirano A. Aspects of the ultrastructure of amyotrophic lateral sclerosis. In: Rowland LP, ed. Human Motor Neuron Diseases. New York, Raven, 1982;75–88

30 Garruto RM, Yanagihara R, Gajdusek DC. Disappearance of high-incidence amyotrophic lateral sclerosis and parkinsonism-dementia on Guam. Neurology 1985;35:193–198

31 Tandan R, Bradley WG. Amyotrophic lateral sclerosis: Part 1. Clinical features, pathology and ethical issues in management. Ann Neurol 1985;18:271–280

32 Gajdusek DC, Salazar AM. Amyotrophic lateral sclerosis and parkinsonian syndromes in high incidence among the Auyu and Jakai people of West New Guinea. Neurology 1982;32:107–126

33 Yase Y. Neurological disease in the Western Pacific Islands, with a report on the focus of amyotrophic lateral sclerosis found in the Kii Peninsula, Japan. Am J Trop Med Hygiene 1970;19(1):155–166

34 Kiloh LG, Lethlean AK, Morgan G, Cawte JE, Harris M. An endemic neurological disorder in tribal Australian aborigines. J Neurol Neurosurg Psychiat 1980;43:661–668

35 Palo J, Jokelainen M. Geographic and social distribution of patients with amyotrophic lateral sclerosis. Arch Neurol 1977;34:724

36 Whiting MG: Toxicity of Cycads: Implications for Neurodegenerative Diseases and Cancer. Transcripts of four cycad conferences. 1st cycad conference 1962;16–17. New York, Third World Medical Research Foundation, 1988

37 Kurland LT. An appraisal of the neurotoxicity of cycad and the etiology of amyotrophic lateral sclerosis on Guam. Sixth International Cycad Conference. 1972;31(5):1540–1542

38 Yase Y. The pathogenesis of amyotrophic lateral sclerosis. Lancet 1972;August:292–296

39 Tan N, Kakulas BA, Masters C, Gajdusek DC, Garruto RM, Chen KM, Gibbs CJ Jr. Observations on the clinical presentations and the neuropathological findings of amyotrophic lateral sclerosis in Australia and Guam. Ann Acad Med 1986;15(1):62–66

40 Chen L. Neurofibrillary change on Guam. Arch Neurol 1981;38:16–18

41 Whiting MG. Toxicity of Cycads: Implications for Neurodegenerative Diseases and Cancer. Transcripts of four cycad conferences. 1st cycad conference 1962;55. New York, Third World Medical Research Foundation, 1988

42 Anderson FH, Richardson EP Jr., Okazaki H, Brody JA. Neurofibrillary degeneration on Guam: Frequency in Chamorros and non-Chamorros with no known neurological disease. Brain 1979;102:65–77

43 Calne DB, McGeer E, Eisen A, Spencer P. Alzheimer's disease, Parkinson's disease, and motoneuron disease: Abiotropic interaction between ageing and environment? Lancet 1986;November:1067–1070

44 Kurland LT. Amyotrophic lateral sclerosis and Parkinson's disease com-

plex on Guam linked to an environmental neurotoxin. TINS 1988;11(2):51–54

45 Ganrot PO. Metabolism and possible health effects of aluminum. Environ Health Perspec 1986;65:363–441

46 Perl DP, Good PF. Uptake of aluminum into central nervous system along nasal-olfactory pathways. Lancet 1987;May:1028

47 Crapper DR, Krishnan SS, Quittkat S. Aluminum, neurofibrillary degeneration and Alzheimer's disease. Brain 1976;99:67

48 Crapper DR, Karlik S, DeBoni U. Aluminum and other metals in senile (Alzheimer) dementia. In: Katzman R, Terry RD, Bick KL, eds. Alzheimer's Disease: Senile Dementia and Related Disorders, Vol. 7: Aging. New York, Raven Press, 1978;471–495

49 Lipman JJ, Colowick SP, Lawrence PL. Aluminum induced encephalopathy in the rat. Life Sci 1988;42(8):863–875

50 Yase Y. The role of aluminum in CNS degeneration with interaction with calcium. Neurotoxicology 1980;1:101–110

51 Yase Y. Environmental contribution to the amyotrophic lateral sclerosis process. In: Serratice G, et al, eds. Neuromuscular Diseases. New York, Raven Press, 1984;335–337

52 Yoshimasu F. Nebayashi Y, Yase Y, Iwata S, Sasajima K. Studies on amyotrophic lateral sclerosis by neutron activation analysis. Folia Psychiat Neurol Japon 1976;30:49–55

53 Yanagihara R, Garruto RM, Gajdusek DC, Tomita A, Uchikawa T, Konayaya Y, Chen K-M, Sobue I, Plato C, Gibbs CJ. Calcium and vitamin D metabolism in Guamanian Chamorros with amyotrophic lateral sclerosis and parkinsonism-dementia . Ann Neurol 1984;15:42-48

54 Garruto RM, Yanagihara R, Gajdusek DC, Arion DM. Concentrations of heavy metals and essential minerals in garden soil and drinking water in the Western Pacific. In: Chen KM, Yase Y, eds. Amyotrophic Lateral Sclerosis in Asia and Oceania. Taipei, National Taiwan University, 1984;265–330

55 Nieboer E, Richardson DHS. The replacement of the nondescript term 'heavy metals' by a biologically and chemically significant classification of metal ions. Environ Pollut Ser Bull 1980;1:3–26

56 Feinroth M, Feinroth MV, Friedman EA, Berlyne GM. Effect of parathyroid hormone and acute renal failure on aluminum absorption in rat everted gut sacs. Clin Res 1980;28:656

57 Mayor GH, Sprague SM, Hourani MR, Sanchez TV. Parathyroid hormone-mediated aluminum deposition and egress in the rat. Kidney Int 1980;17:40–44

58 Long JF, Nagode LA, Kindig O, Liss L. Axonal swellings of Purkinje cells in chickens associated with high intake of 1,25-(OH)$_2$D$_3$ and elevated

dietary aluminum including X-ray microanalysis. Neurotoxicol 1980;1:111–120

59 Farnell BJ, Crapper McLachlan DR, Baimbridge K, DeBoni U, Wong L, Wood PL. Calcium metabolism in aluminum encephalopathy. Exp Neurol 1985;88:68–83

60 Farnell BJ, De Boni U, Crapper McLachlan DR. Aluminum neurotoxicity in the absence of neurofibrillary degeneration in CAl hippocampal pyramidal neurons *in vitro*. Exp Neurol 1982;78:241–258

61 Siegel N, Haug A. Aluminum interaction with calmodulin. Evidence for altered structure and function from optical and enzymatic studies. Biochim Biophys Acta 1983;744:36–45

62 Siegel N, Haug A. Calmodulin dependent formation of membrane potential in barley root plasma membrane vescicles – A biochemical model of aluminum toxicity in plants. Physiol Plant 1983;59:285–291

63 VanBerkum MFA, Wong YL, Lewis PN, McLachlan Crapper DR. Total and poly (A) RNA yields during an aluminum encephalopathy in rabbit brains. Neurochem Res 1986;11(9);1347–1359

64 McLachlan Crapper DR, Lukiw WJ, Wong AL, Bergeron C, Bech-Hansen NT. Selective messenger RNA reduction in Alzheimer's disease. Mol Brain Res 1988;3:255–262

65 McLachlan Crapper DR, Baimbridge KG, Wong AL, Bergeron C, Bech-Hansen NT. Calmodulin and callbindin D_{28} in Alzheimer's disease. Alzheimer Disease and Associated Disorders 1987;1(3):171–179

66 Klatzo I, Wisniewski H, Streicher E. Experimental production of neurofibrillary degeneration: Light-microscopic observations. J Neuropathol Exp Neurol 1965;24:187–199

67 Terry RD, Pena C. Experimental production of neurofibrillary degeneration 2: Electromicroscopy, microscopy, phosphatase, histochemistry and electron probe analysis. J. Neuropathol Exp Neurol 1965;24:200–210

68 Tronscoso JC, Sternberger LA, Sternberger NH, Hoffman PN, Prince DL. Immunocytochemical studies of neurofilament antigens in the neurofibrillary pathology induced by aluminum. J Neuropath Exp Neurol 1985;44:332(abstr 77)

69 Bizzi A, Crane RC, Autilio-Gambetti, Gambetti P. Aluminum effect on slow transport – A novel impairment of neurofilament transport. J Neurol Sci 1984;4:722–731

70 Sternberger NH, Sternberger LA, Ulrich J. Aberrant neurofilament phosphorylation in Alzheimer's disease. Proc Nat Acad Sci (USA) 1982;82:4274–4276

71 Johnson GVM, Jope RS. Cytoskeletal protein phosphorylation is altered in the brains of aluminum-treated rats. 17th Annual Meeting, Society for Neurosciences, New Orleans, 1987;13:abstr 366.10

72 Rasool CG, Abraham C, Anderton BH, Haugh M, Kahn J, Selkoe DJ. Alzheimer's disease: Immunoreactivity of neurofibrillary tangles with anti-neurofilament and anti-paired helical filament antibodies. Brain Res 1984;310:249–260

73 Perry G, Rizzuto N, Autilio-Gambetti L, Gambetti P. Paired helical filaments from Alzheimer's disease patients contain cytoskeletal components. Proc Nat Acad Sci (USA)1985;82:3916–3920

74 Yen S, Gaskin F, Man S. Neurofibrillary tangles in senile dementia of the Alzheimer's type share an antigenic determinant with intermediate filaments of the vimentin class. Am J Pathol 1983;113:373–381

75 Mori H, Kondo J, Ihara Y. Ubiquitin is a component of paired helical filaments in Alzheimer's disease. Science 1987;235(March):1641–1644

76 Grundke-Iqbal I, Iqbal K, Quinlan M, Turg Y-C, Zaidi MS, Wisniewski HM. Microtubule-associated protein tau: A component of Alzheimer paired helical filament. J. Biol Chem 1986;261:6084–6089

77 Grundke-Iqbal I, Iqbal K, Turg Y-C, Quinlan M, Wisniewski HM, Binder LI. Abnormal phosphorylation of the microtubule-associated protein tau in Alzheimber cytoskeletal pathology. Proc Nat Acad Sci (USA)1986;83:4193–4917

78 Wischik CM, Novak M, Edwards PC, Tichelaar W, Klug A, Crowther RA. Structural characterization of the core of the paired helical filament of Alzheimer's disease. Proc Natl Acad Sci (USA) 1988;85:4484–4888

79 Nairn AC, Hemmings HC, Greengard P. Protein kinases in the brain. Ann Rev Biochem 1985;54:931–976.

80 Johnson GVW, Jope RS. Aluminum alters cyclic AMP and GMP levels but not presynaptic colonergic markers in rat brain in vivo. Brain Res 1987;403:1–6

81 Muma NA, Troncoso JC, Hoffman P, Koo EH, Price D. Aluminum neuro-toxicity – altered expression of cytoskeletal genes. Mol Brain Res 1988;3:115–122

82 McLachlan Crapper DR, Lewis PN, Lukiw WJ, Sima A, Bergeron C, De-Boni U. Chromatin structure in dementia. Ann Neurol 1984;15:329–334

83 McLachlan Crapper DR, Lukiw WJ, Kruck TPA. Aluminum, altered tran-scription, and the pathogenesis of Alzheimer's disease. Environ Geochem and Health, in press, 1988

84 Lukiw WJ, Kruck TPA, McLachlan Crapper DR. Alterations in human linker histone-DNA binding in the presence of aluminum salts in vitro and in Alzheimer's disease. Neurotoxicology 1987;8:291–302

85 Davidson TJ, Hartmann HA, Johnson PC. RNA content and volume of motor neurons in amyotrophic lateral sclerosis. I. The cervical swelling. J. Neuropathol Exp Neurol 1981;40(1):32–36

86 Davidson TJ, Hartmann HA. RNA content and volume of motor neurons

in amyotrophic lateral sclerosis. II. The lumbar intumescence and nucleus dorsalis. J Neuropathol Exp Neurol 1981;40(2):187–192

87 Davidson TJ, Hartmann HA. Base composition of RNA obtained from motor neurons in amyotrophic lateral sclerosis. J Neuropathol Exp Neurol 1981;40(2):193–198

88 Trapp GA. Plasma aluminum is bound to transferrin. Life Sci 1983;33:311–316

89 Edwardson JA, Candy JM. Aluminum and the pathogenesis of senile plaques: Studies in Alzheimer's disease and chronic renal failure. Aluminum and Health Workshop, Oslo, Norway, Paper No. 6, Section III, Toxicology, 1988

90 McLachlan Crapper DR, McLachlan CD, Krishnan B, Krishnan SS, Dalton AJ, Steele JC. Aluminum and calcium in Guam, Palau and Jamaica: Implications for amyotrophic lateral sclerosis and parkinsonism-dementia syndromes of Guam. Environ Geochem and Health 1989; 11:45–53

91 Tipton IH, Cook MJ, Steiner RL, Foland JM, McDaniel KK, Fentress SD. Oakridge National Laboratory Reports, Central Files No. 57-2-4(a), 57-2-4(b), 57-11-33(c), 1957

92 Roberts E. Alzheimer's disease may begin in the nose and may be caused by aluminosilicates. Neurobiol of Aging 1986;7:561–567

93 Zakour RA, Boultman H. Evolution of drosophila mitochodrial DNAs – analysis of heteroduplex molecules. Biochem Biophys Acta 1979;564(2): 342–351

94 Donaldson J, Labella FS, Gesser D. Enhanced autoxidation of dopamine as a possible basis of manganese neurotoxicity. Neurotoxicology 1981;2:53–64

95 Donaldson J, McGregor D, LaBella FS. Manganese neurotoxicity: A model for free-radical mediated neurodegeneration. Can J Physiol Pharmacol 1982;60:1398–1405

96 Donaldson J, Barbeau A. Manganese neurotoxicity: Possible clues to the etiology of human brain disorders. In: Gabay S, Harris J, Ho BT, eds. Metal Ions in Neurology and Psychiatry. Neurology and Neurobiology, Vol. 15. New York, Liss, 1985;259–285

97 Florence TM, Stauber JL, Fardy JJ. Ecological studies of manganese on Groote Eylandt. Research on Manganese and Metabolism – Groote Eylandt, Northern Territory. Proceedings of a conference held at Health House, Darwin, NT, 1987;23–35

98 Cawte J, Hams G, Kilburn C. Manganism in a neurological ethnic complex in Northern Australia. Lancet 1987;May:61

99 Bradley WG, Krasin F. A new hypothesis of the etiology of amyotrophic lateral sclerosis: The DNA hypothesis. Arch Neurol 1982;39:677–680

100 Tandan R, Robison SH, Munzer JS, Bradley WG. Deficient DNA repair in amyotrophic lateral sclerosis cells. J Neurol Sci 1987;79:189–203

101 Kurland LT, Molgaard CA. Guamanian ALS: Heredity or acquired? In: Rowland LP, ed. Human Motor Neuron Diseases. New York, Raven Press, 1982;165–171

102 Plato C, Garruto R, Fox K, et al. Amyotrophic lateral sclerosis and parkinsonism-dementia on Guam: A 25 year prospective case-control study. Am J Epidemiol 1986;124:643–656

103 Whiting MG. Toxicity of cycads. Econ Bot 1963;17:271–303

104 Fosberg FR. Résumé of the Cycadaceae. Third Conference on Toxicity of Cycads. Fed Proc 1964;Nov–Dec:1340–1341

105 Birdsey MR. A brief description of the cycads. Sixth International Cycad Conference. Fed Proc 1972;31(5):1467–1469

106 Whiting MG. Food practices in ALS foci in Japan, the Marianas, and New Guinea. Third Conference on Toxicity of Cycads. Fed Proc 1964;Nov–Dec: 1343–1345

107 Ressler C. Neurotoxic amino acids of certain species of Lathyrus and vetch. Third Conference on Toxicity of Cycads. Fed Proc 1964; Nov–Dec: 1350–1353

108 Hirano A, Llena JF, Streifler M, Cohn DF. Anterior horn cell changes in a case of neurolathyrism. Acta Neuropathol (Berl.) 1976; 35:277–283

109 Spencer PS. ALS: Toxic hypotheses old and new. VIth Intern Congr Neuromuscular Disease. Muscle & Nerve 1986; July:56 (abstr K-03)

110 Spencer PS, Nunn PB, Hugon J, Ludolph A, Roy DN. Motorneurone disease on Guam: Possible role of a food neurotoxin. Lancet 1986;April:965

111 Kurland LT. Introductory remarks. Third Conference on Toxicity of Cycads. Fed Proc 1964;Nov–Dec: 1337–1339

112 Dossaji SF, Herbin GA. Occurrence of macrozamin in the seeds of Encephalartos hildebrandtii. Sixth International Cycad Conference. Fed Proc 1972;31(5):1470–1472

113 Polsky FI Nunn PB, Bell EA. Distribution and toxicity of α-amino-β-methylaminopropionic acid. Sixth International Cycad Conference. Fed Proc 1972;31(5):1473–1475

114 Mickelsen O, Campbell E, Yang M. Mugera G, Whitehair CK. Studies with cycad. Third Conference on Toxicity of Cydads. Fed Proc 1964;Nov–Dec:1363–1365

115 Levene CI, Duban S, Hughes RH. Effects of cycasin and cycad meal. Third Conference on Toxicity of Cycads. Fed Proc 1964;Nov–Dec: 1366–1367

116 Spencer PS, Ohta M, Palmer VE. Cycad use and motor neurone disease in Kii Peninsula of Japan. Lancet 1987; December: 1462–1463

117 Ross SM, Spencer PS. Specific antagonism of behavioral action of 'uncommon' amino acids linked to motor-system diseases. Synapse 1987;1:248–253

118 Dastur DK. Cycad toxicity in monkeys: Clinical, pathological, and bio-

chemical aspects. Third Conference on Toxicity of Cycads. Fed Proc 1964; Nov–Dec:1368–1369.

119 Vega A, Bell EA, Nunn PB. The preparation of L- and D-α-amino-β-methyl-aminopropionic acids and the identification of the compound isolated from *Cycas circinalis* as the L-isomer. Phytochemistry 1968;7:1885–1887

120 Nunn PB, Seelig M, Zagoren JC, Spencer PS. Stereospecific acute neuron-otoxicity of 'uncommon' plant amino acids linked to human motor-system diseases. Brain Res 1987;410:375–379

121 Huck S, Grass F, Hörtnagl H. The glutamate analogue α-aminoadipic acid is taken up by astrocytes before exerting its gliotoxic effect *in vitro*. J. Neurosci 1984;4(10):2650–2657

122 Schwarcz R, Foster AC, French ED, Whetsell WO Jr, Köhler C. Current topics II. Excitotoxic models for neurodegenerative disorders. Life Sci 1984;35(1):19–32

123 Ohata M, Fredericks WR, Sundaram U, Rapoport SI. Effects of immobili-zation stress on regional cerebral blood flow in the conscious rat. J Cere-bral Blood Flow Metab 1981;187–194

124 Carlsson C, Hägerdal M, Siesjö BK. Increased cerebral oxygen uptake and blood flow in immobilization stress. Acta Physiol Scand 1975;95:206–208

125 Carlsson C, Hägerdal M, Kaasik AE, Siesjö BK. A catecholamine-mediated increase in cerebral oxygen uptake during immobilization stress in rats. Brain Res 1977;119:223–231

126 Stensaas SS, Stensaas LJ. The reaction of the cerebral cortex to chronically implanted needles. Acta Neuropathol (Berl) 1976;35:187–203

127 Abbot NJ. The neuronal microenvironment. TINS 1986;Jan:3–6

128 Coyle JT, Molliver ME, Kuhar MJ. *In situ* injection of kainic acid: A new method for selectively lesioning neuronal cell bodies while sparing axons of passage. J Comp Neurol 1978;180:301–324

129 Ben-Ari Y, Repressa A, Tremblay E, Nitecka L. Selective and non-selective seizure related brain damage produced by kainic acid. In: Schwarcz R, Ben-Ari Y, eds. Excitatory Amino Acids and Epilepsy. New York, Plenum, 1985;647–686

130 Spencer PS, Nunn PB, Hugon J, Ludolph AC, Ross SM, Roy DN, Robert-son RC. Guam amyotrophic lateral sclerosis – parkinsonism-dementia linked to a plant excitant neurotoxin. Science 1987;237:517–522

131 Baskys A, Grima E, McLachlan DR, Carlen PL. Acute effects of the neuro-toxin β-N-methylamino-L-alanine on CA_1 cells in the hippocampus. Sub-mitted for publication, 1988

Western Pacific Amyotrophic Lateral Sclerosis: Putative Role of Cycad Toxins

PETER S. SPENCER, STEPHEN M. ROSS,
GLEN KISBY, AND DWIJENDRA N. ROY

The Western Pacific parkinsonism-dementia (PD) complex is considered a clinical variant of a form of familial amyotrophic lateral sclerosis (ALS) that has occurred in high but declining prevalence among three population groups [1] (Fig. 1): (a) Chamorros of the Mariana islands of Guam and Rota [2] and others who have adopted their life-style; (b) Auyu and Jaqai linguistic groups of the southern lowlands of Irian Jaya (western New Guinea) [3]; and (c) Japanese in the northern Kii Peninsula of Honshu island [4]. In Guam, where the declining incidence of ALS has been tracked for over 30 years, there has been an increase both in the relative proportion of parkinsonian cases and in the mean age at onset of ALS and PD [1, 5, 6]. Preliminary studies suggest similar trends are occurring in the neurodegenerative disease epicentre of Irian Jaya [7]. While the brains of affected subjects in this remote region have yet to be examined post-mortem, neuropathological study of Chamorro and Japanese cases in the 1960s revealed widespread neurofibrillary degeneration of the Alzheimer type [8, 9]. Later studies showed tangles in an extraordinary 70% of 302 brains of Chamorros who had died after the age of 35 with no recognized neurological disease [10]. Remarkably, recent autopsies have revealed not only widespread neurofibrillary degeneration but also numerous senile plaques comparable to those seen in Alzheimer disease (D. Perl, personal communication). Another recent finding in Guam ALS/PD is the common presence of eye-movement disorders comparable to those of progressive supranuclear palsy (PSP) (J. Steele, personal communication). Taken in concert, therefore, the three foci of Western Pacific ALS/PD provide a unique opportunity not only to explore the etiology of motor neuron disease but also to probe for the fundamental causation

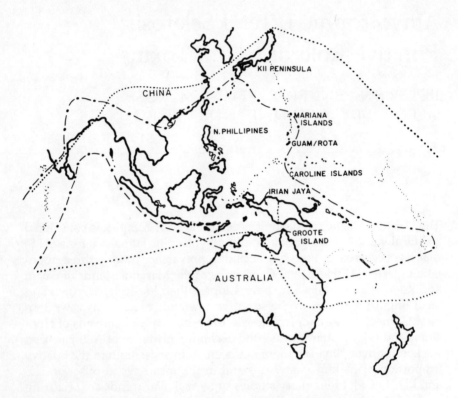

Figure 1. Location of high-incidence foci of ALS in Guam and Rota, Kii Peninsula (Japan), and Irian Jaya (Indonesia), shown in relation to distribution of *Cycas* spp., members of the cycad group of ancient plants. Area contained within the dotted lines shows earlier distribution; that within the broken punctuated lines depicts present *Cycas* distribution. *Cycas revoluta* is used as an ornamental in the Kii Peninsula of Japan, and seed of this plant is imported from the southerly island of Amami-O-Shima for use in the Kii Peninsula as an oral folk medicine as described in the text. Reproduced with permission from Spencer et al. 1987 [41].

of certain neurodegenerative diseases and the factors that regulate their variable clinical expression.

The Search for Causation

Since the incidence of motor neuron disease is declining in all three zones of Western Pacific ALS/PD [1], and inherited and viral factors have been virtually ruled out, the search for etiology has focused on non-transmissible environmental factors that are disappearing as the susceptible population groups acculturate to modern ways. Deficient nutritional intake of calcium, associated with absorption and neuronal deposition of aluminum and other cations, has been advanced as causal [1], but in Guam, calcium concentrations in river water and indigenous food plants are unremarkable [11; J. Steele, personal communication]. The most recent epidemiological study showed that preference for traditional Chamorro food was the only one of 23 tested variables significantly associated with an increase risk for PD [12]. This is consistent with the hypothesis that seed of the neurotoxic cycad plant (Fig. 2) – a traditional source of food and medicine for the Chamorro people – plays an important role in the etiology of Western Pacific ALS/PD [13]. It is also noteworthy that Guamanian folklore links *lytico* (ALS) to the handling and consumption of *Cycas circinalis* , the indigenous cycad of Guam [14].

Originally proposed by Whiting [14] more than a quarter of a century ago and subsequently championed by Kurland [15], the cycad hypothesis was intensively investigated in the 1960s and then abandoned for two reasons: the plant was found not to be used for food in the Japanese and New Guinea ALS foci, and experimental induction of a lookalike motor-system disorder in animals fed cycad products was considered to have failed. The fascinating story of the early work on cycads and neurodegenerative disease may be followed in reports of six international conferences held between 1962 and 1972 to consider their relationship; four of these were published for the first time in 1988 [16]. In 1981, one of us (PSS) began an ongoing series of collaborative field and laboratory investigations that have marshalled new evidence in support of a modified cycad hypothesis, namely that heavy exposure to the neurotoxic seed of this plant plays a leading (but not necessarily exclusive) role in triggering the ALS/PD complex in all three geographic zones. The goal of this work is to identify the structure of the culpable chemical agents in cycad seed, as well as their molecular and cellular mechanisms of action. Information of this type is expected to lead to the search for

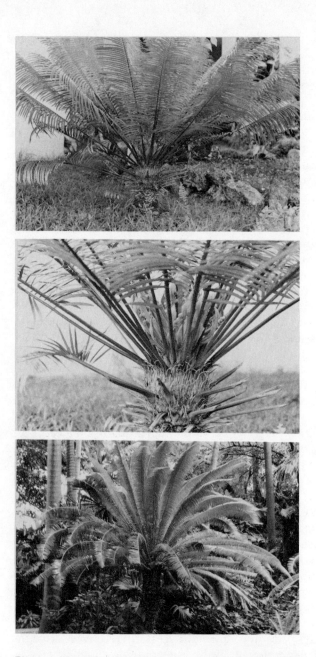

Figure 2. Upper: An immature *Cycas circinalis* plant from Rota in the Mariana Islands. Centre: Adorning the top of the stem is a crown of fronds bearing immature seed. In the past, ripened cycad seed served as an important source of food and topical medicine for the Chamorro people. Lower: A mature cycad tree.

related chemical substances in other environments that may have an etiological relationship with ALS.

The cycads are an ancient group of non-flowering plants of tropical and subtropical climes that have been widely used throughout human history primarily for food and medicine [14, 17]. The distribution of *Cycas* spp. includes all regions in the Western Pacific zone known to have had ALS in high incidence (Fig. 1). Farm animals (cattle, sheep) grazing on cycad leaves develop a poorly characterized, delayed-onset, hindlimb locomotor disorder (neurocycadism) associated with a stiff-legged gait followed by weakness, an associated loss of muscle bulk, and collapse of the hindquarters (Fig. 3) [18, 19]. Neuropathological descriptions of this condition are essentially restricted to the spinal cord where distal degeneration of long tracts has been observed (Fig. 4) [18, 20]. Specific description of motor neurons is unavailable, and the possibility of basal ganglia involvement is unexplored. In addition to hindquarter weakness and unsteadiness, cattle with neurocycadism characteristically display drooping or absent horns, presumably resulting from alterations of connective tissue in the basal growth zone. That cycads may plausibly harbour an agent capable of disrupting connective tissue homeostasis is relevant to (a) the former high frequency of multiple bony exostoses (diaphyseal aclasia) in Chamorros [21]; (b) skin changes in ALS cases in Guam [22] and elsewhere, as well as in a macaque with arm weakness and motor neuron degeneration experimentally induced by ingestion of cycad flour [23]; and (c) the apparent acceleration of skin healing in experimental rodents (and humans) by direct application of crushed cycad seed [24].

Medicinal use of the raw neurotoxic seed of *Cycas* spp. in all three high-incidence zones of Western Pacific ALS/PD is the cardinal common finding to emerge from our recent field studies. Although earlier noted in passing by Whiting during her nutritional survey of cycad usage on Guam [16], little significance was attached at that time to the Chamorro practice of using the crushed pulp and poisonous exudate of the seed kernel of *C. circinalis* as a poultice for the topical treatment of various skin lesions. In 1987, we discovered a comparable use for *Cycas* seed among Auyu people living in the Irian Jaya focus of neurodegenerative disease (Fig. 5) [7]. As in Guam, the cycad poultice is prepared daily and applied to open wounds (of individuals of all ages) for one or more weeks. Absorption and systemic distribution of cycad chemicals must occur throughout the period of poultice application. We also discovered, in 1987, heavy systemic exposure of individuals to untreated cycad seed in the Kii Peninsula (Japan) focus of ALS/PD; here the neurotoxic seed of *C. revoluta* (locally known as *sotetsu*) has been employed as an oral herbal medicine for the treatment of various ailments, including diar-

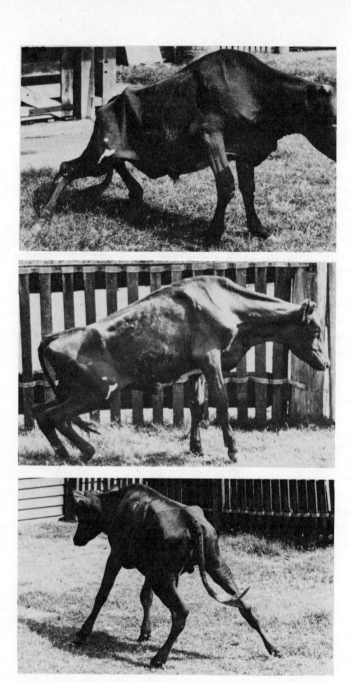

Figure 3. Neurocycadism in domestic farm animals. Note the predominant hindlimb weakness and atrophy [18]. Previously unpublished figure; printed here by kind permission of Dr M.D. McGavin.

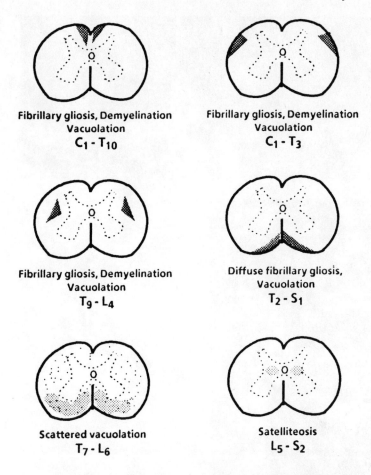

Fibrillary gliosis, Demyelination
Vacuolation
$C_1 - T_{10}$

Fibrillary gliosis, Demyelination
Vacuolation
$C_1 - T_3$

Fibrillary gliosis, Demyelination
Vacuolation
$T_9 - L_4$

Diffuse fibrillary gliosis,
Vacuolation
$T_2 - S_1$

Scattered vacuolation
$T_7 - L_6$

Satelliteosis
$L_5 - S_2$

Figure 4. Diagram of the pathological changes observed at different levels of the spinal cord in cattle grazing on *Cycas revoluta.* 'Demyelination' refers to loss of myelin staining. Modified from Yasuda et al 1984 [20].

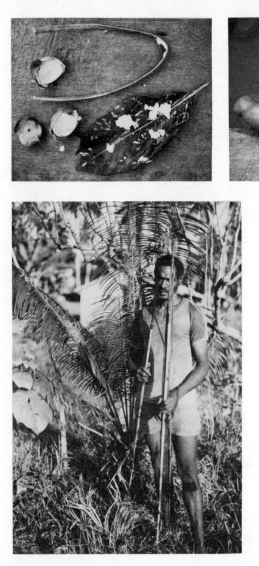

Figure 5. Epicentre of ALS in Irian Jaya, Indonesia. Left: Native hunter standing by a solitary Cycas tree near river Ia. Top left: For topical treatment of
various types of open skin lesions, scrapings of the white kernel of the cycad
seed are crushed, the resulting pulp immersed in the poisonous milky exudate,
and the sodden mass applied directly to the lesion on a leaf which is strapped
to the skin. Top right: Healed skin lesion following treatment with a cycad
seed poultice. Reproduced with permission from Spencer et al, 1988 [25].

rhea, dysmenorrhea, and tuberculosis [25, 26]. Even today, herbal prescriptions listing sotetsu are occasionally issued to patients (including P.S.S.!) by traditional healers (*kitoshi*) and filled by local pharmacists (Fig. 6). Thus, while our recent studies confirm that cycad seed is not used for food in either the Japanese or Irian Jaya focus of ALS/PD, there is nonetheless heavy exposure of selected persons who use the raw, dried seed for medicine. Furthermore, in these regions, preliminary studies have established in individual cases a direct link between medicinal use of cycad seed and the later appearance of ALS [7, 25, 26, and unpublished data].

Although medicinal use of unprocessed cycad seed is currently the prime focus of our experimental investigation, ingestion of improperly detoxified cycad seed flour is also of considerable potential etiological importance [13]. As noted above, seed of *C. circinalis* is a traditional source of food for the Chamorros, and the possible relationship between the heavy wartime utilization of cycad seed for food (and topical medicine) and the subsequent phenomenally high incidence of ALS has been proposed elsewhere [13, 27]. Supporting this proposition is the reported experimental induction of unilateral arm weakness with neuropathological evidence of upper and lower motor neuron degeneration in a single macaque fed cycad flour that was prepared as described below [23] (Fig. 7). Recent neuropathological evaluation of 7 macaques fed cycad flour revealed 'various forms of cerebral and spinal cord degeneration, including the presence of a few neuritic plaques in most cycad-fed animals and an excessively large number in one 10–11 year old monkey' (D.B. Dastur, personal communication).

For use as food in the Marianas, the poisonous cycad seed kernel is typically sliced into two or more pieces, soaked in water (replaced daily) to leach out the toxic principles, and dried, stored, and later ground to powder (Fig. 8). The resulting flour contains small and variable concentrations of chemicals endogenous to, and derived from, the cycad seed. Several factors, including seed maturity, kernel segment size, solvent properties (pH, temperature, etc.), and especially the duration of aqueous leaching, likely affect the degree to which chemicals are removed. Of special note is the great range in the number of days (1–30) considered by Guamanians to be optimal for cycad seed detoxification. Adequate sun-drying of the washed seed is also required to prevent spoiling and the consequent generation of a foul odour. Prolonged leaching and proper drying are likely to remove most relevant chemical factors, and carefully processed (including fermentation) *Cycas revoluta* seed kernel has been employed for food in other Pacific communities (e.g. Amami-O-Shima, Ryukyu Islands, Japan) where high-incidence ALS/PD disease has not been recognized [but see 28].

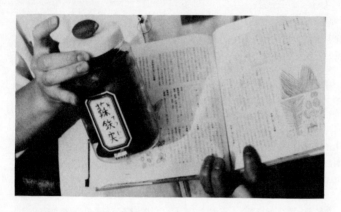

ザクロノハナ _____ 6和

ウメズリソウ _____ 8夕

ソテツの実 _____ 1ケ

当帰 _____ 2夕

サンダイリ _____ 2夕

Figure 6. High-incidence zone of ALS, Kii Peninsula, Japan. Pharmacist's bottle containing dried (but otherwise untreated) seed of *Cycas revoluta* (upper) used to fill herbal medicine prescriptions written by practitioners of folk medicine known locally as *kitoshi* (lower). Line 3 of the prescription states '*sotetsu, one seed.*' Cycad seed is imported into the region from the southern Japanese island of Amami-O-Shima (Ryukyu Islands). Reproduced with permission from Spencer et al, 1987 [7].

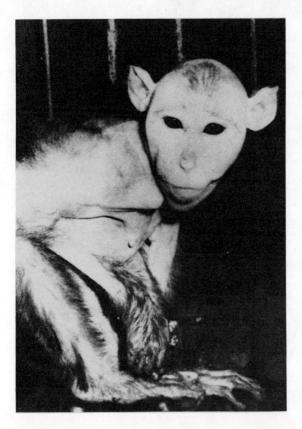

Figure 7. Macaca mulatta with severe weakness and wasting of one arm that developed after months of consuming a diet of flour prepared from *Cycas circinalis* seed. Post-mortem examination reportedly revealed evidence of upper- and lower-motor-neuron degeneration [23], limb muscle atrophy, skin atrophy with collagen degeneration, and mild changes in the liver. Previously unpublished figure; published by permission of the study's author, D.B. Dastur.

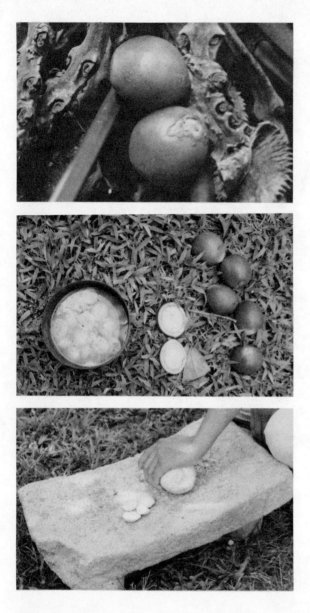

Figure 8. Chamorro food use of *Cycas circinalis* seed in the Mariana Islands. Upper: Two mature seeds of the type used to prepare flour. Centre: Mature seed and split seed showing the starchy white kernel (right); the latter is removed and soaked in water (left) to leach out water-soluble poisonous principles. Lower: Traditional method of grinding the washed and sun-dried cycad seed to produce flour used in tortillas and other local foodstuffs. Reproduced with permission from Spencer 1987 [13].

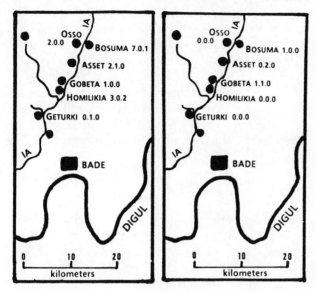

Figure 9. Epicentre of the ALS focus in southeastern Irian Jaya. Map showing confirmed cases of ALS, parkinsonism, and 'poliomyeloradiculitis' (●) found during surveys in 1962–80 by D.C. Gajdusek and colleagues [3] (left) and in 1987 by Spencer et al 1987 [25] (right). Since the population is largely stable, the 1987 observations suggest the incidence of ALS has declined while (as on Guam) the relative prevalence of parkinsonism to ALS has increased. Reproduced with permission from Spencer et al 1988 [25].

Declining Cycad Utilization and ALS Incidence

While cycad seed was an important source of food and medicine for the beleaguered Chamorro people of Guam and Rota during part of World War II [16], their progressive post-war acculturation to the food and medicine practices of the continental United States has resulted in a decline in cycad use that has marched in step with the steadily reducing incidence of ALS among Chamorros on those islands [13]. Similarly, motor neuron disease is now uncommon among Japanese residents in the Kii Peninsula ALS/PD focus, and the folk medicinal use of cycad seed appears to be restricted to a few remaining elderly *kitoshi* who have been replaced in recent decades by practitioners of Western and/or traditional Chinese medicine. The apparent decline of ALS prevalence in Irian Jaya (Fig. 9) can also be putatively linked to reduced reliance on natural sources of medicine. The Auyu people were forest dwellers who depended exclusively on natural products for food (notably, sago from

Metroxylon spp.) and medicine (e.g. *Cycas* seed) prior to their settlement in riverside villages by Dutch missionaries operating in the area from the 1930s. While the Auyu retain many of their traditional ways, the introduction of Dutch and Indonesian education, and the availability of relatively modern methods of medical treatment, are likely to be reducing their use of cycad seed. Thus, the declining patterns of utilization of cycad seed in the three communities at risk for ALS/PD fulfil the criterion of a disappearing environmental factor required as an etiological link to ALS/PD *(vide supra)*.

Timing of Cycad Exposure

From the vantage point of clinical expression Western Pacific ALS/PD appears to be a long-latency, environmentally triggered disorder in which the culpable agent(s) either act slowly (e.g., 'slow toxins') [13] or combine their neurotoxic action with age-related cellular attrition to reduce the target cell populations sufficiently to overcome functional reserve and to precipitate overt neurological dysfunction [29]. For obvious reasons, the latter is unable to account for onset of ALS at an early age. If cycad is the principal trigger for this neurodegenerative disorder, when does the critical exposure occur, and do the timing and degree of intoxication influence the expression of the resulting clinical compromise? While the answers to these important questions are unknown, some clues link motor neuron disease in the Western Pacific loci with cycad exposure at an early age – in some instances, in the first post-natal years of life. One is the presence of multinucleated and misplaced neurons in the cerebellum and vestibular nuclei of some Japanese and Guamanian subjects with ALS/PD (Fig. 10) [9, 30]. This suggests exposure during the later phases of brain development (up to the age of 1 year) to an agent that arrests the mitotic and migratory responses of neurons; one such substance known from experimental rodent studies to display this property is the neuroteratogen methylazoxymethanol (MAM), the aglycone of the cycad glucoside cycasin (Fig. 11). Administration of MAM to newborn rats results in cerebellar microplasia associated with misplaced and multinucleated neurons [31]. A second, more direct, link is our documentation of the oral use of cycad medicine (for treatment of diarrhea) in a 5-year-old Japanese female who developed the first signs of ALS at the age of 18 [25, 26, unpublished observations]. Similarly, in Irian Jaya, a 15-year-old male reportedly applied a cycad poultice for 1 month to an open ankle sore and noticed progressive motor weakness from ALS beginning less than 14 years later [7, 25]. This is consistent

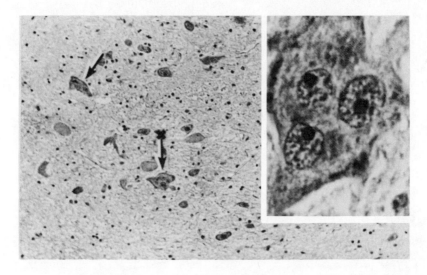

Figure 10. Vestibular nucleus: two multinucleated nerve cells (arrows). Inset: magnified view of one of the nerve cells indicated by arrow. Reproduced with permission from Shiraki and Yase 1975 [9].

with the observation that some Chamorros developed ALS 1–34 years after leaving Guam; based on age of migration, the minimum exposure for these subjects to the Guam environment to have acquired disease susceptibility was the first 18 years of life [32]. Additionally, according to longitudinal data for the incidence of Chamorro neurodegenerative disease [1], the apparent peak for ALS among males in 1955 followed approximately 10 years after the period estimated for maximum reliance on cycad for food and medicine, while that for PD occurred 5–10 years later. Moreover, among male Chamorros, the incidence of ALS was twice that of PD in the early 1950s, whereas 20 years later the relative proportion of such cases was inverted [1, 27]. While comparable data are unavailable for Kii Peninsula ALS/PD, a similar proportional decrease ofALS (relative to parkinsonism) may be occurring in the epicentre of the Irian Jaya disease focus [7] (Fig. 9). Additionally, teenage cases of ALS are no longer seen in any of the high-incidence disease areas and, on Guam, the mean ages for onset of ALS and PD (seen in older subjects) have increased over the past 30 years [6]. Since use of cycad in Guam and elsewhere has decreased in recent decades, these several pieces of data are consonant with the proposal that degree of intoxication is a

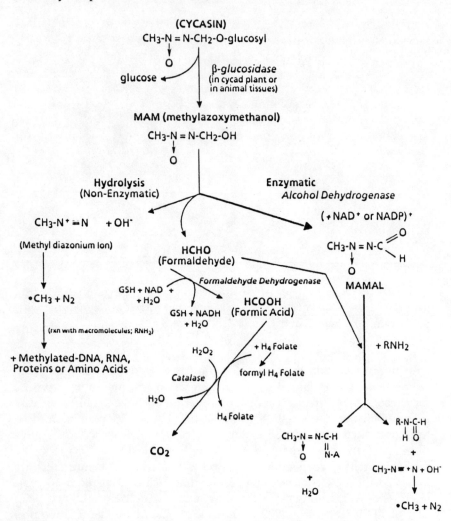

Figure 11. Proposed metabolism of cycasin [46, 47].

critical factor dictating both the age of onset and the clinical characteristics of the resultant disease. Specifically, we have suggested [13] that
heavy exposure precipitates ALS by lethally damaging motor neurons
that appear highly susceptible to at least one of the cycad neurotoxins
(vide infra). The heavily exposed subject also sustains some damage to
the apparently less-susceptible nigrostriatal pathway – demonstrable
only by fluorodopa positron emission tomography (D.B. Calne et al, personal communication) and neuropathologically – but the lesion is insufficient to cause the clinical expression of parkinsonism, and the
individual dies apparently with pure ALS. Other subjects who are less
heavily intoxicated (or who have a lower degree of susceptibility), it is
proposed, may survive for many years with motor neuron compromise
and eventually develop parkinsonism with ALS as a consequence of the
additive effects of toxic damage and age-related attrition of nigrostriatal
neurons. A further possibility is that dementia represents the late effects
of the lowest clinically significant level of cycad exposure, while the
majority of elderly Chamorro subjects with subclinical neurofibrillary
tangles comprise those with extremely low exposure or an unusually
high tolerance. The latter would suggest a role for genetic and gender
factors that modify bioavailability of cycad toxins. In summary, therefore,
we have suggested the various forms of Western Pacific neurodegenerative disease are individual points on a dose-response curve for plant
toxicity [13]. The corollary of this hypothesis is the existence within the
nervous system of differential regional vulnerability to the culpable
agent(s) within, or derived from, cycad seed.

Chemical Principles in Cycad Seed

Two neurotoxic agents have been identified in *Cycas* seed: cycasin(s), the
active form of which is MAM (Fig. 11), and beta-N-methylamino-L-ala-
nine (BMAA) [33] (Fig. 12). The latter may be quantified in plant and
animal tissue after derivatization of amino acids with fluorenylmethyl
chloroformate (FMOC), separation by high-performance liquid chromatography, and detection by fluorescence [34] (Fig. 13). While BMAA
is present in low concentrations (0.02%) relative to that of cycasin in
cycad seed kernel, what constitutes a significant dose of these compounds has yet to be established. Recent studies from our laboratory
show that BMAA increases in concentration with time after crushing the
seed kernel of *Cycas circinalis*, and that cycasin in cycad leachate diminishes in concentration prior to that of BMAA (G. Kisby et al, unpublished
data). Thus, individuals ingesting seed kernel that has been soaked in
water for only a few days would likely receive doses of both MAM and

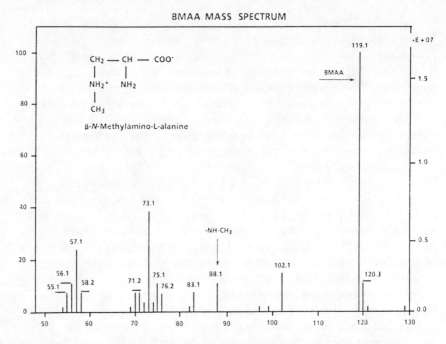

Figure 12. Mass spectrum and chemical formula of beta-N-methylamino-L-alanine (BMAA). BMAA was synthesized by D.N.R. and analysed by S.F. Sears. Reproduced by kind permission of S.F. Sears, R. McCullen, and I. Einhorn.

BMAA. However, larger doses of both compounds would probably be absorbed/generated in subjects with an open wound treated topically with a cycad poultice; this practice provides continuous 24 hr/day, subcutaneous exposure for several weeks, with daily replacement by fresh plant material.

The agent responsible for induction of motor weakness in animals grazing on cycad leaves has not been identified. Seeds of some neurotoxic genera are said to lack BMAA, but the possibility of endogenous generation of this or other neurotoxic amino acids from the methylating action of MAM (*vide supra*) has yet to be tested. MAM displays carcinogenic properties in experimental rodents [35], an observation that earlier suggested this was not the culpable neurotoxic agent. Additionally, as noted above, clinical and neuropathological evidence of motor neuron disease has been reported in macaques chronically fed *C. circinalis* flour lacking detectable concentrations of cycasin (Fig. 8) [23]. However, the animal also showed evidence of skin and liver changes, the latter being

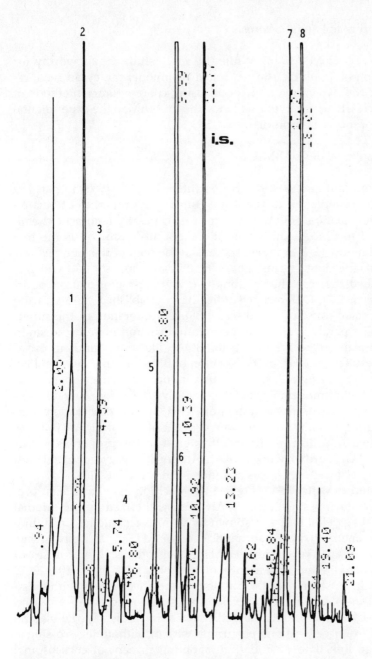

Figure 13. Chromatogram of an aqueous extract of *Cycas circinalis* seed from Guam diluted 2:1. 1, glutamine; 2, aspartate + serine; 3, glutamic acid; 4, glycine; 5, alanine; 6, GABA; i.s., internal standard; 7, unidentified BMAA-like peak; 8, BMAA. Reproduced with permission from Kisby et al, 1988 [34].

a known effect of MAM [16]. While this early study is noteworthy for its prediction of a non-cycasin neurotoxic component in cycad seed, re-creation of the experimental protocol using contemporary methods of analysis is clearly required to rule out a role for MAM in the experimental induction of motor neuron disease.

Neurotoxic Properties of BMAA

Non-protein plant amino acids created interest in the 1960s in part be-cause of the observation of the acute convulsive properties of beta-N-oxalylamino-L-alanine (BOAA), a non-protein plant amino acid chemi-cally related to BMAA. This unusual compound is present as the free amino acid in low (1–2%) concentrations in the seed of the legume *Lath-yrus sativus* (chickling or grass pea) [36], excessive ingestion of which is an established cause of the predominantly upper-motor-neuron disor-der, lathyrism [37]. Our recent studies have established BOAA as the likely proximate cause of this disease [38]. Consideration of the super-ficially similar paralytic effects of neurolathyrism and neurocycadism in grazing animals led to the search for BOAA-like compounds in cycad seed and resulted, in 1967, in the isolation of BMAA from *Cycas* spp. [39]. Like BOAA, large single doses of BMAA induced convulsive behaviour in rodents, but administration of subconvulsive doses for several weeks failed to elicit signs of motor-system disease [33]. This observation, cou-pled with the presence of rather low concentrations of BMAA in *Cycas* seed, resulted in a discontinuance of interest in the properties of this amino acid [33]. Further work on BMAA, MAM, and cycad, in relation to Western Pacific ALS/PD, was abandoned in the 1970s [13].

Recent studies with BMAA suggest this decision may have been pre-mature. For our investigations, BMAA was synthesized by the original method of Vega et al [40] and shown by various techniques (including mass spectrometry) to be the authentic compound (Fig. 12). Daily gavage of cynomolgus monkeys with very large subconvulsive oral doses of BMAA resulted in the appearance of neurological deficits after 2–12 weeks [41]. In most animals, the forelimbs were affected first, with wrist-drop, clumsiness, and difficulty picking up small objects. Muscle weak-ness and loss of muscle bulk followed. Many animals displayed unilateral or bilateral extensor hindlimb posturing, with or without leg-crossing, a primate sign linked to toxic or traumatic impairment of corticospinal function. After 1 month of BMAA administration, several animals exhib-ited a stooped posture, unkempt coat, tremor in and weakness of upper or all four extremities, and a reduction or loss of characteristic aggressive behaviour. More prolonged BMAA dosing led to periods of immobility with an expressionless face and blank stare, a crouched posture, and a bradykinetic, shuffling, bipedal gait performed with the legs flexed and the rump close to the ground. Animals (2 of 2) treated with an oral anti-parkinsonian drug showed selective recovery of marked facial movement and spontaneous activity. These clinical signs – obviously suggestive of motor-neuron, extrapyramidal, and behavioural dysfunction – were accompanied by conduction deficits in the principal motor pathway and by neuropathological evidence of chromatolytic and degenerative changes (but not loss) principally of Betz cells and smaller pyramidal neurons in the motor cortex and, to a lesser degree, of a few large motor neurons in the anterior spinal cord (Figs. 14, 15). A single animal maintained for 13 weeks on BMAA showed isolated neuritic swellings in the pars compacta of the substantia nigra [13]. Otherwise, the basal ganglia, hippocampus, and cerebellum of all sampled animals were similar to those of controls. In summary, therefore, there was a hierarchy of neuronal vulnerability to BMAA: viz. Betz cell (most affected), anterior horn cell, substantia nigra, and hippocampus (detectably unchanged). Subsequent studies have demonstrated BMAA in serum and cerebrospinal fluid of macaques treated orally with the compound [34].

While this constellation of clinical, electrophysiological, and neuro-pathological findings in animals receiving BMAA is potentially highly relevant to the etiology of Western Pacific ALS/PD, the findings are considered to be insufficient to refer at present to the primate disorder as a model of the human disease. We will only use this appellation if and when BMAA in isolation or in combination with other cycad chemicals (or other pertinent environmental agents) elicits in primates evidence of motor neuron loss, pyramidal-tract degeneration, and denervation atrophy of muscle, coupled with clear-cut compromise of selected regions of basal ganglia. Nevertheless, the possibility that BMAA plays a role in the occurrence of ALS/PD has encouraged study of its site of action and mechanisms of selective neuronal compromise.

Site of Action of BMAA

The primate motor-system neurotoxicity of BMAA was predicted from the observation in macaques that subconvulsive doses of BOAA elicited corticomotoneuronal dysfunction with hindlimb extensor posturing [38] and from the superficially similar stereospecific neuronotoxic actions of BOAA and BMAA in mouse CNS explants [42, 43]. Micromolar concentrations of both compounds rapidly induced post-synaptic dendritic vacuolation and dense neuronal changes comparable to those seen with

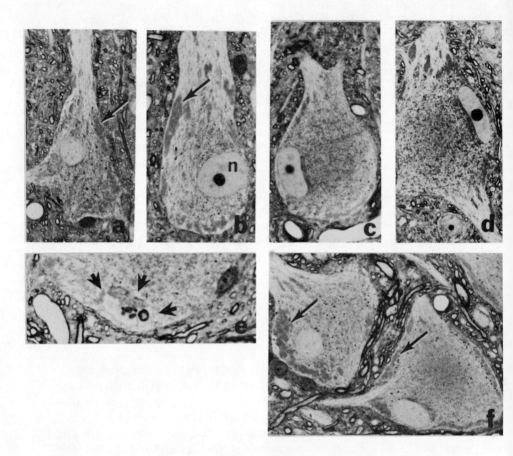

Figure 14. Motor cortex (a through e) and lumbar spinal cord (f) of *Macaca fascicularis* with prominent clinical signs of BMAA-induced motor-system disease. a: Early chromatolysis of pyramid-shaped Betz cell, with partial peripheral displacement of Nissl substance (arrow). b: Later chromatolysis with globular enlargement of perikaryon and apical dendrite (clear spaces correspond to increased neurofilaments) and peripheral displacement of nucleus (n). c: Advanced chromatolysis showing a markedly eccentric nucleus in a globular perikaryon. d: Extreme chromatolysis with increased density of perikaryal cytoplasm (corresponding to numerous mitochondria and multivesicular, vacuolar, and dense bodies). e: Large intranuclear body (arrowheads) in chromatolytic Betz cell perikaryon. f: Severe chromatolysis of a pair of anterior horn cells with partial peripheral displacement of Nissl substance (arrows). Toluidine-blue-stained one-micrometre epoxy-sections of tissues fixed by whole-body perfusion with phosphate-buffered 5% glutaraldehyde and post-fixed with 2% Dalton's chrome osmium tetroxide. a–d: ×200. e and f: ×250. Reproduced with permission from Spencer et al 1987 [41].

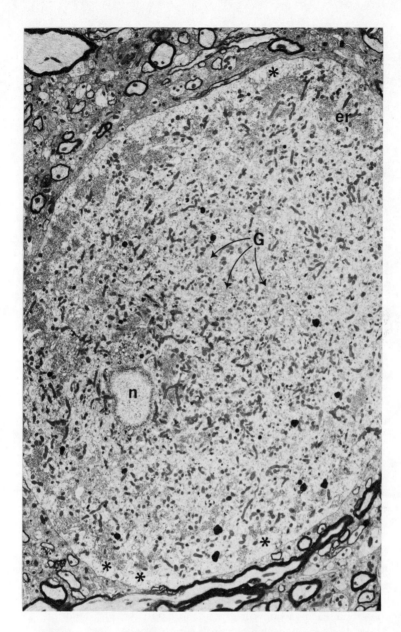

Figure 15. Motor cortex (leg region) of a severely affected macaque after oral dosing with BMAA. Note eccentrically placed nucleus (n) peripherally laden with nuclear pores, circumferentially distributed ribosome-studded endoplasmic reticulum (er), large amounts of Golgi (G), and edematous patches (*) located beneath the neuronal plasma membrane. These are unlikely to be artefactual since the quality of tissue preservation is very high. Transmission electron micrograph of a thin epoxy section stained with alcoholic uranyl acetate and aqueous lead citrate. ×2900.

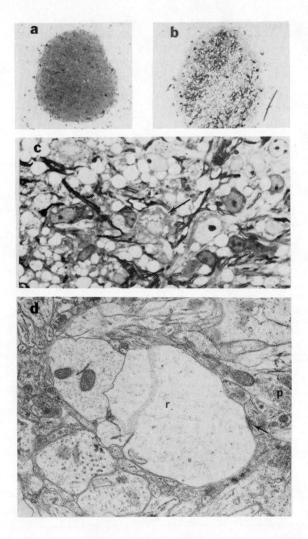

Figure 16. Mouse spinal cord *in vitro*. a: Low magnification of control ventral cord culture. ×96. b: Same magnification, following exposure to BOAA for 1 hour. Note patchwork of vacuoles. c: Higher magnification of BOAA-treated ventral cord culture showing numerous small, rounded, clear edematous vacuoles in the neuropil. Each vacuole corresponds to a post-synaptic dendritic swelling. Arrow denotes a neuronal perikaryon with several intracytoplasmic vacuoles. ×760. a–c: Toluidine-blue-stained one-micrometre epoxy-sections of tissues fixed in Millonig's-buffered 2.5% glutaraldehyde and post-fixed with Millonig's-buffered 1% osmium tetroxide. d: Transmission electron micrograph of dorsal cord explant treated with BMAA for 3 hours shows a grossly edematous post-synaptic structure (r). Presynaptic structures (p) and synaptic clefts (e.g., at arrow) are preserved. ×9600. Thin epoxy section stained with alcoholic uranyl acetate and aqueous lead citrate. Reproduced with permission from Nunn et al 1987 [42].

GLUTAMATE
ASPARTATE

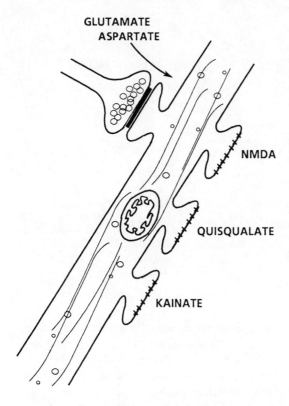

NMDA

QUISQUALATE

KAINATE

Figure 17. Crude representation of axo-dendritic synapse employing glutamate or aspartate as excitatory neurotransmitter, with additional synaptic glutamate-receptor sites responding preferentially to N-methyl-D-aspartate (NMDA), quisqualate, or kainate. Under normal circumstances, neurotransmitter is released presynaptically to activate one or more post-synaptic receptors and to depolarize the dendritic membrane. However, in the presence of potent excitotoxic amino acids (such as BOAA), there is sustained depolarization which is believed to lead to energy failure resulting in the accumulation of fluid in large, post-synaptic swellings (see Fig. 16d). Affected neurons commonly undergo degeneration. Pharmacological and electrophysiological studies demonstrate that BOAA is a direct-acting quisqualate agonist [44], while BMAA reproduces the pattern of discharge induced by BMAA and appears to act directly on the NMDA-receptor complex (C. Allen, personal communication).

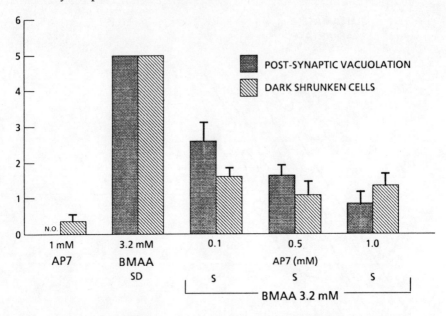

Figure 18. Concentration-dependent inhibition of acute BMAA-induced neuronotoxicity by pretreatment with AP7. Positive control, BMAA, and negative control, AP7, are illustrated on the left. Explants treated with AP7 alone were indistinguishable from untreated cultures. N.O., not observed; S, post-synaptic vacuolation restricted to the superficial layers of the cortex; SD, superficial and deep layers of the cortex. Five to ten explants were used to collect data for each concentration point. Reproduced with permission from Ross et al, 1987 [44].

potent glutamate analogues such as kainate (Figs. 16, 17). BMAA was less potent and slower-acting than equimolar concentrations of BOAA, and the differential neuronotoxic (excitotoxic) actions of these compounds could be delineated by pretreatment of the explant with drugs active at the glutamate receptor subtypes [44]. Glutamate receptors have been classified into three subtypes, based on the depolarizing neuronal membrane response initiated by selective agonists (Fig. 17). Whereas the neuronotoxic action of BMAA was concentration-dependently attenuated by 2-amino-7-phosphonoheptanoic acid (AP7) (Fig. 18), a selective antagonist for the N-methyl-D-aspartate (NMDA) receptor, BOAA neuronotoxicity was similarly impaired by pretreatment with piperidine dicarboxylic acid (PDA), a non-specific antagonist that blocks the action of the excitotoxic amino acids kainate and quisqualate [44]. Additional studies with mouse cortical explants demonstrated modulation of NMDA and

BMAA (but not BOAA) neurotoxicity by glycine and magnesium (S. Ross et al, unpublished data), and blockade of the neuronotoxicity of the methylated amino acids by pretreatment of the CNS explant with MK-801 [41], a potent blocker of the NMDA-associated ion channel. These data suggested the neurotoxic action of BMAA (or a metabolite) was mediated directly or indirectly via the NMDA receptor complex.

Comparable observations were made by measuring in young CD-1 mice changes in the duration of hyperexcitability induced by BMAA or BOAA administered by intracerebroventricular (icv) microinjection (45). BMAA caused a transient hyperexcitable state followed by long-lasting whole-body shaking and wobbling. Pretreatment of mice icv with AP7 provided complete protection against this BMAA-induced behaviour. AP7 also showed a non-significant trend for protection of the early, transient hyperexcitable state caused by injection of BMAA. By contrast, PDA had no effect on BMAA-induced hyperexcitability, although this drug was dose-dependently active in attenuating the seizuregenic responses triggered by administration of BOAA icv [45]. These results confirmed the differential acute neurotoxic actions of BOAA and BMAA, as well as suggesting once again that the acute neurotoxic action of BMAA (or a metabolite) was mediated directly or indirectly via the NMDA receptor complex.

These neuropharmacological studies have been supplemented and extended by measuring electrophysiologically the time-course and patterns of depolarization of synaptically interconnected mouse hippocampal cells grown in primary cell culture (C. Allen et al, unpublished data). Voltage-clamp recordings made using the whole-cell configuration of the patch-clamp technique have shown similar waveforms of currents activated by BOAA and quisqualate. In comparable studies, pressure injection onto the cell surface of either NMDA or BMAA in a solution elicited similar patterns of depolarization. Under the same conditions, both the NMDA and the BMAA currents were blocked by APV (Fig. 19). Taken in concert, therefore, these studies suggest that, whereas BOAA preferentially and reversibly binds to the quisqualate receptor, BMAA acts in its parent form at a site possibly associated with the NMDA complex.

Although the different neuronal receptors targeted by BOAA and BMAA may be etiologically linked to the distinct patterns of neuronal vulnerability in human lathyrism (cortical motor neuron) and Western Pacific ALS (upper and lower motor neurons, substantia nigra, and hippocampus), the two motor-system disorders show another clinical distinction that appears to be cardinally important to an understanding of their underlying pathogeneses: whereas lathyrism is a largely *self-limiting* disorder that appears subacutely in individuals who consume excessive

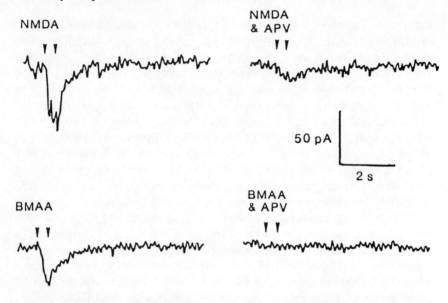

Figure 19. Voltage-clamp recordings from cultured hippocampal neurons (6–14 days in culture) made using the whole-cell configuration of the patch-clamp technique. Currents activated by NMDA and BMAA (500 micromolar) are both blocked by the selective NMDA-antagonist APV. Reproduced by permission of Dr C.N. Allen.

amounts of BOAA-containing grass for several months, ALS/PD is likely to be a long-latency neurotoxic disorder which is triggered years or decades prior to the clinical appearance of a *progressive* disease. Since the onset of Western Pacific ALS in teenagers cannot be explained by concurrence of toxic damage to motor neurons and age-related attrition of the same cellular population, it seems likely that cycads contain factors which are able to penetrate neurons and to establish irreversible changes that trigger their progressive downfall. Since changes of this type are unlikely to be mediated via the cell surface, it will be important to determine whether BMAA or other cycad toxins are able to enter selected neurons and interfere with a cellular function that is critical for long-term neuronal survival.

Conclusion

Western Pacific ALS/PD is associated with oral or percutaneous exposure to untreated *Cycas* seed kernel in all three geographic regions where the disease has been demonstrated to occur in high incidence. *Cycas* spp.

elicit a poorly defined locomotor disorder in grazing animals, although the culpable neurotoxic agent has yet to be identified. At least two compounds with differential neurotoxic properties have been previously isolated from *Cycas* seed: BMAA and MAM; others may exist and additional neurotoxic compounds may form endogenously from the interaction of physiological fluids with cycad components such as MAM. MAM is a proven experimental hepatotoxin, carcinogen, and neuroteratogen: the compound arrests rodent cerebellar neuronal migration and mitosis during development, and multinucleated and displaced neurons in some cases of ALS/PD may represent a biological marker of early exposure to this compound. BMAA is a weak excitant neurotoxin in rats, a neurotoxin in mouse cord and cortex explants, and neuropharmacological and neurophysiological studies indicate the depolarizing, excitotoxic, and neuronotoxic actions of BMAA are possibly mediated directly or indirectly by the NMDA-receptor complex. While BMAA produces an interesting constellation of motor-neuron, extrapyramidal, and behavioural dysfunction in cynomolgus monkeys repeatedly fed huge subconvulsive oral doses of the pure (99%) authentic compound, insufficient neuropathological changes have been generated to merit description of the primate response as an animal model of Western Pacific ALS/PD. We are at present studying the role of BMAA, MAM, and other factors in the etiology of this important disorder. Epidemiological studies and other evidence strongly suggest that human exposure to cycad toxins may precede by years or decades the onset of clinical ALS or PD, the nature of the clinical disease possibly being determined by dose and host susceptibility. The mechanism underlying the proposed long-latency adverse effects of cycad exposure is believed to represent the single most important question in elucidating the pathogenesis of this neurodegenerative disorder. An understanding of the chemical factors that trigger the Western Pacific motor-system disease is expected to lead to the identification in other environments of comparable chemical factors. Thus, experience with this disease demonstrates the rationality of searching for exogenous or endogenous chemical factors that might have a role in triggering some forms of motor neuron disease, parkinsonism, and even presenile dementia. A search of this type should not be restricted to chemical components in plants used for medicine or food but take into account the wider potential for chemical exposure associated with the occupational and general environment.

Acknowledgments

The authors thank Richard Robertson, Mary Seelig, Joseph Ragusa, and Linda Baboukis for expert technical assistance, and Monica Fenton for assistance in the preparation of this manuscript. This study was supported by US Public Health Service grant NS19611.

References

1 Garruto RM, Yase Y. Neurodegenerative disorders of the Western Pacific: The search for mechanisms of pathogenesis. Trends Neurosci 1986;9:368–374

2 Elizan TS, Hirano A, Abrams BM, et al. Amyotrophic lateral sclerosis and parkinsonism-dementia complex on Guam. Neurological reevaluation. Arch Neurol 1966;14:356–368

3 Gajdusek DC. Motor-neuron disease in natives of New Guinea. New Eng J Med 1963;268:474–476

4 Yase Y. Neurologic disease in the Western Pacific islands, with a report on the focus of amyotrophic lateral sclerosis found in the Kii Pensinsula, Japan. Am J Trop Med 1970;19:155–166

5 Garruto RM, Yanigahara R, Gajdusek DC. Disappearance of high-incidence amyotrophic lateral sclerosis and parkinsonism-dementia on Guam. Neurology 1985;35:193–198

6 Rodgers-Johnson P, Garruto RM, Yanagihara R, et al. Amyotrophic lateral sclerosis and parkinsonism-dementia on Guam: A 30-year evaluation of clinical and neuropathological trends. Neurology 1986;36:7–13

7 Spencer PS, Palmer V, Herman A, Asmedi A. Cycad use and motor neurone disease in Irian Jaya. Lancet 1987;ii:1273–1274

8 Hirano A, Malamud N, Kurland LT. Parkinsonism-dementia complex, an endemic disease on the island of Guam. II. Pathological features. Brain 1958;84:622–679

9 Shiraki H, Yase Y. ALS in Japan. In: Vinken PJ, Bruyn GW, eds. Handbook of Clinical Neurology, Vol 22. Systems Disorders and Atrophy, Part 2. New York, American Elsevier, 1975;353–419

10 Chen K-M, Yase Y. Parkinsonism-dementia, neurofibrillary tangles, and trace elements in the Western Pacific. In: Hutton JT, Kenny AD, eds. Senile Dementia of the Alzheimer Type. New York, Alan R Liss, 1985:153–173

11 Zolan WJ, Ellis-Neill L. Concentrations of aluminum, manganese, iron and calcium in four southern Guam rivers. University of Guam, Aganna Technical Report No. 64, June 1986

12 Reed D, Labarthe D, Chen K-M, Stallones R. A cohort study of amyotrophic lateral sclerosis and parkinsonism-dementia on Guam and Rota. Am J Epidemiol 1987;125:92–100

13 Spencer PS. Guam ALS/parkinsonism-dementia: A long-latency neurotoxic disorder caused by 'slow toxin(s)' in food? Can J Neurol Sci 1987;14:345–357

14 Whiting MG. Toxicity of cycads. Econ Bot 1963;17:271–302

15 Kurland LT. An appraisal of the neurotoxicity of cycad and the etiology of amyotrophic lateral sclerosis on Guam. Fed Proc 1972;31:1540–1542

16 Whiting MG. Toxicity of Cycads: Implications for Neurodegenerative Diseases and Cancer. Transcripts of Four Cycad Conferences. New York, Third World Medical Research Foundation, 1988. *See also* Proceedings of the Third Conference on the Toxicity of Cycads. Fed Proc 1964;23:1337–1387. Sixth International Cycad Conference. Fed Proc 1972;31:1465–1538

17 Thieret JW. Economic botany of cycads. Econ Bot 1958;12:3–41

18 Hall WTK, McGavin MD. Clinical and neuropathological changes in cattle eating the leaves of *Macrozamia lucida* or *Bowenia serrulata* (family: Zamiaceae). Path Vet 1968;5:26–34

19 Hooper PT. Cycad poisoning. In: Keeler RF, Tu AT, eds, Handbook of Natural Toxins. I. Plant and Fungal Toxins. New York, Dekker Marcell, 1983;463

20 Yasuda N, Kono I, Shimizu T, et al. Pathological studies on poisoning of grazing cattle due to ingestion of cycad, *Cycas revoluta* Thunb. The lesions and their distribution in the spinal cord. Kagoshima U Bull Agric Arts & Sci 1984;34:131–137

21 Krooth RS, Macklin MT, Hilbish TF. Diaphysial aclasis (multiple exostoses) on Guam. Am J Human Genet 1961;13:340–347

22 Fullmer HM, Siedler HD, Krooth RS, Kurland LT. A cutaneous disorder of connective tissue in amyotrophic lateral sclerosis. A histochemical study. Neurology 1960;10:707–724

23 Dastur DK. Cycad toxicity in monkeys: Clinical, pathological and biochemical aspects. Fed Proc 1964;23:1368–1369

24 O'Gara RW, Brown JM, Whiting MG. Induction of hepatic and renal tumors by topical application of aqueous extract of cycad nut to artificial skin ulcers in mice. Fed Proc 1972;31:1383

25 Spencer PS, Palmer V, Ohta M, Herman A. Cycad, a suspect etiological factor for Guam ALS/PD, is associated with motor neuron disease in Irian Jaya, Indonesia, and Kii Peninsula, Japan. In: Tsubaki T, Yase Y, eds. Amyotrophic Lateral Sclerosis. Amsterdam, Elsevier Science Publishers, 1988;35–40

26 Spencer PS, Ohta M, Palmer V. Cycad use and motor neurone disease in Kii Pensinsula of Japan. Lancet 1987;ii:1462–1463

27 Spencer PS. Western Pacific ALS/parkinsonism-dementia: A model of neuronal aging triggered by environmental toxins. In: Calne DB, et al, eds. Parkinsonism and Aging. New York, Raven Press 1989;133–153

28 Kondo K, Tsubaki T, Sakamoto F. The Ryukyuan muscular atrophy. An obscure hereditable neuromuscular disease found in the islands of southern Japan. J Neurol Sci 1970;11:359–382

29 Calne DB, Eisen A, McGeer E, Spencer PS. Alzheimer's disease, Parkinson's disease, and motoneurone disease: Abiotrophic interaction between ageing and environment? Lancet 1986;ii:1067–1070

30 Yase Y. The pathogenesis of amyotrophic lateral sclerosis. Lancet 1972;ii:292–296

31 Jones M, Yang M, Mickelsen O. Effects of methylazoxymethanol glucoside and methylazoxymethanol acetate on the cerebellum of the postnatal Swiss albino mouse. Fed Proc 1972;31:1508–1511

32 Garruto RM, Gajdusek DC, Chen K-M. Amyotrophic lateral sclerosis among Chamorro migrants from Guam. Ann Neurol 1980;8:612–619

33 Polsky FI, Nunn PB, Bell EA. Distribution and toxicity of α-amino-β-methylaminopropionic acid. Fed Proc 1972;31:1473–1475

34 Kisby GE, Roy DN, Spencer PS. Determination of β-N-methylamino-L-alanine (BMAA) in plant (Cycas circinalis L.) and animal tissue by precolumn derivitization with 9-fluorenylmethyl chloroformate (FMOC) and reversed-phase high performance liquid chromatography. J Neurosci Methods 1988;26:45–54

35 Laqueur GL, Matsumoto H. Neoplasms in female Fischer rats following intraperitoneal injection of methylazoxymethanol. J. Natl Cancer Inst 1966;37:217

36 Roy DN. Toxic amino acids and proteins from Lathyrus plants and other leguminous species: A literature review. Nutr Abst & Rev: Ser A 1981;51:691–707

37 Ludolph AC, Hugon J, Dwivedi MP, Schaumburg HH, Spencer PS. Studies on the aetiology and pathogenesis of motor neuron diseases. 1. Lathyrism: Clinical findings in established cases. Brain 1987;110:149–165

38 Spencer PS, Roy DN, Ludolph A, Hugon J, Dwivedi MP, Schaumburg HH. Lathyrism: Evidence for the role of neuroexcitatory amino acid BOAA. Lancet 1986;ii:1066–1067

39 Bell EA, Vega A, Nunn PB. A neurotoxic amino acid in seeds of Cycas circinalis. In: Whiting MG, ed. Toxicity of Cycads: Implications for Neurodegenerative Diseases and Cancer. Transcripts of Four Conferences. Fifth Conference 1967;XI-1–XI-7. New York, Third World Medical Research Foundation, 1988

40 Vega A, Bell EA, Nunn PB. The preparation of L- and D-alpha-amino-beta-methylaminopropionic acids and the identification of the compound isolated from Cycas circinalis as the L-isomer. Phytochem 1968;7:1885–1887

41 Spencer PS, Nunn PB, Hugon J et al. Guam amyotrophic lateral sclerosis–parkinsonism-dementia linked to a plant excitant neurotoxin. Science 1987;237:517–522

42 Nunn PB, Seelig M, Spencer PS. Stereospecific acute neuronotoxicity of

'uncommon' plant amino acids linked to human motor-system diseases. Brain Res 1987;410:375–379

43 Spencer PS, Hugon J, Ludolph A, Nunn PB, Ross SM, Roy DN, Schaumburg HH. Discovery and partial characterization of primate motor-system toxins. In: Bock G, O'Connor M, eds. Selective Neuronal Death. Chichester, Wiley (Ciba Foundation Symposium), 1987;221–238

44 Ross SM, Seelig M, Spencer PS. Specific antagonism of excitotoxic action of 'uncommon' amino acids assayed organotypic mouse cortical cultures. Brain Res 1987;425:120–127

45 Ross SM, Spencer PS. Specific antagonism of behavioral action of 'uncommon' amino acids linked to motor-system diseases. Synapse 1987;1:248–253

46 Morgan RW, Hoffmann GR. Cycasin and its mutagenic metabolites. Mutation Res 1983;114:19–58

47 Feinberg A, Zedeck MS. Production of highly reactive alkylating agent from the organospecific carcinogen methylazoxymethanol by alcohol dehydrogenase. Cancer Res 1980;40:4446–4450

Latent Neuro-abiotrophies:
A Clue to Amyotrophic Lateral Sclerosis

ANDREW A. EISEN AND DONALD B. CALNE

In this chapter we shall expand upon a recent hypothesis proposing that ALS and other abiotrophies result from the interaction of prior exposure to nutritional, infective, or other environmental agents and normal ageing [1, 2]. Several conditions are now recognized in which considerable evidence for this hypothesis has accumulated (Table 1); others may surface. These conditions are characterized by progessive degeneration of functionally related cells (abiotrophy) and become clinically overt in later life. A prerequisite for the hypothesis is that attrition of the neuronal populations in question is relatively linear or, more likely, exponential over time (Fig. 1). In addition it should be possible to demonstrate evidence for prior toxicity before the disease is recognized clinically.

Normal Ageing

Much of the evidence indicating that a given cell population declines steadily over life, rather than undergoing rapid attrition in old age, is indirect. Actual cell counts, for example, from the zona compacta of the substantia nigra or anterior horn cells in the spinal cord are diffficult to obtain in sufficient numbers to be statistically relevant. Some neuronal populations, for example those in the cortex, the motor neurons of the external ocular muscles, and the cells of the facial nucleus, have a fairly normal complement until late in life [2]. Others, however, and in particular those relevant to the present discussion, namely the cells of the substantia nigra and anterior horn cells as well as those of the medical basal forebrain, do appear to fall out in a linear fashion throughout life. In these, maturation and senescene appear to be in continuum (Fig. 1).

TABLE 1
Age-related abiotrophies due to prior environmental influences

Disease	Environmental influence
Guamanian ALS/PD	Cycad ingestion (BMAA) + low dietary Ca
MPTP-induced parkinsonism	MPTP contamination
Post-polio syndrome	Viral + anterior horn cell overload
Post-encephalitic parkinsonism	Viral + nigrostriatal neuronal overload
Pugilistic encephalopathy	Trauma
Lathyrism	BOAA toxicity

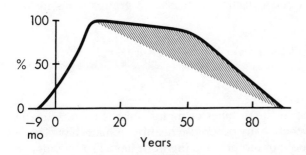

Figure 1. Neuronal ageing and cell attrition could occur predominantly in later life at which time cell loss would be marked (solid thick line). Alternatively cellular maturation and attrition might form a continuum (shaded area). This is probably the case for anterior horn cells and nigrostriatal neurons. If, for example, at the age of 20 there was exposure to an environmental toxin the regression line reflecting cell attrition would be lower and result in early demise.

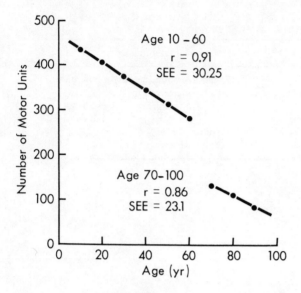

Figure 2. Physiological motor unit estimates indicate a steady attrition of anterior horn cells throughout life. The data are derived from a variety of different studies [3, 4, 5, 7].

Evidence supporting a linear decline of these cell groups is briefly reviewed below.

Age-Related Changes of the Lower Motor Neuron

Motor Units

The age-related decline in the number of motor units is most dramatic by the age of 60 years when many otherwise healthy humans have fewer than one-half of the quota of motor units in youth have [3–6]. Evidence for this comes mainly from electrophysiological estimates using the McComas technique of incremental stimulation [4, 5, 7] or modifications thereof [3, 8]. These studies indicate that loss over an average life span is linear (Fig. 2). Over the first six decades the loss is steady but modest; thereafter attrition is much steeper and by the age of 70 there may be a motor unit loss in excess of 25% of that at age 20 [9]. Anatomical counts of human motor units in relation to age, although rare, also indicate a steady decline from the second decade onwards [1]. A similar age-related reduction in motor units has been documented in rodents, where physiological and motor unit counting can be applied more directly [10–12] and accurately and can be related to morphological changes of muscle fibres which show gradual adaptive conversion of Type II 'fast twitch' to Type I 'slow twitch' fibres [13, 14]. These findings have recently been confirmed in man using a method developed for studying whole human muscle in cross-section [15, 16]. This technique has shown that whole-muscle 'hypotrophy' typical of old age is due to muscle fibre loss rather than, as previously suggested, to reduction in size of individual muscle fibres [17].

Ongoing re-innervation, by collateral or terminal sprouting, and muscle hypertrophy normally compensate for motor unit and muscle fibre loss [17, 18] so that atrophy and weakness may not be apparent until there has been a loss of between 30% and 90% of motor units [3, 5]. The factors limiting these important compensatory mechanisms, which are continually in force throughout life, remain unclear. These changes are reflected in age-related increases in the duration and amplitude of motor unit potentials [19] as well as fibre density as measured using single fibre electromyography [20] (Fig. 3).

Neuromuscular Junction

The neuromuscular junctional apparatus is dynamic, undergoing re-modelling throughout life. There is a continual sprouting and withdrawal of terminal axons, possibly related to function [21]. This balance changes with age and the pre- and post-synaptic remodelling shifts in favour of denervation with increasing age [22, 23]. In older subjects the number and length of preterminal axons increase and the end plate has a greater number of smaller acetylcholine receptors than in younger persons [24]. These characteristics change linearly with age (Fig. 4).

Nerve

Peripheral nerve shows morphological changes with age. Total axon populations, but not axonal diameter or myelin thickness, decrease with age. This is also true of the optic nerve [25]. There is an age-related slowing of both motor and sensory conduction velocities which is linear so that conduction velocity decreases between 5 and 10 m/sec between the third and seventh decades [26–30] (Fig. 5).

Muscle

Decreased muscle mass and strength are prominent features of ageing [31]. Ageing muscle has a reduced number of muscle fibres [32], affecting preferentially Type II fibres [15, 16]. This could explain the increased

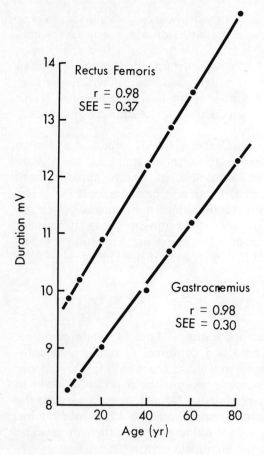

Figure 3. Motor unit duration. The regression lines indicate a linear increase in motor unit potential duration for the rectus femoris and gastrocnemius muscles with increase in age. Data derived from ref. 19.

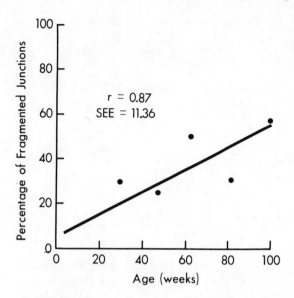

Figure 4. Age-related changes in rat soleus neuromuscular junction. The junction becomes more complex with age. The changes occur in a linear fashion from birth onwards [see 21, 22].

contraction time characteristic of elderly human muscle [31]. An alternative explanation for the latter observation would be a uniform loss of fibres accompanied by progressive slowing of the twitch with age. The reduction in the number of muscle fibres, although accompanied by fibre hypertrophy, is unable to compensate for the decreased functional capacity of the ageing muscle. This is partly due to the reduction in fibre length and sarcomere number that goes hand in hand with the reduction in the number of muscle fibres. These changes in muscle fibres occur in a linear fashion, commencing early in life but becoming considerably more exaggerated from the sixth decade onwards.

In summary, then, there is good evidence to indicate that all components of the lower motor neuron change over a life span and that these changes are for the most part linear although certainly the fastest change occurs after the age of 60.

Nigrostriatal Ageing

Deterioration in the integrity of the nigrostriatal pathway, as measured by a variety of indices, has been recently reviewed, the conclusion being

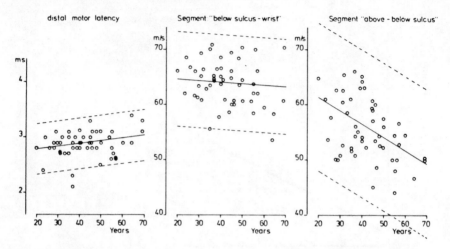

Figure 5. Conduction velocity and distal latency slow and increase respectively with age (modified from ref. 30). In the left panel the distal ulnar nerve motor latency measured in msec increases linearly with age. Middle and right panels are ulnar nerve motor conduction velocities (m/sec) measured from below the elbow to wrist and across the elbow respectively. Both show linear slowing with age.

that steady attrition occurs in the course of ageing, the rate of which is increased in the elderly [33]. The most convincing evidence is derived from morphometric studies showing attrition of nigral neurons that is directly proportional to age [34]. There is an approximate decline in the number of neurons of 1.4% per decade up to the age of 65; thereafter this exceeds 11% per decade[35].

Alteration of enzyme content of the nigrostriatal system is an indirect reflection of its cell count. Tyrosine hydroxylase and dopa decarboxylase levels have been shown to decline throughout life, apparently rather precipitously over the first two decades [34, 36]. In contrast, dopamine concentrations seem to remain relatively stable until the age of 60, and thereafter a dramatic decrease occurs [37].

Post-mortem studies [38] and *in vivo* measurements using positron emission tomography [39] of dopamine receptors have also shown a somewhat linear fall in spiperone binding and methylspiperone striatal binding, respectively. However, given that some dopamine receptors are post-synaptic and some are presynaptic, it is difficult to infer accurately changes in nigral neuron counts from measurements of receptors.

Evidence of Subclinical Lesions in the Abiotrophies – The ALS/PD Complex

A prerequisite for the hypothesis is documentation of pathology some-time before a specific clinical syndrome becomes recognizable. Below are described a number of such conditions and the evidence for early, pre-clinical, lesions.

The Cycad Hypothesis

Evidence derived from toxicological and epidemiological studies can be cited in favour of the ALS/PD complex of Guam being due to environ-mental agent(s). Until the mid-1960s Guam shared with the Kii Peninsula of Japan and western New Guinea a prevalence of ALS that was about 100 times that of the rest of the world. The incidence, in Guam, has dropped dramatically since then so that today it is the same as or even lower than elsewhere [40]. Furthermore, the typical slight predominance of affected males compared to females, seen in the Western world, has steadily reversed on Guam and now men and woman are affected about equally [40]. The reduced incidence of ALS-PD on Guam began in the mid-1960s some 20 years after the end of the World War II when Western foods began to be imported in plenty, coinciding with the steadily re-duced ingestion of cycad.

The long time interval between reduced use of cycad flour on Guam (about 1940) and the dramatic decrease in incidence of ALS/PD (1960) is in keeping with the concept of prior exposure to a long-latency toxin [42]. It has long been suggested that Guamanian ALS/PD is due to in-toxication from ingestion of the cycad seed (*Cycas circinalis*). As early as the 1880s the native Chamorros of Guam, descendants of migrants from the Malay Archipelago, had used the cycad seed to prepare flour from which 'fadang,' a type of tortilla, was made. This became a dietary staple and during the Japanese occupation of Guam during the Second World War its use predominated in the southern villages of Umatac and Merizo. These were the villages in which later ALS/PD had the highest incidence. For a time the inhabitants had been cut off from other food supplies and fadang was used in excess. It is of interest that the Japanese occupation forces must have had knowledge of the potential danger of cycad, or they did not find fadang palatable; in any event ALS/PD among Japanese soldiers was rare.

The Chamorros recognized acute toxicity resulting from ingestion of unwashed cycad. Before the cycad nut was ground into flour for preparing the fadang, it was washed in water for several days. The nut was deemed safe if chickens fed the absorbent water survived. The extent of washing varied, ranging from a few days to a week or two, this being determined by custom of a particular family. Not surprisingly, some families had a much higher incidence of ALS/PD than others, which erroneously led to the assumption that the disease was genetically determined.

The cycad hypothesis was originally proposed by Dr. Marjorie Whiting [43] and Dr Leonard Kurland [44]. The toxic ingredient was considered to be methylazoxymethanol (MAM). However, although toxic and carcinogenic, this substance at best induces a cerebellar syndrome in animals quite unlike that of ALS/PD [45, 46]. As a result the cycad hypothesis lost appeal, although Kurkland and Mulder [see 47, 48] remained convinced that the cycad plant was very relevant in the etiology of Guamanian ALS/PD.

Recently, the role of cycad has once more become central to the issue of ALS-PD on Guam mainly as a result of the efforts of Spencer (see the previous chapter in this volume). It was appreciated that the cycad nut contains α-amino-β-methylaminopropionic acid (BMAA), an amino acid closely related to α-amino-β-oxalylaminopropionic acid (BOAA). This latter substance is found in the seeds of *Lathyrus sativus*, consumption of which produces a chronic motor system disease characterized by progressive spastic paraparesis, lathyrism (*vide infra*). In 1981 Spencer and Schaumburg (see Spencer et al, this volume), recognized the relationship between BOAA and BMAA and the motor system syndromes for which they might be responsible. Primate models were subsequently developed [49–51].

The Calcium Deficiency Hypothesis

Attractive as the cycad hypothesis might be, and in particular the role of BMAA, it appears that the story on Guam may be more complicated. In 1972 Yase [52] and later Gajdusek and colleagues [53] proposed that Guamanian ALS/PD was due to mineral deficiency and resulting metal intoxication. It was argued that calcium and magnesium concentrations of Guamanian drinking water were low. This resulted in a state of early age, chronic hyperparathyroidism. Higher than normal levels of hydroxy-vitamin D occurred with deposition of calcium in neurons as hydroxyapatite [54]. Disruption of the neuronal cytoskeleton induced excessive neurofilament production and accumulation in turn initiated production of neurofibrillary tangles so characteristic of Guamanian ALS/PD [55]. Disturbance of axoplasmic flow would follow and likely be responsible for the proximal axonal swelling typical of all forms of ALS

[56]. New application of wave-length spectrometry and computer-controlled electron-beam x-ray micro-analysis allows precise quantitative imaging of metal in neurons and has confirmed neuronal calcium deposition [54].

However, there are aspects of this hypothesis that are problematic [57]. Present-day concentrations of calcium and magnesium in the soil of, for example, Umatac, the village with the highest incidence of ALS/PD on Guam, are the same as or even higher than found elsewhere in Guam [58]. This does not preclude previously low concentrations. Also ALS is rarely seen in patients with overt hyperparathyroidism [59]. It may be that most patients with clinically overt hyperparathyroidism, who are usually beyond the pediatric range, are treated before there has been time for significant deposits of hydroxyapatite to occur. A recent report of a primate model developing a motor system disease after being subjected to prolonged (4 years) deficient dietary calcium supports the hypothesis [60]. It is also of interest that there has been recent evidence correlating parkinsonism with early-age exposure to rural environment and drinking well water that may be mineral deficient [61].

The cycad and mineral hypotheses are not necessarily mutually exclusive. It might be that early, childhood, mineral deficiency and its effects set the stage for later toxicity by BMAA or other toxins. One could reasonably speculate that variations in these two interacting factors might in fact be the determinant in developing Guamanian ALS rather than PD or in developing predominant upper, instead of lower, motor neuron ALS.

Migration Studies

The other important line of evidence indicating that ALS/PD of Guam is environmental derives from the study of migrants. Guamanians who spent their childhood and youth on Guam and migrated to the United States, Japan, Germany, or Korea have developed the disease 1–34 years after leaving the island [62]. A few Filipino immigrants who had lived on Guam for more than 15 years and had adopted the Chamorro lifestyle developed ALS/PD [62]. The many thousands of transients through Guam have not been at risk [42]. The long latent period is in keeping with our hypothesis of prior exposure to an environmental agent(s) and interaction with subsequent cellular ageing [2]. It is likely that those, on Guam, developing ALS, parkinsonism, or dementia in the future will have the Western variety of these diseases. We have recently seen a 54-year-old white woman who has spent many years on Guam, and indeed still lives there, who has developed classical ALS but has never ingested cycad.

Subclinical Guamanian ALS/PD

Is there evidence for Guamanian ALS/PD prior to development of overt clinical disease? We have recently studied several Guamanians using positron emission tomography (PET). Some with clinical ALS but who have neither parkinsonism nor dementia had abnormal dopa PET scans. The scans clearly indicate disordered metabolism of the basal ganglia. One would anticipate that in due course these patients will develop overt parkinsonism. By contrast, dopa scans on a few Western ALS patients have not shown abnormality in the region of the basal ganglia. These findings do not necessarily rule out an association of Western ALS with Parkinson's disease or dementia and may merely reflect the short median survival of Western ALS patients, 4 years, a time which may preclude development of either of the other diseases.

Evidence, then, would seem sufficient to suggest that ALS on Guam is due to toxicity, possibly cycad ingestion in combination with a background of calcium deficiency in early life. The latent period between exposure and clinical disease is measurable in years or often decades and is coincident with a time when attrition of anterior horn cells can no longer be compensated for by sprouting.

Previous Toxic Exposure and Western ALS

The background knowledge learned from Guamanian ALS/PD prompted us to seek evidence for early toxic exposure being responsible for Western ALS [63]. From a population base of 312 patients with a variety of motor neuron diseases, seen prospectively by one of us (A.E.) between the years 1980 and 1987, 121 fulfilled our minimal criteria of adult-onset ALS with clinical evidence of upper and lower motor neuron deficit and corroborative electrophysiological testing. Cases of spinal muscular atrophy, primary lateral sclerosis, monomelic motor neuron disease, and juvenile ALS were excluded. Seventy-two patients were seen in follow-up. These and any new referrals seen subsequent to January 1987 were specifically asked about their activities 15–30 years prior to onset of clinical symptoms. In particular they were asked to seek information regarding casual acquaintances and work-mates who may also have developed ALS after a similar time interval.

Four such pairs of patients have thus far been identified from among the 72 follow-ups (Table 2). The first pair lived on the same street for almost 3 decades, prior to their both developing ALS within 2 years of each other. The second pair, aged 32 and 36, lived on the same street for 3 years before developing ALS within 2 years of each other; both

TABLE 2
Development of ALS in patient pairs who shared a previous common environment

Sex/age at clinical onset (year)	Period of prior acquaintance	Longest possible latent period to disease (years)
M/65 (1977)	1949–79	28
F/56 (1979)		30
M/36 (1986)	1982–86	4
M/32 (1987)		5
M/56 (1980)	1959–60	21
F/63 (1986)		27
M/61 (1985)	1953–54	32
M/58 (1980)		27

were bus drivers. The third pair lived within one block of each other from 1959 to 1960. They recalled significant social interaction, but moved apart and did not meet again until after they had both developed ALS. The last pair had spent 2 years together in the Canadian navy. At that time the Canadian navy had fewer than 20,000 personnel. We have preliminary but unconfirmed evidence that the prevalence of ALS in the Canadian navy personnel who served between 1945 and 1950 may be as high as it was in Guam. We would speculate that each pair of patients shared exposure to some, as yet unidentified, environmental agent, relevant in the cause of their ALS.

One other patient in our data base was born in Indonesia and moved to Holland at the age of 3 months. When he was between 11 and 14 years old he and his family moved to western New Guinea, a high-incidence focus of ALS [16]. He developed ALS when aged only 36. It might be speculated that he was exposed to whatever is (are) the environmental agent(s) responsible for ALS in western New Guinea, and, if so, there was a latent period of about 22 years to the onset of clinical disease.

Pugilist's Encephalopathy

This is an example of a post-traumatic abiotrophy. The chronic neurological syndrome affecting professional boxers which becomes clinically apparent a few years, or more usually many years, after termination of the boxer's professional career is well recognized [64, 65]. It is characterized by progressive dementia and extrapyramidal and cerebellar signs.

There may be also be associated neuropsychiatric features manifested by amnesia, morbid jealousy, rage reactions, and psychosis.

Recently described pathological changes include neurofibrillary tangles in the absence of senile plaques involving parts of the hippocampus and mediotemporal cortex, loss of Purkinje cells on the inferior surface of the cerebellum, and degeneration of the substantia nigra [66]. Magnetic resonance imaging is at present the most sensitive method of detecting evidence of brain trauma but its use has not been reported in pugilistic encephalopathy. It remains to be determined what the time course of cellular attrition is in this syndrome, but it seems likely that cell loss subsequent to single or repeated trauma is at first steady and then subsequently becomes more rapidly progessive at a time when attrition associated with ageing becomes prominent.

Post-Polio Syndrome

It is estimated that there are approximately 300,000 patients in North America with post-polio syndrome. Symptoms usually develop insidiously 20–45 years following the initial acute illness, often after the patient has functioned normally and has been capable of considerable physical activity [67, 68; see Dalakas, this volume].

Typically weakness and sometimes pain in the form of muscle cramps occur in an extremity that was previously involved by polio though it is not uncommon for the symptoms to occur in an apparently previously normal limb. It is this involvement of a previously unaffected limb that initially raised the question of associated or newly developing ALS [11]. Recent pathological studies have shown that abnormalities are restricted to the anterior horn cells without involvement of corticospinal tracts or upper motor neurons and clearly indicate that there is no relationship to ALS [68]. In most patients the time course is quite unlike that of ALS, being slow and relatively benign with only gradual progression from the time of onset. The disease runs over a long period, often more than 10–15 years. Furthermore, although the occasional electromyographic study has demonstrated active denervation with fibrillation and positive sharp waves or runs of complex high-frequency discharges, the majority of electrophysiological studies are in keeping with chronic partial reinnervation [69, 70]. Post-polio syndrome exemplifies a disease in which functional compensation, achieved through collateral sprouting, is eventually subjected to overload and the compensatory mechanisms fail. As natural neuronal ageing and attrition are added to the previous loss of cells, the burden of responsibility of surviving anterior horn cells increases exponentially and they too fail.

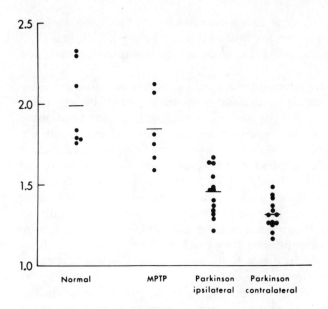

Figure 6. Putamen cerebellum activity ratios deriving from fluoro dopa PET. Compared to normal, asymptomatic subjects who were exposed to MPTP but who were clinically normal had activity lying between normal and parkinsonism.

MPTP-Induced Parkinsonism

It is now well established that 1-methyl-4-phenyl-1,2,5,6-tetrahydropyr-idine (MPTP) induces parkinsonism in both man and a variety of animals [71]. Studies using positron emission tomography (PET) have shown abnormal dopa scans in the basal ganglia of patients who received MPTP but who were clinically normal [72] (Fig. 6). It seems possible that many, if not most, of these will eventually develop parkinsonism, and they are at present being followed [73].

A primate model has recently been used to study unilateral parkin-sonism. By injecting small doses of MPTP into one carotid artery it is possible to induce unilaterally abnormal dopa PET scans in the absence of clinically overt parkinsonism [74].

Post-Encephalitic Parkinsonism

Encephalitis lethargica (Von Economo's disease) was prevalent in the early part of this century, peaking in 1920 and 1924. About a third of the patients died with the acute illness and half of the survivors were left with severe neurological or psychiatric deficits. However, about a third appeared to recover completely, some of whom subsequently developed parkinsonism [75].

There has been little information regarding the natural history of post-encephalitic parkinsonism, especially after middle life. The scant evidence mostly suggests that the parkinsonian deficit remained stationary and did not deteriorate [8, 76]. One of us (D.C.) has had an opportunity recently to evaluate 11 patients who were the sole survivors of about 300 patients originally hospitalized for von Economo's encephalitis and its sequelae between 1925 and 1935 [77]. The findings of the study clearly indicate, after a long period of stability, that there is deterioration of motor function in patients who had encephalitis lethargica in childhood or young adulthood. Progression in some was sufficiently severe to render them bedridden by the time they reached their mid-60s, which indicates that the decline in motor function exceeded that anticipated by normal ageing of the nervous system.

One explanation, akin to that pertaining to the post-polio syndrome, is late dying-back and loss of neurons which were previously capable of maintaining relatively normal function through collateral sprouting. When a critical number of additional cells is lost deterioration will be clinically obvious and might progress rather rampantly. Attrition in the nigrostriatal pathway, like that of anterior horn cells, can reach 80% before clinical features become obvious [77].

Careful analysis of this syndrome reveals that in many ways it is the nigrostriatal counterpart of the post-polio syndrome. In the initial outbreak many patients either succumbed from a devastating encephalitis or, after a transient period of obvious parkinsonism, passed into coma and death. Others recovered completely, but a group remained who developed moderate evidence of parkinsonism. They were able to maintain relatively independent daily activities until late-life, when progression of the motor deficit began.

Lathyrism

There is considerable evidence that human lathyrism, which is manifested by progressive paraparesis, results from prior ingestion of *Lathyrus sativus* (the chickling pea). The active ingredient is β-N-oxalylamino-L-alanine (BOAA). This substance is an excitotoxic amino acid [42, 49, 50]. Lathyrism is prevalent in parts of India, Bangladesh, and Ethiopia, especially during times of famine when the chickling pea becomes a dietary staple [78, 79]. A primate model of lathyrism has been developed in which animals are fed BOAA. A motor system disease, having considerable similarity to human lathyrism, results [49].

An outbreak of lathyrism was described in World War II prisoners following consumption of chickling peas [78]. Several to many years after the war when they had migrated to Israel and been followed for as long as 40 years, several developed progressive weakness after many years of apparent stability. This situation is very reminiscent of the post-polio syndrome.

We conclude that amyotrophic lateral sclerosis and other abiotrophies are the result of exposure to a variety of environmental agents years or decades prior to development of clinical symptoms. The additional component of normal cellular attrition, which is linear throughout life, eventually reaches a stage when compensatory mechanisms fail and disease becomes overt. This typically occurs after age 55 years, when the rate of cellular attrition cannot be matched by neuronal sprouting. Variations in the extent and progression of a given syndrome are probably dependent on dose and time. It cannot be assumed that a specific toxin is necessarily responsible for a given abiotrophy; it is just as likely that several environmental agents are interactive.

References

1 Calne DB, Langston JW. Aetiology of Parkinson's disease. Lancet 1983; ii:1457–1459

2 Calne DB, Eisen A, McGeer E, Spencer P. Alzheimer's disease, Parkinson's disease, and motorneurone disease: Abiotropic interaction between ageing and environment? Lancet 1986;ii:1067–1070

3 Brown WF. Functional compensation of human motor units in health and disease. J Neurol Sci 1973;20:199–209

4 McComas AJ, Fawcett PRW, Campbell MG, Sica REP. Electrophysiological estimation of the number of motor units within human muscle. J Neurol Neurosurg Psychiat 1971;34:121–131

5 McComas AJ, Sica REP, Campbell MJ, Upton ARM. Functional compensation in partially denervated muscles. J Neurol Neurosurg Psychiat 1971;34:453–460

6 Tomlinson BE, Irving D. The numbers of limb motor neurons in the human lumbosacral cord throughout life. J Neurol Sci 1977;34:213–219

7 Campbell MJ, McComas AJ, Petito F. Physiological basis of ageing muscles. J Neurol Neurosurg Psychiat 1973;36:174–182

8 Howard RS, Lees AJ. Encephalitis lethargica. A report of four recent cases. Brain 1987;110:19–33

9 Stalberg E, Hilton-Brown P, Rydin E. Capacity of the motor neuron to alter its peripheral field. In: Dimitrijevic MR, Kakulas BA, Vrbova G, eds. Recent Achievements in Restorative Neurology, 2. Progressive Neuromuscular Diseases. Basel, Karger, 1986;237–253

10 Eisen A, Karpati G, Carpenter S, Danon J. The motor unit profile of the rat soleus in experimental myopathy and reinnervation. Neurology 1974;878–884

11 Eisen A, Karpati G, Carpenter S. The motor unit profile in two experimental chronic myopathies. Neurology 1975;25:807–812

12 Peyronnard JM. An experimental evaluation of the motor unit counting technique. Can J Neurol Sci 1975;2:332

13 Caccia MR, Harris JB, Johnson MA. Morphology and physiology of skeletal muscle in ageing rodents. Muscle & Nerve 1979;2:202–212

14 Rowe RWD. The effect of senility on skeletal muscles in the mouse. Exp Gerontol 1969;4:119–126

15 Lexell J, Henriksson-Larsen K, Winblad B, Sjöström M. Distribution of different fibre types in human skeletal muscles: Effects of aging studied in whole muscle cross sections. Muscle & Nerve 1983;6:588–595

16 Lexell J, Henriksson-Larsen K, Sjostrom M. Distribution of different fibre types in human skeletal muscles. 2. A study of cross-sections of whole m. vastus lateralis. Acta Physiol Scand 1983;117:115–122

17 Jennekens FGI, Tomlinson BE, Walton JN. Histochemical aspects of five limb muscles in old age. An autopsy study. J Neurol Sci 1971;14:259–276

18 Wolfart G. Collateral regeneration from residual motor nerve fibres in ALS. Neurology 1957;7:124–134

19 Buchthal F, Rosenfalck P. Action potential parameters in different human muscles. Acta Psychiat Scand 1955;30:125–131

20 Stalberg E, Fawcett PRW. Macro EMG in healthy subjects of different ages. J Neurol Neurosurg Psychiat 1982;45:870–878

21 Cardasis CA, Padykula HA. Ultrastructural evidence indicating reorganization at the neuromuscular junction in the normal rat soleus. Anat Rec 1981;200:41–59

22 Cardasis CA, LaFontaine BA. Aging rat neuromuscular junction: A morphometric study of cholinesterase-stained whole mounts and ultrastructure. Muscle & Nerve 1987;10:200–213

23 Fagg GE, Scheff SW, Cotman CW. Axonal sprouting at the neuromuscular junction of adult and aged rats. Exp Neurol 1981;74:847–854

24 Oda K. Age changes of motor innervation and acetycholine receptor distribution on human skeletal muscle fibers. J Neurol Sci 1984;66:327–338

25 Johnson BM, Miao M, Sadun AA. Age-related decline of human optic nerve axon populations. Age 1987;10:5–9

26 Behse F, Buchthal F. Normal sensory conduction in the nerves of the leg in man. J Neurol Neurosurg Psychiat 1971;34:404–414

27 Dorfman LJ, Bosley TM. Age-related changes in peripheral and central nerve conduction in man. Neurology 1979;29:38–44

28 LaFratta CW, Canestrari RE. A comparison of sensory and motor nerve conduction velocities as related to age. Arch Phys Med Rehab 1966;47:286–290

29 Norris AH, Shock NW, Wagman IH. Age changes in maximum conduction velocity of motor fibers of human ulnar nerves J Appl Physiol 1953;5:589–593

30 Rosenfalck A, Rosenfalck P. Electromyography, sensory and motor conduction: Findings in normal subjects. Laboratory of Clinical Physiololgy, Copenhagen, 1975; publication from the Rigshospital

31 McDonagh MJN, White MJ, Davies CTM. Different effects of ageing on the mechanical properties of human arm and leg muscles. Gerontology 1984;30:49–54

32 Howard JE, McGill KC, Dorfman LJ. Age effects on properties of motor unit action potential: ADEMG analysis. Ann Neurol 1988;23 (in press)

33 Calne DB, Peppard RF. Aging of the nigrostriatal pathways in humans. Can J Neurol Sci 1987;14:424–427

34 McGeer PL, McGeer E, Suzuki JS. Aging and extrapyramidal function. Arch Neurol 1977;34:33–35

35 Mann DMA. Dopamine neurons of the vertebrate brain: Some aspects of anatomy and pathology. In: Winslow W and Markstein R, eds. The Neurobiology of Dopamine Systems. Manchester, Manchester University Press, 1984;87–103

36 Cote LJ, Kremzner LT. Biochemical changes in normal aging in human brain. In: Mayeux R and Rozen WD, eds. Advances in Neurology, Vol. 38, The Dementias. New York, Raven Press, 1983;19–30

37 Carlsson A, Nyberg P, Winblad B. The influence of age and other factors on the concentrations of monoamines in normal aging and dementia. Umea Univ Med Dissertations, Sweden, 1984;53–84

38 Severson JA, Marcusson J, Winblad B, et al. Age-correlated loss of dopaminergic binding sites in human basal ganglia. J Neurochem 1982;39:1623–1631

39 Wong DF, Wagner HN Jr, Dannals RF, et al. Effects of age on dopamine and serotonin receptors measured by positron tomography in the living human brain. Science 1984;226:1393–1396

40 Garruto, RM, Yanagihara R, Gajdusek DC. Disappearance of high-incidence

amyotrophic lateral sclerosis and parkinsonian-dementia on Guam. Neurology 1985;35:193–198

41 Reed D, Labarthe D, Chen K-M, Stallones R. A cohort study of amyotrophic lateral sclerosis and parkinsonism-dementia on Guam and Rota. Am J Epidemiol 1987;125:92–100

42 Spencer PS. Guam ALS/parkinsonism-dementia: A long latency neurotoxic disorder caused by 'slow toxin(s)' in food. Can J Neurol Sci 1987;14:347–357

43 Whiting MG. Toxicity of cycads. Econ Bot 1963;17:271

44 Kurland LT. An appraisal of the neurotoxicity of cycad and the etiology of amyotrophic lateral sclerosis on Guam. Sixth Internat Cycad Conf, Chicago. Fed Proc 1972;31:1540–1542

45 Hirano A, Jones M. Fine Structure of cycasin-induced cerebellar alterations. Fed Proc 1972;31:1517–1519

46 O'Gara RW, Brown JM, Whiting MG. Induction of hepatic and renal tumours by topical application of aqeuous extract of the cycad nut to artificial skin ulcers in mice. Third Conf on the Toxicity of Cycads, Chicago. Fed Proc 1964;23:1383–1385

47 Kurland LT, Molgaard CA. Guamanian ALS: Hereditary or acquired? In: Rowland LP, ed. Human Motor Neuron Diseases. New York, Raven Press, 1982;165–171

48 Kurland LT, Mulder DW. Overview of motor neuron disease. Proc Int Meeting Motor Neuron Diseases, Bangalore, 1984

49 Spencer PS, Ludolph A, Dwivedi MP, et al. Lathyrism: Evidence for the role of the neuroexcitatory amino acid BOAA. Lancet 1986;ii:1066–1067

50 Spencer PS, Hugon J, Ludolph A, et al. Discovery and partial characterization of primate motor-system toxins. In: Bock G and O'Connor M, eds. Selective Neuronal Death. Ciba Foundation Symposium No. 126. Chichester, Wiley, 1987;221–238

51 Spencer PS, Nunn PB, Hugon J, et al. Guam amyotrophic lateral sclerosis–parkinsonism-dementia due to a plant excitant neurotoxin. Science 1988;237:517–522

52 Yase Y. The pathogenesis of amyotrophic lateral sclerosis. Lancet 1972;11:292–296

53 Yanagihara R, Garruto RM, Gajdusek DC, et al. Calcium and vitamin D metabolism in Guamanian Chamorros with amyotrophic lateral sclerosis and parkinsonism-dementia. Ann Neurol 1984;15:42–47

54 Yoshimasu F, Yasui M, Yase Y, et al. Studies on amyotrophic lateral sclerosis by neutron activation analysis. 3. Systematic analysis of metals on Guamanian ALS and PD cases. Folia Psychiat Neurol Jpn 1982;36:173–179

55 Hirano A. Some current concepts of amyotrophic lateral sclerosis. Neurol Med (Tokyo) 1976;4:43–52

56 Carpenter S. Proximal axonal enlargement in motor neuron disease. Neurology 1968;18:842–851

57 Rowland LP. Motor neuron disease and amyotrophic lateral sclerosis: Research progress. Trends Neurosci 1987;10:393–398

58 Steele JC, Guzman T. Observations about amyotrophic lateral sclerosis and the parkinsonism-dementia complex of Guam with regard to epidemiology and etiology. Can J Neurol Sci 1987;14:358–362

59 Patten BM, Pages M. Severe neurological diseases associated with hyper-parathyroidism. Ann Neurol 1984;15:453–456

60 Shanker SK, Garruto RM, Amyx HL, et al. Possible role of low dietary calcium in the evolution of motor neuron disease: A primate model. Ann Neurol 1987;22:119

61 Rajput AH, Uitti RJ, Stern W, et al. Geography, drinking water chemistry, pesticides and herbicides and the etiology of Parkinson's disease. Can J Neurol Sci 1987;14:414–418

62 Garruto RM, Gajdusek DC, Chen K-M. Amyotrophic lateral sclerosis among Chamorro migrants from Guam. Ann Neurol 1980;8:612–619

63 Buchman A, Eisen A, Hoirch M, et al. Epidemiology of ALS in British Columbia: Evidence for prior environmental toxic exposure. Neurology 38 (in press)

64 Corsellis JAN, Bruton CJ, Freeman-Browne D. The aftermath of boxing. Psychol Med 1973;3:270–303

65 Critchley M. Medical aspects of boxing particularly from a neurological standpoint. Br Med J 1957;1:357–362

66 Jordan BD. Neurological aspects of boxing. Arch Neurol 1987;44:453–459

67 Campbell AMG, Williams ER, Pearce J. Late motor neuron degeneration following poliomyelitis. Neurology 1969;19:1101–1106

68 Fishman PS. Late-convalescent poliomyelitis. Arch Neurol 1987;44:98–100

69 Nelson KR, Harman M. EMG and clinical evaluation of delayed polio weakness. Muscle & Nerve 1987;10:660

70 Petajan JH, Currey K. Late oneset muscle weakness and atrophy from undiagnosed poliomyelitis. Muscle & Nerve 1987;10:665

71 Crossman AR, Clarke CE, Boyce S, et al. MPTP-induced parkinsonism in the monkey: Neurochemical pathology, complications of treatment and pathophysiological mechanisms. Can J Neurol Sci 1987;14:428–435

72 Calne DB, Langston JW, Martin WRW, et al. Positron emission tomography after MPTP: Observations relating to the cause of Parkinson's disease. Nature 1985;317:246–248

73 Langston JW. MPTP and Parkinson's disease. Trends Neurosci 1985;8:79–83

74 Guttman M, Young VW, Sim SU. Asymptomatic unilateral MPTP lesions visualized in vivo by fluordopa positron emission tomographic scans in cynomologus monkeys. Ann Neurol 1987;22:172

75 Duvoisin RC, Yahr MD. Encephalitis and parkinsonism. Arch Neurol 1965;12:227–239

76 Gibb WRG, Lees AJ. The progression of idiopathic Parkinson's disease is

not explained by age related changes. Clinical and pathological comparisons with post-encephalitis parkinsonian syndrome. Acta Neuropathol (in press)

77 Calne DB, Lees AJ. Late progression of post-encephalitic Parkinson's syndrome. Can J Neurol Sci (in press)

78 Cohn DF, Steifler M. Human neurolathyrism. A follow up study of 200 patients. Part 1. Arch Suisses Neurol Neurochir Psychiat 1981;128:151–156

79 Gebre-Ab T, Wolde Gabriel Z, Maffi M, et al. Neurolathyrism: A review and a report of an epidemic. Ethiop Med J 1978;16:1–11

Cycad Toxicity Not the Cause of High-Incidence Amyotrophic Lateral Sclerosis / Parkinsonism-Dementia on Guam, Kii Peninsula of Japan, or in West New Guinea

D. CARLETON GAJDUSEK

Guamanian patients with amyotrophic lateral sclerosis (ALS) and with parkinsonism-dementia (PD) [1] have had onset of their disease while living in Western cities of the continental United States on fully Western diets for as long as one, two, or even three decades after departure from Guam [2]. They have had no contact with cycad for these several decades preceding their disease. There have also been cases of ALS in emigrants from the high-incidence foci in Japan to urban communities, and the same has occurred in an immigrant to the city of Merauke who had left the high-incidence hyperendemic Ia River village of her Auyu kinsmen in West New Guinea 14 years before the onset of her ALS [3].

These 'delayed effects' demand a continuous subclinical progression of a lethal process or the triggering of a fatal predisposition already 'set' in the first twenty years of life in the hyperendemic foci. The data that no continuous exposure to or triggering by cycad has occurred in these patients are strong [1].

No neurotoxin has yet been demonstrated to give rise to fatal central nervous system disease, neurological signs or symptoms of which first start to be detectable years after exposure to the neurotoxin has ceased. In fact, we have *no* example of *any* toxin producing progressive damage to *any* organ years after last exposure to the substance. We have hypothesized such 'delayed effect' of a chemical agent for many idiopathic chronic CNS diseases; however, thus far, only hypersensitivity disorders, slow infections and genetically timed disorders have given this pattern of long delay. Hypersensitivity reactions such as rheumatic fever, glomerulonephritis, demyelinating allergic encephalitis, von Economo's encephalitis, and perhaps multiple sclerosis are examples of the first type

318 Amyotrophic Lateral Sclerosis

of delayed pathogenesis. Well-known slow infections are caused by bacteria (tuberculosis), spirochetes (syphilis), rickettsia (*R. prowazecki* in Brills disease), yeasts (crytococcosus, histoplasmosis), protozoa (malaria, trypanosomes), helminths (cysticercosis, angylostrongyloidiasis, gnathostomiasis), and conventional viruses (measles, rubella, adenovirus type 31, CMV, herpes simplex, Epstein-Barr virus, JC-papovavirus in progressive multifocal leukoencephalopathy [PML], Russian spring summer encephalitis [RSSE] in Kozhevnikov's epilepsy, human immunodeficiency virus [HIV], human T-lymphotropic virus type I [HTLV-I] and unconventional viruses (kuru, Creutzfeldt Jakob disease, scrapie). With all of these pathogens the presence of the chronic infection can be demonstrated immunologically, histopathologically, and by visualization or isolation of the offending microorganism or demonstration of its subunit proteins or nucleic acid. In these slow infections progressive pathology can be demonstrated during the preclinical phase. Examples of genetically determined delayed onset of degenerative diseases are legion: Huntington's disease, early-onset familial Alzheimer's disease, Friedreich's ataxia, etc.

In the high-incidence foci of ALS/PD on Guam and Kii Peninsula, several laboratories have demonstrated that the neurofibrillary tangle (NFT)–containing neurons in both ALS and PD, and even in normal subjects, born and bred in the area, have enormously high levels of aluminum, calcium, and silicon deposited in the neuronal perikaryon [4–13]. This microenvironmental deficiency in calcium and magnesium [3, 14] has led, in very isolated sedentary populations, to a calcium-sparing adjustment to calcium lack which favours the deposition of the calcium-aluminum-silicon in brain tissue, particularly in neurons [3–17]. Such pathology has been produced in monkeys given oral aluminum after chronic calcium and magnesium deprivation [18–20]. In fact, cynomolgus monkeys on chronic calcium deprivation receiving only normal dietary aluminum develop motor neuron pathology [18, 19].

The thesis that the normal abiotrophy of old age, with progressive loss of neurons and decrease of brain weight, may account for the sudden clinical appearance of ALS and PD has been advanced by Calne et al [21]. Although this seems to account for the apparent late onset and progression of disease in late-poliomyelitis paralysis, pugilistic encephalopathy, and radiation injury in the central nervous system, it does not appear to be a tenable thesis for Guamanian ALS/PD. In Guamanian ALS/PD brain and/or cord atrophy are so massive, with such great loss of grey matter in the course of a year or two, that the clinical disease cannot be only the result of the normal loss of grey matter with age which has made the pre-existing impairment clinically evident. The extensive atrophy of the cord (or brain in PD) is too great to have remained undetected in earlier decades. Not only would it have been clinically evident long before actual onset, but it would have been detectable by modern computerized axial tomography and nuclear magnetic resonance imaging (MRI) techniques and at autopsy in subjects dying earlier from other causes. Furthermore, careful study of Guamanian ALS and PD brains reveals extensive invasion with microglial cells and macrophages which indicate recent neuronal damage and loss.

Epidemiological study of ALS and PD in Chamorros from Guam for over 40 years [22, 23] has located many cases with clinical onset in the United States several decades after leaving Guam, with no exposure to cycad during these years [2, 22]. The motor neuron disease caused by cycad is well documented as a naturally occurring disease of cattle, and it may be reproduced in experimental animals. It does not seem to have been a problem for the millions of people who use cycad as their staple source of carbohydrates and the tens of millions for whom it provides an important dietary supplement. The traditional processing adequately eliminates the neurotoxin. The cycad data presented by Spencer and others [24–26] are not new facts [27–34], and extensive attempts to show that Guamanians ever processed cycad in such a way as to leave neurotoxin in the flour have been negative [1, 31, 35–37]. When cycad does produce the motor neuron disease in foraging cattle it is acute or sub-acute in onset and appears without years of delay after exposure. There is no progression after exposure ceases. The same is true for motor neuron disease produced in laboratory animals with cycad toxin.

The clearly established absence of any exposure to cycad in many patients from all three foci for decades before the onset of their disease leaves us with no precedent in neuropharmacology for hypothesizing such long-delayed effect of a hypothetical toxic exposure in childhood or youth. The recent evidence of damage to the basal ganglia and parkinsonism from dopaminergic neuron destruction by 1-methyl-4-phenyl-1,2,5,6-tetrahydropyridine (MPTP) has led to much speculation in this direction [38]. In fact, all the patients who developed a parkinsonism-like condition from MPTP had a subacute onset. None have had clinical disease appear years after exposure. It is only the data from exposed cohorts who are still clinically well but demonstrate by positron emission tomography dopanergic neuron loss in the basic ganglia (decreased dopamine production) that such a hypothetical extrapolation has been made. Even in this case, impaired physiology is demonstrable before clinical disease intervenes.

Several laboratories have observed that neurofibrillary tangle (NFT)–containing neurons in cases of Guamanian and Japanese PD and ALS have enormously high levels of aluminum, calcium, and silicon deposited in the neuronal perikaryon [4-13, 55]. We have also demonstrated the enormous accumulation of these elements in NFT-containing neurons in *normal* Guamanian subjects who have died from other than neurological causes. These person may have been destined to develop ALS and PD later. The only role I can see for hypothetical cycad toxicity, since no neurotoxin has ever been demonstrated in cycad flour as it was used in the past on Guam, is that extensive neuronal damage produced in infancy at a still subclinical level has resulted in slow mineral deposition in the damaged neuron. It would then be the mineral deposition secondary to acute cycad poisoning that produces the predisposition to later developing clinical disease. However, the conjecture that many infants were ever exposed to significant amounts of undetoxified cycad during the critical period for such calcification of damaged brain is enormously far-fetched.

The exact physiological changes and molecular mechanism leading to calcium, aluminum, and silicon deposition in neurons is unknown. That it has occurred even decades prior to disease is proved. The mechanism of the neuron damage seems to be through neurofibrillary tangle production with the deposition of amyloid fibrils in the tangles. Why the long delay? We may be led to conjecture that it requires decades for such mineral deposition to interfere sufficiently with axonal transport that massive neurofilament accumulation occurs to produce chromatolytic neurons, which eventually die [20, 39–42]. In such pooled or sequestered cytoskeletal deposits (or deposits of cytoskeletal-associated proteins) the amyloid precursor beta protein may also be entrapped and slowly degraded and polymerized into insoluble amyloid fibres, mostly in the form of paired helical filaments, along with other sequestered, copolymerized or adsorbed proteins, to form neurofibrillary tangles. We have shown that the neurofibrillary tangles of Guamanian ALS and PD contain the same amyloid polypeptide [42] as found in Alzheimer's disease and the normal ageing brain [20, 45–53]. Recently we have succeeded in producing a model of neurofibrillary degeneration resembling closely the neuropathology seen in Guamanian ALS/PD to cynomolgus monkeys made chronically deficient to calcium [18–20]. This model may aid in elucidating the molecular mechanism of aluminum and silicon interactions with neuronal metabolism [54–56], especially in the form of montmorillonite clays [53] such as are apparently found in our Guamanian neurons [6] and act as nucleating agents in the centre of some amyloid plaque cores in Alzheimer's disease [56–58].

References

1 Garruto RM, Yanagihara RT, Arion DM, et al. Bibliography of Amyotrophic Lateral Sclerosis and Parkinsonism-Dementia of Guam. NIH Publication 83-2622. Bethesda, Maryland, National Institutes of Health, 1983;167

2 Garruto RM, Gajdusek DC, Chen K-M. Amyotrophic lateral sclerosis among Chamorro migrants from Guam. Ann Neurol 1980;8:612–619

3 Gajdusek DC, Salazar A. Amyotrphic lateral sclerosis and parkinsonian syndromes in high incidence among the Auyu and Jakai people of West New Guinea. Neurology 1982;32:107–126

4 Garruto RM, Fukatsu R, Yanagihara R, et al. Imaging of calcium and aluminum in neurofibrillary tangle-bearing neurons in parkinsonism-dementia of Guam. Proc Nat Acad Sci (USA) 1984;81:1875–1879

5 Garruto RM, Swyt C, Fiori CE, et al. Intraneuronal deposition of calcium and aluminum in amyotrophic lateral sclerosis of Guam. Lancet 1985; ii:1353

6 Garruto RM, Swyt C, Yanagihara R, et al. Intraneuronal colocalization of silicon with calcium and aluminum in amyotrophic lateral sclerosis and parkinsonism with dementia of Guam. New Eng J Med 1986;315:711–712

7 Linton RW, Bryan SR, Griffis DP, et al. Digital imaging studies of aluminum and calcium in neurofibrillary tangle-bearing neurons using secondary ion mass spectrometry. Trace Elements in Med 1987;4:99–104

8 Perl D, Gajdusek D, Garruto RM, et al. Intracellular aluminum (Al) accumulation in neurofibrillary tangle (NFT) – bearing neurons in Guamanian ALS and parkinsonism-dementia (PD). Abstr Ninth International Congr Neuropathol (Vienna), 1982;13:31 (abstr D-1)

9 Perl DP, Gajdusek DC, Garruto RM, et al. Intraneuronal aluminum accumulation in amyotrophic lateral sclerosis and parkinsonism-dementia of Guam. Science 1982;217:1053–1055

10 Yase Y. The pathogenesis of amyotrophic lateral sclerosis. Lancet 1972;ii:292–296

11 Yase Y. The role of aluminum of CNS degeneration with interaction of calcium. Neurotoxicology 1980;1:101–109

12 Yoshimasu F, Yasui M, Yase Y, et al. Studies on amyotrophic lateral sclerosis by neutron activation analysis – 2. Comparative study of analytical results on Guam PD, Japanese ALS and Alzheimer's disease cases. Folio Psychiat Neurol Japon 1980;34:75–82

13 Yoshimasu F, Yasui M, Yoshida H, et al. Aluminum in Alzheimer's disease in Japan and parkinsonism-dementia in Guam. XII World Congress of Neurol 1985;abstr 15.07.02

14 Garruto RM, Yanagihara R, Gajdusek DC, Arion DM. Concentrations of heavy metals and essential minerals in garden soil and drinking water in

the Western Pacific. In: Chen KM, Yase Y, eds. Amyotrophic Lateral Sclerosis in Asia and Oceania. Taipei, National Taiwan University Press, 1984;265–329

15 Gajdusek DC. Environmental factors provoking physiological changes which induce motor neurone disease and early neuronal ageing in high incidence foci in the Western Pacific. In: Rose FC, ed. Research Progress in Motor Neuron Disease. Progress in Neurology Series. London, Pitman Books, 1984;44–69

16 Yanagihara R. Heavy metals and essential minerals in motor neuron disease. In: Rowland LP, ed. Advances in Neurology, Vol. 36, Human Motor Neuron Diseases. New York, Raven Press, 1982;233–237

17 Yanagihara RT, Garruto RM, Gajdusek DC, et al. Calcium and vitamin D metabolism in Guamanian Chamorros with amyotrophic lateral sclerosis and parkinsonism-dementia. Ann Neurol 1984;15:42–48

18 Garruto RM, Shanker SK, Yanagihara RT, et al. Low calcium, high aluminum diet-induced motor neuron pathology in cynomolgus monkeys. Acta Neuropathol 1989;78:210–219

19 Garruto RM, Yanagihara R, Shanker SK, et al. Experimental models of metal-induced neurofibrillary degeneration. In: Tsubaki T, Yase Y, eds. Amyotrophic Lateral Sclerosis. Amsterdam, Elsevier Science Publishers, 1988;41–50

20 Yanagihara R, Garruto RM, Shanker SK, et al. Cellular and molecular biology of neurofibrillary degeneration in amyotrophic lateral sclerosis and parkinsonism-dementia of Guam. In: Tsubaki T, Yase Y, eds. Amyotrophic Lateral Sclerosis. Amsterdam, Elsevier Science Publishers V, 1988;103–111

21 Calne DB, Eisen A, McGeer E, Spencer P. Alzheimer's disease, Parkinson's disease, and motoneurone disease: Abiotrophic interaction between ageing and environment. Lancet 1986;ii:1067–1070

22 Garruto RM, Yase Y. Neurological degenerative disorders of the Western Pacific: The search for mechanism of pathogenesis. Trends Neurosci 1986;9:368–374

23 Yanagihara RT, Garruto RM, Gajdusek DC. Epidemiological surveillance of amyotrophic lateral sclerosis and parkinsonism-dementia in the Commonwealth of the Northern Marianas Islands. Ann Neurol 1983;13:79–86

24 Spencer PS, Nunn PB, Hugon J, et al. Guam amyotrophic lateral sclerosis/parkinsonism-dementia linked to a plant excitant neurotoxin. Science 1987;237:517–522

25 Spencer PS, Ohta M, Palmer VS. Cycad use and motor neurone disease in the Kii Peninsula of Japan. Lancet 1987;ii:1462–1463

26 Spencer PS, Palmer VS, Herman A, Asmedi A. Cycad use and motor neurone disease in Irian Jaya. Lancet 1987;ii:1273–1274

27 Dastur DK. Cycad toxicity in monkeys: Clinical, pathological, and biochemical aspects. Proc. Third Conference on Toxicity of Cycads, Chicago, April 17. Fed Proc 1964;23:1368–1369

28 Duncan MW Kopin IJ, Garruto RM, et al. 2-Amino-3(methylamino)-propionic acid in cycad-derived foods is an unlikely cause of amyotrophic lateral sclerosis/parkinsonism. Lancet 1988;ii:631–632

29 Duncan MW, Marini AM, Kopin IJ, Markey SP. BMAA and ALS-PD: A causal link? Internatl ALS-MND Update 1989; 2Q89:31

30 Hirano A, Jones M. Fine structure of cycasin-induced cerebellar alterations. Proc. Sixth Conference on Toxicity of Cycads, Chicago, April 17. Fed Proc 1972;31:1517–1519

31 Hirono I, Shibuya C. Induction of neurological disorder by cycasin in mice. Nature 1967;216(5122):1311–1312

32 Kurland LT. An Appraisal of the neurotoxicity of cycad and the etiology of amyotrophic lateral sclerosis on Guam. Proc Sixth Internat Cycad Conference, Chicago, April 17. Fed Proc 1967;315:1504–1507

33 Whiting MG. Food practices in ALS foci in Japan, the Marianas, and New Guinea. Proc Third Conference on Toxicology of Cycads, Chicago, 17 April. Fed Proc 1964;23(6):1343–1344

34 Whiting MG. Toxicity of cycads – A literature review. Econ Bot 1963;17:270–302

35 Polsky RI, Nunn PB, Bell EA. Distribution and toxicity of α-amino-β-methyl-aminoproprionic acid. Fed Proc 1972;31:1473–1475

36 Sieber SM, Correa P, Dalgard DW, et al. Carcinogenicity and hepatotoxicity of cycasin and its aglycone methylazoxymethanol acetate in nonhuman primates. J Natl Cancer Inst 1980;65:177–189

37 Yang MG, Mickelson O, Campbell ME, et al. Cycad flour used by Guamanians: Effects produced in rats by long-term feeding. J Nutrit 1966;90:153–156

38 Markey SP. MPTP: A new tool to understand Parkinson's disease. Discussions in Neuroscience. Geneva, Foundation pour l'Etude du Système Nerveau (FESN), 1986;3(4):1—51

39 Gajdusek DC. Hypothesis: Interference with axonal transport of neurofilament as a common pathogenetic mechanism in certain diseases of the central nervous system. New Eng J Med 1985;312:714–719

40 Gajdusek DC. Calcium aluminum silicon deposits in neurons lead to paired helical filaments identical to those of AD and Down's patients. Neurobiol Aging 1986;7:555–556

41 Gajdusek DC. On the uniform source of amyloid in plaques, tangles and vascular deposits. Neurobiol Aging 1986;7:453–454

42 Guiroy DC, Miyazaki M, Multhaup G, et al. Amyloids of neurofibrillary

tangles of Guamanian parkinsonism dementias and Alzheimer's disease share identical amino acid sequence. Proc Natl Acad Sci (USA) 1987;84:2073–2077

43 Glenner GC, Wong CV. Alzheimer's disease and Down's syndrome: Sharing of a unique cerebrovascular amyloid fibril protein. Biochem Biophys Red Comm 1984;122:1131–1135

44 Goldgaber D, Lerman M, McBride W, et al. Characterization and chromosomal localization of a cDNA clone encoding brain amyloid of Alzheimer's disease. Science 1989;235:877–880

45 Goldgaber D, Teener JW, Gajdusek DC. Multiple forms of amyloid β-protein precursor mRNAs. In: Brown P, Bolis L, Gajdusek DC, eds. Molecular Mechanisms in Neurodegenerative Disorders. Discussions in Neuroscience. Geneva, Foundation pour l'Etude du Système Nerveau (FESN), 1988;5(3):40–46

46 Kang J, Lemaire H-G, Unterbeck A, et al. The precursor of Alzheimer's disease amyloid A4 protein resembles a cell-surface receptor. Nature 1987;325:733–736

47 Masters CL, Multhaup G, Simms G, et al. Neuronal origin of a cerebral amyloid: Neurofibrillary tangles of Alzheimer's disease contain the same protein as the amyloid of plaque cores and blood vessels. EMBO J 1985;4:2757–2763

48 Masters CL, Simms G, Weinman NA, et al. Amyloid plaque core protein in Alzheimer's disease and Down's syndrome. Proc Natl Acad Sci (USA) 1985;82:4245–4249

49 Robakis NK, Ramakrishna N, Wolfe G, Wisniewski HM. Molecular cloning and characterization of a cDNA encoding the cerebral vascular and neuritic plaque amyloid peptides. Proc Natl Acad Sci (USA) 1987;84:4190–4194

50 Svedmyr A, Shankar SK, Miyazaki M, et al. Cytoskeletal proteins forming amyloid-like structures in vitro. Neurology 1987;37(suppl 1): abstr PP297, p 204

51 Tanzi RE, Gusella JF, Watkins PC, et al. Amyloid β protein gene: cDNA, mRNA distribution, and genetic linkage near the Alzheimer locus. Science 1987;235:880–884

52 Tanzi RE, McClatchey AI, Lamperti ED, et al. Protease inhibitor domain encoded by an amyloid protein precursor mRNA associated with Alzheimer's disease. Nature 1988;331:528–530

53 Weis A. Replication and evolution in inorganic systems. Angew Chem (Eng) 1981;20:850–860

54 Austin JH. Silicon levels in human tissues. In: Bendz G, Lindqvist I, eds.

Biochemistry of Silicon and Related Problems. New York, Plenum, 1978;255–268

55 Iler RK. Hydrogen-bond complexes of silica with organic compounds. In: Bendz G, Lindqvist I, eds. Biochemistry of Silicon and Related Problems. New York, Plenum, 1985;53–76

56 McLachlan DRC. Aluminum and Alzheimer's disease. Neurobiol of Aging 1986;7:525–532

57 Candy JM, Klinowski RH, Perry EK, et al. Alumino-silicates and senile plaque formation in Alzheimer's disease. Lancet 1986;i:354–356

58 Perl DP. Pathologic association of aluminum in Alzheimer's disease. In: Reisberg B, ed. Alzheimer's Disease: The Standard Reference. New York, Free Press, 1983;116–121

59 Piccardo P, Yanagihara RT, Garruto RM, et al. Histochemical and X-ray microanalytical localization of aluminum in amyotrophic lateral sclerosis and parkinsonism-dementia of Guam. Acta Neuropathol 1988;77:1–4

Post-poliomyelitis Motor Neuron Disease: What Did We Learn in Reference to Amyotrophic Lateral Sclerosis?

MARINOS C. DALAKAS

Neurologists have been aware for years that some patients with old polio may experience later in life progressive muscle weakness in their already weak muscles [1–6]. Although isolated cases of post-polio weakness have been described since 1870 [1–2], during the last 6–7 years an increasing number of patients who had suffered an acute episode of paralytic poliomyelitis and subsequently recovered have been showing up in doctor's offices all over the world complaining of a variety of new symptoms. The patients themselves coined the term *post-polio syndrome* [7–9] to describe a variety of new difficulties with daily living that they started to experience many years later. Because of our interest in motor neuron diseases, this emerging symptomatology of post-polio patients became a subject for our study since acute paralytic poliomyelitis itself is a motor neuron disease of viral origin.

Early in 1982, and before the post-polio syndrome was publicized or accepted as a clinical entity, the following observations were apparent when we started to examine a few self-referred newly symptomatic post-polio patients [7–9]:

1 The patients were devastated and overwhelmed by fear of a recurring poliomyelitis.
2 They had visited multiple doctors including internists, gastroenterologists, orthopedists, neurologists, physiatrists, nutritionists, psychiatrists, and holistic medical therapists and they had been given several diagnoses. They had been confused, angered, and frustrated because their symptoms had not been explained.
3 Other patients were told that they developing amyotrophic lateral sclerosis, which caused additional fear and uncertainty.
4 Within the self-coined term 'post-polio syndrome' the patients had

included a variety of diverse symptoms such as muscle pains, fatigue, weakness, paresthesias, headaches, constipation, back pain, neck pain, changes in sleeping patterns, breathing difficulties, hot and cold flashes, bladder difficulties, or gastrointestinal complaints [10–14].

Definition

Since our early studies [15, 16], we were able to distinguish two subsets of post-polio patients based on their symptomatology: one group with predominantly *musculoskeletal* symptoms and another with new *muscle weakness* that we termed post-poliomyelitis progressive muscular atrophy (PPMA)[15, 16]. Nowadays, the term post-polio syndrome has prevailed [8, 11] and appears to be universally popular in describing all the new difficulties that the post-polio patients experience.

Post-polio syndrome, as I define it, includes only the *new neuromuscular symptoms* that some patients develop 25–35 years after reaching maximum recovery form acute paralytic poliomyelitis [8, 9, 11]. These symptoms are unrelated to any other neurologic, orthopedic, psychiatric, or systemic medical illness and consist of:

1 *musculoskeletal complaints,* as an indirect result of the late effects of polio such as joint pain, fatigue, decreased physical endurance, back pains, and early symptoms of wear and tear in biomechanically disadvantaged joints [7–16];
2 the *post-poliomyelitis progressive muscular atrophy (PPMA)* which describes the new muscle weakness affecting certain muscle groups (including rarely the bulbar and respiratory muscles) with or without muscular atrophy or pain [7–16]; or
3 *a combination of 1 and 2.*

In this chapter we will review the clinical, electrophysiological, immunological, virological, muscle biopsy, and spinal cord morphological characteristics of patients with PPMA, making a distinction between PPMA and ALS.

ALS is the prototype of motor neuron disease of unknown cause. PPMA is the new low motor neuron deterioration that occurs in patients with long-standing lower motor neuron deficit caused originally by a known virus. Although at the cellular level both ALS and PPMA have in common the dysfunction of the lower motor neurons, they differ in several clinical, histological, and electrophysiological parameters [16–26]. Comparison therefore of ALS with PPMA is not only clinically useful, especially when there is an overlapping of symptoms and signs, but is also of special neurobiological interest. It could provide information about the life span of an overfunctioning motor neuron that has been stressed to reinnervate and maintain for years very large motor units – as compared to the pathologically shortened life span of ALS neurons – or about the long-term viability and function of a scarred motor neuron that survived an acute viral insult such as polio virus [16–26].

Patient Selection

All patients with PPMA were studied at the National Institutes of Health after giving informed consent. The criteria which are a prerequisite for consideration of a referred patient for evaluation of PPMA have been previously described [7–22]. In brief:

1 Every patient has to have a history of acute paralytic poliomyelitis which occurred in childhood or adolescence. We tried to establish this history by a careful review of records to document the clinical occurrence of an acute febrile illness followed by paralysis. We checked for neighbourhood and school epidemics and selected patients who were affected in the United States, particularly during the late epidemics when the diagnosis of poliomyelitis was probably made with more accuracy.
2 Partial recovery of motor function after polio and functional stability or recovery for at least 15 years.
3 Residual muscle atrophy, weakness, and areflexia in at least one limb but with normal sensation.
4 Development of new muscle weakness (PPMA).
5 No history of any known medical, neurological, orthopedic, or psychiatric illness that could explain their new symptoms. Although we have excluded such patients from our initial study, which was aimed to define the new symptoms and understand the pathogenetic mechanisms involved, we have subsequently evaluated patients with PPMA who have, in addition, a coexisting cardiovascular disease, diabetes, mild alcoholic neuropathy, or history of recent falls and injuries. Assignment of the cause of current disability in toto to PPMA can be difficult in such cases, as we have previously discussed [11].

Only patients who were less than 60 years old at the initial visit (mean age 42.7, range 24–59) were entered into the study of PPMA. This was done to exclude patients who were subject to loss of motor neurons due to the normal ageing process. As we have previously described, patients with old polio are subject to compression neuropathies, radiculopathies, and injuries. For this reason, we have excluded from the studied patients those whose new symptoms were related to a compression neuropathy from the use of crutches or wheelchairs or from lumbar or cervical radiculopathy.

The group of PPMA patients selected as described above was compared with a large number of patients with ALS that we have examined at the NIH during the last 10 years. In general, patients with ALS had a progressive disease with often a combination of upper and lower motor neuron involvement. None of the ALS patients that we studied had a history of a prior paralytic disease such as poliomyelitis.

All the post-polio patients included in the comparative study had the following detailed examination [10–16, 16]

1 Serial clinical neurological examinations during the initial and subsequent follow-up visits to assess degree and rate of progression of neurological signs and symptoms. All the patients were examined neurologically and their muscle strength quantitated according to the scale of the Medical Research Council [27]. In addition to our objective quantitative muscle study, the patient's own description of functional decline in their muscle strength was recorded. For recording in numerical fashion the muscle strength of every patient, we used the following previously described formula [9–11]. We considered the total normal strength of the four limbs as 100 points of neuromuscular function and assigned 25 points to each of the four limbs. The 25 points were equally distributed among five major muscle groups. (For example, in the leg 5 points each were assigned to the foot extensors, foot flexors, knee extensors, knee flexors, and hip flexors and extensors.) Five points of neuromuscular function for each of the major muscle groups corresponded to a '5' (normal) rating on the Medical Research Council scale. Weaker muscle groups that rated 4, 3, 2, 1, and 0 on the MRC scale received 4, 3, 2, 1, and 0 points respectively. These calculations provided an automatic estimate of the cumulative total strength of every limb recorded at each revisit, as previously described [9–11].

2 Routine blood chemistry tests, including determination of muscle enzymes, CBC, vitamin levels, serology, toxicology, quantitative immunoglobulins, and immunoelectrophoresis.

3 Examination of the lymphocyte subsets using monoclonal antibodies that identify surface membrane markers as previously described [23–29].

4 Search for circulating antineuronal antibodies to spinal cord neurons using the immunoperoxidase and immunofluorescene technique as reported previously [30–32].

5 Determination of antibodies to poliomyelitis virus, herpes, cytome-

galovirus, measles, and human lymphotropic virus type I and III (HTLV-I and HIV) in both serum and spinal fluid. Specific IgG viral synthesis in the spinal fluid was also calculated as we have previously reported [16, 29, 33–36]. Search for antibodies to the polio virus was performed by neutralization plaque assay and by ELISA in both the serum and the CSF as described (15, 16, 35, 36). Titres of neutralizing antibody to polio virus type I (Mahoney strain type II), mouse embryo fibroblast strain, and type III (Saukett strain) were examined. The extent of the production of polio virus antibody inside the blood/brain barrier was determined by making correction for blood/brain barrier permeability using the ratio of CSF to serum albumin [35, 36].

6 Examination of the spinal fluid for oligoclonal bands by high-resolution agarose gel electrophoresis and immunofixation electrophoresis as previously described [33, 34].

7 Open muscle biopsies. These were performed on 27 patients with new muscle weakness and 5 asymptomatic post-polio patients who served as controls [18, 21–23]. Post-polio muscles at different stages of residual deficit were studied. This included newly symptomatic or asymptomatic muscles that had fully or partially recovered after the original illness or muscles originally spared according to available clinical description, old photographs, or medical records. None of the biopsied muscles had a known history of injury or needle insertions for at least six months prior to the biopsy. Open muscle biopsies were performed according to standard techniques and processed for muscle enzyme histochemistry as previously described [21, 37]. Serial muscle biopsy sections were also stained with trichrome, acid phosphatase, and esterase to characterize the type of the inflammatory cells present [28, 37]. Eight post-polio patients who initially presented with new muscle weakness were re-biopsied several years later to assess changes in the muscles during progression of the disease [10]. Thus, 40 muscle biopsies were available for review. In ALS patients, muscle biopsy was often performed from a minimally involved or preferably from a non-clinically affected muscle to determine subclinical involvement of motor neurons in a disease that is thought to be generalized. End-stage muscles or muscles with severe deficit and significant atrophy were infrequently biopsied.

8 Electromyographic studies including quantitative studies of the voluntary motor units and spontaneous activity, performed as described [19, 11, 32, 38]. Single fibre EMG using standard techniques [39] was also utilized. Data from single fibre studies were analysed for fibre density, which is the average number of muscle fibres recorded by the needle during a single placement; for jitter, which is the mean con-

secutive difference in the intervals between the activation of two muscle fibres in the same motor unit; for blocking, which is the failure of a muscle fibre to activate when its motor unit is activated; and for neurogenic jitter, which is the sequence variation of at least two muscle fibres with respect to the third that must be due to an abnormality of the nerve rather than the neuromuscular junction.

9 Histology of the spinal cord from patients with classic ALS and post-polio patients. Paraffin-embedded sections of spinal cords were processed for routine histological stains [24–26]. The post-polio spinal cords were from patients with PPMA or asymptomatic post-polio state that died from non-neurological conditions [24–26].

10 Positron emission tomography (PET) scan of the brain measuring the utilization of [^{18}F]-2-fluoro-2-deoxy-D-glucose (FDG) in the cortex, basal ganglia, and cerebellum [19, 40]. The study was done in 12 ALS patients and 3 PPMA patients in an attempt to find differences in neuronal glucose utilization between patients who have classic ALS with or without upper motor neuron involvement and patients with PPMA who lack upper motor neuron signs. The latter study was specifically designed to examine whether the viability and function of the upper motor neurons are affected when the lower motor neuron target in the spinal cord is severely reduced as occurs in the post-polio state. For these purposes post-polio patients with severe residual disability were selected to match the disability of ALS patients [19, 40].

Results

Clinical Observations

From the patients with post-polio syndrome only those with symptoms characteristic of PPMA were selected for a comparative clinical study. Specifically, we have excluded patients who had radiculopathies, compression neuropathies, back, knee, or joint injury or symptoms related to osteoarthritis. As has been previously emphasized [7–16] post-polio patients with only musculoskeletal symptoms are different from the PPMA group because they often have a poorly defined symptomatology, which includes an overall deterioration of functional capacity expressed as fatigue, decreased endurance, joint pains due to degenerative arthritis, worsening mobility due to long-standing scoliosis, or poor posture and difficulties related to unnatural or unusual mechanics imposed by tendon transfers or shortened limbs and possibly increase in their body weight. These patients often describe vaguely the location of their symptoms with a frustrating degree of variability and fluctuation or, at times, even inconsistently. Emotional difficulties are not uncommon. In contrast, patients with PPMA experience a rather distinct symptomatology which consists of:

(a) *New muscle weakness with or without atrophy* in few muscle groups, more often in muscles that had previously been affected and had fully or partially recovered. In all the patients, the new weakness is characteristically asymmetrical [7–16]. Patients may have increased difficulties in activities such as walking, standing, climbing stairs, ambulating for the same distance as before, transferring from bed to chair, driving, dressing, combing their hair, or shaving. Disabled polio patients maintain for years a high level of performance even on relatively few muscle groups with normal strength. This has been possible because of the scattered nature of their motor deficit even in the same limb and the extraordinary ability to compensate with unconventional use of the healthy muscles in that limb. For such patients, new weakness, even in part of a single muscle, if critical for a specific movement, often leads to disruption of the existing delicate muscle balance with a disproportionate loss of functional skill.

(b) *Muscle pain* of neurogenic type [41] can be present in several PPMA patients but it is only infrequently severe. This myalgia is different from the joint pain or the pain due to osteoarthritis that the patients with musculoskeletal complaints often experience, although some of the PPMA patients also have musculoskeletal complaints in addition to the new weakness. Some PPMA patients describe the pain as a deep ache [42]; some claim it to be similar to the pain they had during acute polio.

(c) *Fasciculations* are often noted in the PPMA patient even in muscles that do not appear to have become weaker, although they are more frequent in the newly weakened muscles.

Weakness in bulbar and respiratory muscle is infrequently noted. As a rule, however, PPMA affects these muscles only in patients with minimal bulbar or respiratory muscle reserves due to significant residual weakness from the original illness [9, 20]. We have now documented by videofluoroscopy asymmetrical weakness in the pharyngeal constrictor muscles not only in PPMA patients who complained of new swallowing difficulties but also in some PPMA patients with new weakness confined to the limbs but who had suffered transient bulbar involvement during acute polio [43]. This suggests that there is subclinical dysfunction of bulbar muscles even in asymptomatic post-bulbar polio patients. Similarly, those PPMA patients who recovered poorly from severe poliomyelitic respiratory muscle paralysis or had been left with partial residual respiratory muscle weakness can now experience new respiratory difficulties which could be either due to new weakness of the respiratory muscles or due to a combination of kyphoscoliosis, emphysema, cardio-vascular disease, or poor posture especially in wheelchair-bound patients. Patients therefore who were functioning for years with a very low vital capacity may now require ventilatory assistance, especially at night, when their late-onset ventilatory insufficiently compromises further their already low respiratory muscle reserves [44]. At times, these patients can experience sleep disturbances such as sleep apnea [11, 44, 45]. Sleep apnea, however, appears to affect only those patients who had bulbar disease originally and had been left with residual bulbar difficulties requiring some kind of ventilatory assistance during the early months of recovery [11, 44, 45].

The progression of the PPMA patient is generally very slow, estimated to be 1% per year of the total neuromuscular function with often many years of relative stability, varying from 1 to 10 years [9–13]. The new weakness is generally so slowly progressive that it could not be appreciated on a year-to-year basis but only on cumulative periods that overall average 3 years (range 1–10) [9–13]. A representative course and progression for PPMA patients is shown in Figure 1. Some patients have a stepwise progression of weakness with intermittent periods of relative stability, whereas others have a slow, continuous decline in strength. As shown in Figure 1, in five patients (nos. 5, 6, 7, 8, 9) new muscle weakness had increased but remained almost confined to muscles that were weak upon first examination; in three others (nos. 1, 3, 12) new weakness had appeared in additional muscles. Three patients (nos. 7, 10, 11) who had severe residual disability developed more generalized weakness causing significant new disability and needed electric wheelchairs (whereas 10 years earlier they had required only crutches) even though the new decline in strength was very minimal in each muscle group. Two patients (nos. 3, 4), followed for 13 and 11 years, respectively, had only minimal generalized weakness which interfered little with specific functions or everyday activities. It is now clear that the functional effect of the new disability in PPMA patients depends on the baseline neurological status and degree of residual deficit they had at the onset of new symptoms; the more the residual deficit, the greater the functional impact of PPMA on the patient's neuromuscular functions [46].

PPMA patients do not have or develop upper motor neuron signs although very rarely an occasional isolated Babinski sign has been seen [7–16]. The presence of such isolated Babinski signs, however, in post-polio patients with such a chronic and extensive denervation does not necessarily imply a coexisting upper motor neuron involvement [5]. As in other chronic peripheral nerve diseases, such a sign can be due to unequal degree of paralysis in the foot muscles and their uneven degree

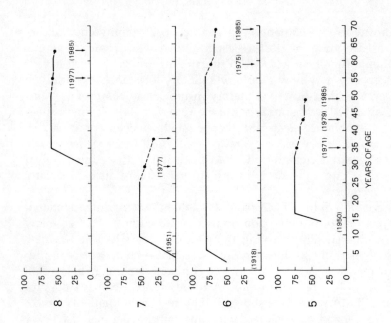

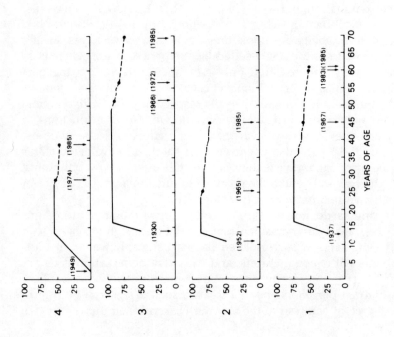

Figure 1. Progression of muscle weakness in 12 patients with post-poliomyelitis muscular atrophy, expressed as total points of estimated neuromuscular function at various years of age. Numbers on the left refer to individual patients. Points of muscular function (100 points is the normal strength in all four limbs), as reported before [3, 21], are on the ordinate. The continuous line represents the patients' course after the attack of acute polio and their progressive partial recovery with subsequent long stabilization, as determined from information provided by the patients or early records. The interrupted line represents the course of new muscle weakness from onset until the latest follow-up evaluation. Arrows with the year in parentheses represent time of the acute polio attack (first arrow), the time of the first examination after the manifestation of new weakness (second arrow), and subsequent examinations (third and fourth arrows). A decline in muscular strength that was either continuous or that occurred in a stepwise fashion took place in all the patients between the first and last evaluations.

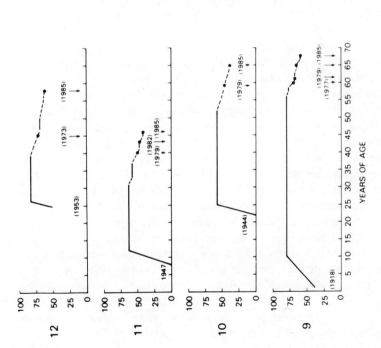

of innervation [11]. Although spasticity has been reported by some [47], we have not seen it in any of our PPMA patients who did not have any other concomitant neurological disorder. In fact, none of our patients that we have thoroughly examined and followed (now up to 80 patients) had or developed ALS [48].

In contrast to the above description of PPMA, ALS patients may start focally but when they are examined signs of a more generalized disease are found or develop in a very short period. The progression of ALS is much faster, as shown in Figure 2 for five ALS patients and one PPMA patient that we followed up for the same period of time during an experimental therapeutic trial with interferon [49]. In contrast with PPMA, the progression of ALS is most of the time more linear (Fig. 2), bulbar and respiratory muscle involvement is invariably present or develops, and the disease is always fatal. As a general rule, in PPMA the severity of the new symptoms in reference to the resulting new disability depends on the residual deficit the patients had at their 'starting point.' For example, a post-polio patient who has been left with severe residual deficit of bulbar or respiratory muscles can experience new respiratory symptoms if PPMA develops and affects these muscles. In such a patient, however, the symptoms should not be interpreted as ALS. In contrast, we have not seen any of our large number of PPMA patients who had residual deficits confined only to the limbs to develop bulbar or respiratory muscle weakness resembling ALS as a manifestation of PPMA. This was not present even during our long, careful follow-up study [9–12]. Based on our experience, therefore, the incidence of ALS is not higher in post-polio patients, contrary to some older reports [50, 51]. Furthermore, the clinical symptomatology of PPMA is different from that of ALS not only in the rate of progression and final disability but also in the distribution of the new weakness. ALS is a generalized motor neuron disease affecting both upper and lower motor neurons. PPMA remains predominantly focal or multifocal affecting certain muscle groups but sparing the upper motor neurons. The average period after the acute polio that new symptoms develop in PPMA is about 30–35 years and both sexes are affected with same frequency [7–16, 42]. In ALS, a 2:1 male predominance appears to be commonly reported [52].

Epidemiological surveys showing the exact prevalence of PPMA are not available. The data from mail surveys without examinination of the patients [42, 53] are not accurate, as we have repeatedly emphasized [7–16]. What has been remarkable in all the clinical studies, however, is the period of onset of the post-polio symptoms, which has been rather consistent, with an average range of 25–38 years after recovery from the original polio [7–16, 42, 53]. Factors often associated with the develop-

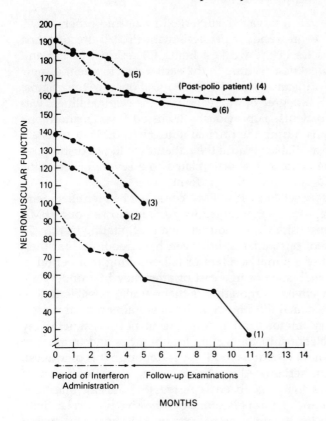

Figure 2. Course of five patients (nos. 1, 2, 3, 5, 6, in parentheses) with ALS and one patient (no. 4) with PPMA during a trial with administration of interferon, as previously reported [22]. Total neuromuscular score in this study was the sum of a functional score (normal 60) based on the patients' neuromuscular function and a motor examination score (normal 176) as reported [22]. The course of the ALS patients during the 14 months of observation after interferon administration is clearly different from that of the PPMA. All ALS patients substantially worsened. At the end of the 14-month period, patient 1 became quadriplegic on the respirator; patient 2 became quadriplegic and developed bulbar signs; patient 3 became quadriplegic, with severe bulbar and respiratory involvement, and expired; patient 5 became quadriplegic with bulbar involvement; and patient 6 developed bulbar signs and needed assistance to ambulate. In contrast, patient 4 with PPMA remained essentially unchanged or perhaps was only slightly worse.

ment of PPMA at *shorter* intervals documented by us and others [7–16, 42, 53] include: (1) severe residual paralysis with PPMA affecting first and more often muscles in the weakest limbs, (2) residual bulbar and respiratory muscle weakness leading to the earlier development of new bulbar or respiratory difficulties, and (3) older age at onset of the original acute poliomyelitis.The degree of the severity of the original illness was not a factor in our patients, as previously discussed [11]. Furthermore, the degree of paralysis during the original illness was difficult to assess even if records were available because the patients could not distinguish if the severity of the acute illness was related to a severe encephalitic form of the disease or a severe paralytic form.

Recent risk factors associated with PPMA could not be identified. Similar difficulties are repeatedly mentioned for ALS. In most of our PPMA patients the onset was insidious without known precipitating factors [7–16]. A small number of our patients, however, have reported that their symptoms started after a minor accident or fall, resulting in a period of immobilization of a limb such as in a cast or after they had undergone weight gain from inactivity. Although it is theoretically possible to lose some distal terminal axonal intramuscular branches after a local muscle injury and secondary immobilization resulting in new weakness, any direct cause/effect relationship connecting local injuries and traumas to the development of new weakness in PPMA is doubtful. It is of interest, however, that in some series of ALS patients, an increased frequency of injuries or physical activity has been reported [54], raising questions about the role of insidious neuronal trauma or excessive physical activity as a predisposing factor in some cases. Even in ALS, however, such a cause/effect relationship remains tenuous and doubtful.

Chemistry and Virology in the Serum and CSF

Routine blood chemistries are normal in both ALS and PPMA patients. The serum CK can be elevated up to 1000 units (normal up to 200) in some PPMA and ALS patients. Caution should be exercised not to confuse such a finding as a sign of possible inflammatory myopathy especially since inflammation can be seen in the muscle biopsies of patients with PPMA [7–22]. The elevated CK is probably consistent with the secondary 'myopathic' features noted in a long-standing denervating disease [21, 55, 56]. The elevated CK is of no prognostic or diagnostic significance. The clinical and serological characteristics of and differences between PPMA and ALS are summarized in Table 1.

The total serum immunoglobulins and immunoelectrophoresis in PPMA patients are normal. This is in contrast to ALS patients, who rarely have an associated monoclonal gammopathy, of unknown significance

TABLE 1
Clinical characteristics of PPMA and ALS

Muscle weakness	Fasciculations	Pain	CK	Long tract signs	Bulbar and respiratory symptoms	Progression
PPMA Focal and asymmetrical; it does not spread to previously normal bulbar or respiratory muscles	Sparse	Common	Can be elevated	Absent	Absent, except in patients with severe residual deficit and minimal reserves in these muscle groups	Very slow; estimated loss of function 1% per year
ALS May start focally but becomes generalized and spreads to bulbar and respiratory muscles	Diffuse	Rare	Can be elevated	Present	Present	Rapid; leads to death in 3–5 years in most of the patients

From Dalakas [20]

[57]. Contrary to what has been recently described [57, 58], the IgM monoclonal gammopathy in ALS patients has not been shown to recognize a unique epitope on myelin or axonal proteins [59, 60]. Most important, the majority, if not all, of these patients did not have ALS but a low motor neuron syndrome indistinguishable from an axonal neuropathy [57, 58]. Furthermore, the glycolipid that the IgM of one such patient immunoreacted with was not unique, as reported [8], because the same glycolipid is also an antigen in patients with demyelinating neuropathies, as we have shown [59, 60]. In addition, such patients do not convincingly respond to immunotherapy. One of our patients with IgMκ gammopathy and classic ALS was also unresponsive to a series of plasmapheresis [61].

Viral antibody titres in both serum and CSF are not different in PPMA and ALS patients. The neutralizing antibody titres to polio virus are higher in the serum of PPMA patients; however, there is no specific elevation of polio viral antibodies in the spinal fluid when a correction for blood/brain barrier permeability was made using the ratio of CSF to serum albumin [35, 36]. In fact, the ratio of antibodies to polio virus in the serum and CSF was the same in both ALS and PPMA [19, 20].

Immunology in the Serum and CSF

Analysis of lymphocyte subsets for T suppressor, T helper, and B cell markers with monoclonal antibodies in as many as 28 PPMA patients and up to 20 ALS patients failed to reveal an internally consistent, specific immunoregulatory abnormality. Only rarely have we seen occasional patients with lymphocyte population and mean regulatory ratio above or below the normal range. This is, however, similar to the ratios in our normal volunteers, 2–3% of which may have such irregularities that apparently vary according to recent viral illnesses, common colds, or other undetermined factors (Dalakas, unpublished observations, 1981–1983).

Search for antibodies to neuronal cell components failed to reveal specific binding of the patients' serum to neurons, glial cells, or vascular endothelial cells [7–16]. Spinal fluid analysis for oligoclonal bands revealed the presence of 2–4 weak IgG bands in up to 40% of PPMA patients tested. This was in contrast to the CSF of our patients with classic ALS, where no bands were present [19, 20, 33, 34]. It is of interest that the CSF from five asymptomatic post-polio patients and from four patients that recovered from recent acute poliomyelitis (the latter specimens were sent to us by Dr Ming-Key Chang from Taiwan) did not have oligoclonal bands. Whether an antibody IgG response to neuronal or

TABLE 2
Differences and characteristics in the muscle biopsies of patients with ALS and PPMA

	PPMA	ALS
1 Fibre type grouping of normal sized fibres	Always present even in asymptomatic muscles (large groups, up to 170 fibres per group)	Found in up to 25% of the patients (groups are *much* smaller than those noted in PPMA)
2 Scattered angulated fibres	Present in PPMA (absent in asymptomatic post-polio)	Present
3 Group atrophy	Very rare in the *newly weakening* and previously healthy muscles	Always present in the *weakening* and previously healthy muscles
4 Inflammation	Up to 40% of biopsies	Rare
5 Hypertrophic, moth-eaten, and targetoid fibres	Often present owing to long-standing partial denervation	Rare

From Dalakas [20]

viral component is manifested only in some of the post-polio patients who have new weakness is only speculative. The bands were weak without a concomitant elevation of CSF IgG and, at present, their significance is unknown. Oligoclonal bands in the CSF, often against known viral proteins, are present in other subacute, chronic, or latent viral diseases of the CNS, such as SSPE, herpes, PML, or AIDS encephalopathy. Their presence only in PPMA patients who suffered from a viral motor neuron infection many years earlier and not in patients with ALS who have motor neuron disease but no history of known viral infection could be interpreted to suggest that, if ALS is due to a virus, this virus probably behaves differently from the other *conventional* viruses affecting the human CNS. The nature of these bands remains to be determined.

Muscle Biopsy with Enzyme Histochemistry

The histochemical findings in 35 muscle biopsies of PPMA patients, 5 asymptomatic post-polio patients, and 27 ALS patients are summarized in Table 2. The main features in PPMA muscles in contrast to ALS as previously reported [17–23] include:

(a) *Large* fibre type grouping of *normal* sized fibres, containing up to

170 muscle fibres per group, is present in all PPMA muscles. This suggests that in PPMA the surviving motor neurons have overcompensated for the lost ones by excessive sprouting of their distal axons in an effort to fully reinnervate and control a larger than normal area of muscle function resulting in motor unit sizes of giant proportions. In ALS, however, the fibre type grouping of *normal size* fibres is usually mild, is present only in 25% of the biopsies, and contains on the average not more than 25 muscle fibres per group, as we have previously discussed [11, 19–23, 62]. This suggests that in ALS the degree of compensation via axonal sprouting is incomplete either because of impaired sprouting and reinnervation or because of the shorter life span of motor neurons.

(b) *Scattered angulated fibres and group atrophy.* Angulated fibres, scattered among the normal sized fibres, are always found in PPMA as well as in ALS but not in the asymptomatic post-polio muscles [7–23]. Group atrophy, which is always present in the *atrophic* muscles of patients with post-polio and ALS, is characteristically absent in the newly weakened and previously well-recovered PPMA muscles [7–23]. As PPMA progresses, however, small group atrophy can develop [7–23]. This indicates that in PPMA the ongoing compensation with excessive distal sprouting and motor unit enlargement stresses the neuronal cell body, which after a number of years can no longer support further reinnervation and cannot maintain the metabolic demands of all the distal sprouting, resulting in slow disintegration of some nerve terminals (represented as small, scattered angulated fibres) but not death of a whole motor neuron. In contrast, if major axonal branches or entire neurons were progressively dying as in ALS, atrophic fibres in groups (group atrophy) would have developed very early, resulting in more severe and rapidly progressive muscle weakness.

(c) *Perivascular or interstitial inflammation.* This consists predominantly of lymphocytes and is present in up to 40% of the PPMA biopsies [19–23]. Inflammation is only rarely seen in ALS and other motor neuron diseases but it can be occasionally seen in neuropathies. Such inflammation, especially in areas unrelated to fibre necrosis, could represent an ongoing disease activity similar to the presence of mild inflammation we have seen in the spinal cord of PPMA patients [24–26]. The possibility that in PPMA these lymphocytes represent an ongoing immune response in a form of activated lymphocytes, similar to those seen in other autoimmune neuromuscular diseases such as myasthenia gravis, cannot be excluded. Alternatively, such an inflammatory response may represent mechanical injuries due to extreme stretching or lengthening of these muscles.

TABLE 3
Electrophysiological findings in post-polio state and ALS

	Post-polio*	ALS
Fibrillation and psw	Present (+) including the stable muscles	+ + +
Fasciculations	Frequently present (+), even in stable muscles	+ + +
Giant, potentials, of long duration, polyphasic	Often above 10 mV in amplitude	Rarely above 10 mV in amplitude
Fibre density	Very high	Increased
Jitter and blocking	Increased, even in 'stable' muscles suggestive of ongoing reinnervation (very unstable in weak muscles)	Often increased
Neurogenic jitter	Not often seen, suggestive of instability of distal sprouts and failure of reinnervation of groups	Often found

* No significant differences were found between PPMA and stable post-polio muscles [38]
psw: positive sharp waves
+ to + + +: degree of frequency
From Dalakas [20]

(d) *Hypertrophic fibres with internal nuclei, 'moth-eaten' and targetoid fibres.* These are relatively common findings in PPMA patients, especially in those muscles that have been partially recovered after the original disease [19–25]. They could be the result of the chronic denervating state, reflecting possibly an attempt of the muscle fibre to adapt to increasing work demands from overuse [63]. Such fibres are very rare in ALS probably because of the short life span of the disease and underuse of the remaining muscles as a result of the rapid progression of the weakness.

Electromyographic Findings

The electrophysiological findings and differences between PPMA and ALS are summarized in Table 3. We have examined several PPMA patients with conventional EMG as well as single fibre EMG. Muscles that have been stable or newly weakened have been specifically studied and compared [10, 11, 38].

In PPMA the frequency of fibrillation potentials can be very low and several minutes should be spent at each site in order to be sure of their presence or absence. There is no doubt that the fibrillation that appeared in the acute polio can continue during the early months of recovery and can even persist in the chronic state, 20 or more years after the original illness [10, 11, 38, 64, 65]. The presence of fibrillation in PPMA does not therefore represent a sign of new denervation. Weichers has reported a case where fibrillation was seen 9 years after polio [64]. Our own studies show that fibrillation is present equally in muscles that are strong or weak, stable or deteriorating [10, 11, 38]. As compared to ALS, however, the degree of fibrillation and positive sharp waves in post-polio is not as dramatic as in ALS. In my judgment, ALS muscles show much higher frequency of fibrillation, which is easily detectable after the insertion of the needle except in the very earlier stage of the disease.

It has been believed for years that fibrillation is indicative of acute denervation. In circumstances of acute nerve injury it has been thought that fibrillation lasts at most a year or two and ceases to exist after reinnervation has been completed. Careful review of the literature, however, indicates that this is not always the case. Buchthal and Pinnelli [66] have shown that 20% of patients after nerve injuries might have fibrillation 5 years after the nerve lesion. This was also the experience of Lütschg and Ludin, who saw fibrillation in 3 of 12 patients with nerve injuries 6–16 years before [67]. Fibrillations, therefore, may be an indication of a continuing process of denervation and reinnervation as part of the 'normal process' of repair after nerve injury and do not necessarily indicate active disease. Their presence in post-polio muscles does not appear to have any special diagnostic implication.

In reference to fasciculations, these can also be present in all post-polio muscles regardless of new weakness or stability. Again, this does not appear to have special significance and does not indicate developing motor neuron disease, even if they are associated with muscle cramps [68]. Complex repetitive discharges can also be seen without apparent significance in both stable and post-polio muscles. It is my experience overall that the presence of fasciculations is much more frequent in ALS patients. One has to spend more minutes waiting with the needle inserted in the muscle for the presence of fasciculations in PPMA than in ALS muscles except in the early stage of ALS when there is no apparent difference.

Motor unit action potentials on voluntary activation are very large in amplitude and long in duration in PPMA patients and these abnormalities are seen in most muscles, even in those that are stable or normal [7–23, 38, 64, 65, 69, 70]. Motor unit size correlates with muscle power but not with the presence of recent progression [69, 70]. Motor unit counting by the method introduced by McComas et al can in fact demonstrate loss of motor neurons in post-polio muscle [71]. It has been my experience that giant voluntary motor unit action potentials in post-polio patients can reach up to 20 mV amplitude whereas in ALS the amplitude of the voluntary motor unit is rarely above 10 mV. This observation is consistent with the size of fibre type grouping noted in the muscle biopsies and indicates that in PPMA the motor neurons have been excessively stressed to innervate and have resulted in giant sized motor units. In ALS, in contrast, the process is limited either because the motor neurons do not live long enough for the reinnervating process to reach functional maturity or because their capacity to oversprout is impaired owing to sickness of the cell.

The findings with the single fibre EMG are also informative in comparing PPMA and ALS. The fibre density is very much increased in post-polio muscles but it is also increased in ALS although not to the proportion noted in post-polio [11, 38]. This again reflects the size of the motor units and the degree of reinnervation mentioned above and is the physiological correlate of extensive type grouping seen histologically. A reasonable assessment of the total number of muscle fibres in the whole motor unit is also provided with macro EMG, which shows increased amplitude in both diseases but much more so in post-polio, consistent with the previous data [72]. Jitter, formally termed the 'mean consecutive difference' that measures the time difference of the generation of the muscle action potentials in two or more muscle fibres in successive firings, is increased in all the post-polio muscles, including the clinically stable one. Blocking, which indicates failure of impulse propagation at one of the neuromuscular junctions or one of the axonal branch points, is also increased in post-polio muscles. Both jitter and blocking are also increased in ALS and no difference exists between the two in reference to the frequency and degree of jitter or blocking [10, 11, 38, 65].

The interpretation of the single fibre EMG results is not clear [11]. Jitter reflects instability at the axonal branch points or the neuromuscular junction, which is electrophysiologically normal in post-polio [11, 38]. The general opinion is that jitter at axonal branch points represents an acute process arising from the newly myelinated axonal sprouts. However, as noted above for the presence of fibrillation, we could not correlate jitter or blocking with the presence of recent deterioration. It appears, therefore, that increased jitter can persist indefinitely after acute polio and may represent the presence of a continuing denervation and reinnerveration process. Of interest may be the presence of neurogenic jitter, which is the jitter ascribed to the axonal branch points and not due to instability at the end plate. Neurogenic jitter can be seen in ALS patients, and we have noted it in most of the patients we studied [10, 11, 38]. However, neurogenic jitter was absent in the patients with PPMA that we have examined [10, 11, 38]. While this is a negative observation, it does suggest that in PPMA the presence of pathological findings involves individual axonal twigs rather than the whole nerve, as most likely occurs in ALS because of the drop-out of whole neurons.

Another electrophysiological difference between ALS and PPMA is based on the study of Borg and Borg [73], who examined the properties of single motor action potentials in both post-polio and ALS. In post-polio, there was a reduced proportion of nerve fibres with low conduction velocity as compared to normal. The mean fibre conduction velocity was increased in patients with post-polio but decreased in patients with ALS [73]. In post-polio there was a normal relationship between conduction velocity and refractory period, while in ALS there were abnormally long refractory periods. The conclusion from these studies is that there appear to be differences in the physiology of axons in post-polio and ALS and that in the post-polio state the axons behave more normally. In addition, axons in post-polio tend to be larger than normal, supporting the idea that the remaining functional motor units are all large. This is consistent with the hypothesis that in ALS the whole motor neuron dies whereas in post-polio there is dysfunction of the neuron with disintegration of the distal branches and sprouts.

Spinal Cord Pathology

The pathological findings for the spinal cord in stable post-polio, PPMA, and ALS are summarized in Table 4. We have shown [24–26] loss of motor neurons in the anteromedial and anterolateral groups of the grey matter in all the studied post-polio spinal cords. Several surviving neurons were present throughout the grey matter but some of them had abnormal configuration of their somata consisting of atrophy, accumulation of lipofuscin, and loss of Nissl substance; other neurons were in a chromatolytic state [24–26]. A remarkable finding was the presence of inflammation, which was perivascular in five and parenchymal in six post-polio spinal cords [24–26]. The inflammatory exudates consisting of lymphocytes and plasma cells were present in every post-polio patient, regardless of the presence of new weakness (Table 4), suggesting that abnormalities continue for many years in the spinal cord, the site of the

TABLE 4
Spinal cord examination in post-polio state and ALS

	PPMA or stable post-polio	ALS
Inflammation	Yes, perivascular and in the parenchyma of the grey matter	Absent
Active gliosis	Yes, disproportional to the neuronal loss	Gliosis, proportional to the neuronal loss
Neuronal atrophy	Present, with chromatolysis	Chromatolysis is rare
Axonal spheroids	Yes	Only in rapidly progressive form
Corticospinal tracts	Spared	Always affected

From Dalakas [20]

original viral infection. Meningeal lymphocytic infiltrates were also present in all our cases [24–26]. Gliosis was increased and it was disproportional to the overall degree of neuronal dysfunction. The corticospinal tracts were intact. In contrast, in ALS the spinal cord shows no inflammation, the gliosis is proportional to the loss of neurons, no chromatolysis is present, and degeneration of the corticospinal tracts is almost always present. Another interesting observation was the presence of axonal spheroids that we noted in three PPMA patients [24–26]. Axonal spheroids represent defect in the transport of neuronal material from the neuron down the body of the axon, and they are similar to the axonal swelling seen in IDPN intoxication [74, 75]. Axonal spheroids are only rarely seen in conventional ALS but are found in these patients who have undergone recent (within 6–12 months) neuronal deterioration [74]. Their presence in PPMA neurons supports our view of new, ongoing neuronal dysfunction.

Metabolic Status of Cortical Neurons

The cortical metabolic activity of the ALS and PPMA cortex was studied with the PET scan using [^{18}F]-2-fluoro-2-deoxy-D-glucose as previously reported [19, 40]. In PPMA, as well as ALS patients with disease confined to lower motor neurons, the metabolic activity of the cortex is normal. In contrast, in patients with advanced ALS and upper motor neuron involvement, there is a diffuse hypometabolism, which averages 22% below normal, throughout the cortex and basal ganglia but not the cerebellum [40]. The degree of hypometabolism in ALS patients correlates with the length of disease, as we reported [40]. The apparent difference in the metabolic activity of the cortex between ALS and PPMA adds another dimension to the other differences described above between these two motor neuron diseases. When we recently reanalysed the data on PPMA patients' cortical metabolic activity using a brain size index for correction [76], there was a trend toward somewhat lower metabolic activity in the post-polio patients than in the normals and in the patients with ALS confined to lower motor neurons, but not as low as in the ALS patients with upper motor neuron involvement [76]. Although the significance of this observation is uncertain, it may be due to the fact that during the original polio attack the disease was generalized, causing a degree of encephalitis which may have affected the function of some cortical neurons.

Discussion: The Pathogenesis of PPMA in Reference to ALS

Although both PPMA and ALS are disorders of the motor neuron, their physiological, clinical, and histological features differ in a number of ways as described above. Based on these findings, we formulate the pathogenesis of PPMA as follows. After acute polio, there exist unimpaired motor neurons, motor neurons that have fully or partially recovered and can resume normal or near-normal function, and dying neurons. The terminal axons of the surviving motor neurons sprout in an attempt to reinnervate as many as possible of those muscle fibres orphaned by the death of their parent motor neurons. An uninvolved or recovered anterior horn cell adopts in its motor unit territory additional muscle fibres that could reach as many as 4–5 new muscle fibres for every muscle fibre innervated originally [77]. This process produces very large motor units and is so effective that despite the loss of up to 50% of the original number of motor neurons, the muscle can retain clinically normal strength [77].

After the maximum recovery has been achieved following the acute polio, the reinnervated motor units have not matured and stabilized as was expected. To the contrary, there is evidence of an ongoing denervating/reinnervating process resulting in continuous remodelling of the motor units in all the muscles regardless of the presence of new weakness, as evidenced by the presence of abnormal jitter and blocking in both the clinically stable and the newly weakened muscles. This reflects a continuous effort of the post-polio motor neuron to reinnervate additional muscle fibres via excessive distal sprouting, a process that has been stressing the cell body for a number of years. When the metabolic capability of the motor neuron to maintain such an excessive number of functional sprouts reaches a limit, these hyperfunctioning motor neurons can no longer maintain the metabolic demands of all their sprouts and lose their ability to further reinnervate. This results in slow deterioration affecting the nerve terminals. As each nerve terminal dies, individual muscle fibres become denervated. Some of these individual muscle fibres may be able to be reinnervated a second time but eventually as the neuron loses its ability to keep pace, enough nerve terminals are destroyed and enough reserves are diminished for weakness to appear [10, 11]. This is supported by the increased jitter even in asymptomatic muscles, and is consistent with the fall in the amplitude with macro-EMG and the presence in the muscle biopsy of new scattered angulated fibres which are evident only when this process has reached the level of producing symptoms.

PPMA, therefore, is caused by the death of individual terminals in the motor units that remain after polio rather than by death of the whole units as occurs in ALS. This explains most of the physiological and histochemical features of PPMA, and it is consistent with the focal nature of its weakness and its slow, stepwise, unpredictable progression. As each terminal dies the weakness progresses slowly. Regeneration proceeds muscle fibre by muscle fibre and there is no opportunity to form new groups of fibres. This conclusion is supported by the presence of single, scattered angulated fibres in the muscle biopsy specimens without group atrophy and the observation by single fibre EMG that there is no neurogenic jitter [7–23, 38]. Neurogenic jitter which is characterized by groups of axon potentials that jitter together can be observed in patients with ALS. Its absence in patients with PPMA supports the observation that there is lack of reinnervation of groups [10, 11]. Furthermore, if major axonal branches or entire neurons were progressively dying as in ALS, atrophic fibres in groups (group atrophy) would have developed, resulting in more severe and rapidly progressive muscle weakness. Although no group atrophy was noted in the newly weakened post-polio muscles, as PPMA progresses some adjacent fibres can become atrophic and eventually a small group atrophy will develop as more distal sprouts that belong to the same or neighbouring motor units continue to disintegrate [23]. Finally some of the very scarred neurons with minimal muscle reserves, such as those innervating very few muscle fibres may completely disintegrate, resulting in group atrophy. Group atrophy, therefore, noted more frequently by others [65], is the end stage of this process. Normal ageing alone cannot be responsible for this process, since neuronal loss does not occur in persons younger than 60 [78], and muscle biopsy specimens from normal persons who are younger than 70 rarely show small, scattered angulated fibres [79].

PPMA is not ALS and does not lead to ALS. It is a rather benign, very slowly progressive motor neuron disease, confined to lower motor neurons, and has more differences from than similarities to ALS. Confusion should be therefore avoided, and if clusters of PPMA patients are reported as 'ALS' such a report should be cautiously investigated. At the present time, a post-polio patient appears to have the same chance to develop ALS as the non–post-polio sufferer. An ongoing epidemiological survey that is now being conducted by the Center for Health Statistics (Dalakas MC, personal communication, 1987) should substantiate (or disprove) our contention.

Some points need further clarification. We have seen and heard of very rare post-polio patients who died with respiratory muscle weakness in a fashion resembling ALS. This can happen in those post-polio survivors who have been left with a severe residual respiratory muscle deficit from the original disease and can be due to either medical problems affecting respiratory reserves such as congestive heart failure, intrinsic lung disease, and bronchopneumonias or due to PPMA affecting predominantly the thoracic motor neurons diminishing further the already compromised respiratory muscle reserves. PPMA affecting the respiratory muscles, if it develops, should progress slowly and can be monitored with pulmonary function studies [44]. It should be stressed that we have observed a decline in the respiratory function only in those PPMA patients who had been left with minimal thoracic muscle reserves after the original illness and not in patients who at their onset of PPMA had only limb weakness and adequate-to-normal respiratory function.

It has been reported that rare post-polio patients have spasticity [47]. My approach to these data is as follows: (a) Were other causes of spasticity ruled out? (b) Does the patient have significant scoliosis causing spinal cord compression? (c) Has MRI or myelogram been performed to rule out other concomitant spinal cord disease? If no other disease is found, and the patient has spasticity and new muscle weakness with diffuse atrophy and fasciculations, the possibility of ALS should be considered not because it is more common in a post-polio state but simply because post-polio patients are not immune to developing ALS. Occasionally, positive Babinksi's sign can be seen in PPMA patients [11]. If no other upper motor neuron signs are present, this finding is of uncertain significance. It could represent dysfunction of cortical neurons which were also clinically or subclinically affected during the original illness, or it may be due to unequal degree of paralysis and uneven innervation of the muscles in the foot, as can be occasionally seen in peripheral nerve disorders [11].

From the comparative analysis of the clinical, histological, electrophysiological, metabolic, and histochemical findings described above, we can make some speculations regarding the neurobiology of motor neurons. After a viral insult to the motor neurons (acute polio), there appears to be evidence of an ongoing activity with a continuous effort of the surviving motor neurons to reinnervate and remodel their motor units. Evidence of such a continuous activity was based predominantly on our electrophysiological findings of denervation/reinnervation even in the stable post-polio muscles 5–10 years after polio (Huang, Hallett, Dalakas, unpublished observations) and was supported by one recent case, 2 years after vaccine-associated polio [64]. The presence of continuous activity in the post-polio state is also supported by our observations in the spinal cord, where we have found active gliosis and inflammation many years later, raising the possibility of a smouldering neuronal dysfunction which, although subsided, did not completely cease after the acute viral infection.

PPMA appears to develop in some patients after an average period of 30 years from the original polio attack [7–16, 42, 53]. Since the PPMA motor neurons have been stressed to maintain enlarged motor units for a long time, one wonders if there is a time limit of almost 30 years for the capacity of such hyperfunctioning neurons to maintain fully the metabolic needs of their distal axonal sprouts. Unfortunately, no information exists in a human biological system regarding the life span of a scarred neuron or a normal but hyperfunctioning neuron that has been stressed to oversprout in order to control a larger than normal area of motor function. Spinal cord neurons start to decline in function after the age of 60 through the process of normal ageing [78]. In addition, motor unit decompensation may be accelerated by normal ageing, which has been associated with increased end-plate complexity [80] and reduced terminal sprouting [81]. Therefore, normal ageing or premature ageing brought on by attrition could be contributing factors to the mechanisms of PPMA discussed above.

From the PET scan studies it is evident that ALS is a more generalized disorder extending beyond the corticospinal tract and the motor cortex. It also appears from preliminary data that motor neuron diseases confined to lower motor neurons such as PPMA have relatively normal cortical metabolism. This suggests that the functional integrity of the upper motor neuron does not depend on a signal from its lower motor neuron target via the corticospinal tract. Upper motor neurons therefore behave differently from the lower motor neurons, which disintegrate after their peripheral axon is cut [82].

References

1 Charcot JA, Jottroy A. Cas de paralysie infantile spinale avec lésions des cornes antérieures de le substance gris de la moelle épiniere. Arch Physiol Norm Pathol 1870;3:134

2 Cornil V, Lepine R. Sur un cas de paralysie générale spinale antérieure subaique, suivi d'autopsie. Gaz Méd de Paris 1875;127

3 Campbell AMG, Williams FR, Pearce J. Late motor neuron degeneration following poliomyelitis. Neurology (Minneap) 1969;19:1101–1106

4 Anderson AD, Levine SA, Gellert H. Loss of ambulatory ability in patient with old anterior poliomyelitis. Lancet 1972;ii:1061–1063

5 Mulder DW, Rosenbaum RA, Layton DO Jr. Late progression of poliomyelitis or forme fruste amyotrophic lateral sclerosis. Mayo Clin Proc 1972;47:756–61

6 Hayward S, Seaton D. Late sequelae of paralytic poliomyelitis. A clinical and electromyographic study. J Neurol Neurosurg Psychiat 1979;42:117–122

7 Dalakas MC. Post-poliomyelitis muscular atrophy. In: Laurie G and Raymond J, eds. Proceedings of the 2nd International Poliomyelitis and Independent Living Conference. St Louis, CV Mosby, 1984;18

8 Dalakas MC. Post-polio syndrome. In: Yearbook of Nursing '88. Springhouse, PA, Springhouse Pub, 1988;50–54

9 Dalakas MC. New neuromuscular symptoms after polio (the post-polio syndrome): Clinical studies and pathogenetic mechanisms. In: Halstead LS and Weichers DO, eds. Research and Clinical Aspects of the Late Effects of Poliomyelitis. March of Dimes 1987;23:241–264

10 Dalakas MC, Elder G, Hallett H, Ravits J, Baker M, Papadopoulos N, Albrecht P, Sever J. A long-term follow-up study of patients with post-poliomyelitis neuromuscular symptoms. New Eng J Med 1986;314:959–963

11 Dalakas MC, Hallett M. The post-polio syndrome. In: Plum F, ed. Advances of Contemporary Neurology. PA, Philadelphia, FA Davis, 1988;51–94

12 Dalakas MC. New neuromuscular symptoms in patients with old poliomyelitis: A three year follow-up study. Eur Neurol 1986;25:381–387

13 Dalakas MC. Recent research issues in post-poliomyelitis muscular atrophy (PPMA): Pathogenesis and rate of progression. In: Laurie G, Raymond J, eds. Proceedings of 3rd International Post-polio Conference. St Louis, Gazette International Networking Institute, 1986;39

14 Dalakas MC, Elder G, Sever JL. A 9 year follow-up study of patients with late post-poliomyelitis muscular atrophy. Neurology 1985;35(suppl 1):108

15 Dalakas MC, Sever JLk, Fletcher M, Madden DL, Papadopoulous N, Shekarchi l, Albrecht P. Neuromuscular symptoms in patients with old poliomyelitis: Clinical virological and immunological studies. In: Halstead LS, Wiechers DO, eds. Late Effects of Poliomyelitis Miami, Symposia Foundation, 1984;73–89

16 Dalakas MC, Sever JL, Madden DL, Papadopoulous NM, Shekarchi IC, Albrecht P, Krezlewicz A. Late post-poliomyelitis muscular atrophy: Clinical virological and immunological studies. Rev Infect Dis 1984;6:S562–567

17 Dalakas MC. Future basic research issues for post-poliomyelitis. In: Halstead LS, Weichers DO, eds. Late Effects of Poliomyelitis. Miami, Symposia Foundation, 1984;225–227

18 Dalakas MC. Morphological changes in the muscle of patients with post-poliomyelitis new weakness. A histochemical study of 39 muscle biopsies. Muscle & Nerve 1986;9:117

19 Dalakas MC. How relevant are recent studies of ALS and post-polio progressive muscular atrophy patients regarding PET scanning, polio antigen/antibody, and AIDS virus? Muscle & Nerve 1986;9:56

20 Dalakas MC. ALS and post-polio: Differences and similarities. In: Halstead LS, Wiechers DO, eds. Research and Clinical Aspects of the Late Effects of Poliomyelitis. March of Dimes 1987;23:63–81

21 Dalakas MC. Morphological changes in the muscles of patients with post-poliomyelitis neuromuscular symptoms. Neurology 1988;38:99–104

22 Dalakas MC, Elder G, Sever JL. Morphological changes in the muscles of patients with post-poliomyelitis muscular atrophy (PPMA): Analysis of 38 biopsies. Neurology 1986;36(1):137

23 Dalakas MC, Elder G, Hallett M, Sever JL. Post-poliomyelitis neuromuscular symptoms (a reply). New Eng J Med 1986;315:897–898

24 Pezeshkpour GH, Dalakas MC. Long term changes in the spinal cord of patients with old poliomyelitis: Signs of continuous disease activity. Neurology 1987;37(1):215

25 Pezeshkpour GH, Dalakas MC. Pathology of the spinal cord in post-poliomyelitis muscular atrophy. In: Halstead LS, Wiechers DO, eds. Research and Clinical Aspects of the Late Effects of Poliomyelitis. March of Dimes 1987;23:229–236

26 Pezeshkpour GH, Dalakas MC. Long-term changes in the spinal cord of patients with old poliomyelitis: Evidence of active disease. Arch Neurol 1988;45:505–508

27 Medical Research Council. Aids to the Examination of the Peripheral Nervous System. London, Her Majesty's Stationery Office, 1981;1

28 Dalakas MC, et al. Human peripheral blood lymphocytes bear markers for thymosins (α_1, α_7, β_4). In: Goldstein AL, Chirigos G, eds. Thymic Hormones and Lymphokines. New York, Plenum Press, 1984;111–114

29 Dalakas MC, Stone G, Elder G, et al. Tropical spastic paraparesis: Clinical, immunological, and virological studies in two patients from Martinique. Ann Neuro 1988;23(suppl):S136–S142

30 Dalakas MC, Engel WK. Polyneuropathy with monoclonal gammopathy: Studies of 11 patients. Ann Neuro 1981;10:45–52

31 Dalakas MC, Trapp BT. Thymosin β_4 is a shared antigen between lymphoid

cells and oligodendrocytes of normal human brain. Ann Neurol 1986;19:349–355

32 Dalakas MC, Cunningham G. Characterization of amyloid deposits in biopsies of 15 patients with 'sporadic' (nonfamilial or plasma cell dyscrasic) amyloid polyneuropathy. Acta Neuropathol 1986;69:66–72

33 Dalakas MC, Papadopoulos NM. Paraproteins in the spinal fluid of patients with paraproteinemic polyneuropathies. Ann Neurol 1984;15:590–593

34 Dalakas MC, Houff SA, Engel WK, et al. CSF monoclonal bands in chronic relapsing polyneuropathy. Neurology 1980;30:864–867

35 Albrecht P, et al. Standardization of poliovirus neutralizing antibody tests. Rev Inf Dis 1984;6:S540–554

36 Albrecht P, et al. Intra-blood-brain barrier measles virus antibody synthesis in multiple sclerosis patients. Neurology 1983;33:45–50

37 Dalakas MC, Gravell M, London WT, et al. Morphological changes of an inflammatory myopathy in rhesus monkeys with simian acquired immuno-deficiency syndrome. Proc Soc Exp Biol Med 1987;185:368–376

38 Ravits J, Hallett M, Baker M, Dalakas MC. Clinical and EMG studies of post-poliomyelitis muscular atrophy. Neurology 1987;37(Suppl 1):161

39 Stalberg E. Electrophysiological studies of reinnervation in amyotrophic lateral sclerosis. In: Rowland LP, ed. Human Motor Neuron Diseases. New York, Raven Press, 1982;47

40 Dalakas MC, Hatazawa J, Brooks RA, Di Chiro G. Lowered cerebral glucose utilization in amyotrophic lateral sclerosis. Ann Neurol 1988;22:580–586

41 Glasberg MR, Dalakas MC, Engel WK. Muscle cramps and pains: Histochemical analysis of muscle biopsies in 63 patients. Neurology 1978;28:387

42 Halstead LS, Wiechers DO, eds. Research and Clinical Aspects of the Late Effects of Poliomyelitis, Vol. 23. March of Dimes, 1987

43 Sonies B, Dalakas M. New bulbar symptoms in previously asymptomatic post-polio patients: A dynamic study of oral motor dysfunction with video-fluoroscopy. Neurology 1988;38(suppl):425

44 Fisher DA. Poliomyelitis: Late pulmonary complications and management. In: Halstead LS, Wiechers DO, eds. Late Effects of Poliomyelitis. Miami, Symposia Foundation 1984;185–192

45 Fisher DA. Sleep disordered breathing as a late effect of poliomyelitis. In: Halstead LS, Wiechers DO, eds. Research and Clinical Aspects of the Late Effects of Poliomyelitis. March of Dimes 1987;23:115–120

46 Guilleminault C, ed. Sleeping and Waking Disorders: Indications and Techniques. Menlo Park, CA, Addison-Wesley, 1982

47 Block HS, Wilbourn AJ. Progressive post-polio atrophy: The EMG findings. Neurology 1986;36(suppl):137

48 Dalakas MC. Unpublished observations 1982–1988

49 Dalakas MC. et al. Recombinant α_2 interferon in a pilot trial of patients with ALS. Arch Neurol 1986;43:933–935

50 Poskanzer DC, Cantor HM, Kaplan GS. The frequency of preceding poliomyelitis in amyotrophic lateral sclerosis. In: Norris FH Jr, Kurland LT, eds. Motor Neuron Diseases: Research on Amyotrophic Lateral Sclerosis and Related Disorders. New York, Grune and Stratton, 1969;286–290

51 Zilkha K. Discussion on motor neuron disease. Proc R Soc Med 1962;55:1028–1029

52 Weiner LP. Possible role of androgen receptors in amyotrophic lateral sclerosis. Arch Neurol 1980;37:129–131

53 Halstead LS, Wiechers DO, eds. Late Effects of Poliomyelitis. Miami, Symposia Foundation, 1984

54 Kondo K, Tsubaki T. Case-control studies of motor neuron disease: Association with mechanical injuries. Arch Neurol 1981;38:220–226

55 Drachman DB, Murphy SR, Nigam MP, Hills JR. Myopathic changes in chronically denervated muscle. Arch Neurol 1967;16:14–24

56 Haase GR, Shy GM. Pathological changes in muscle biopsies from patients with peroneal muscular atrophy. Brain 1960;83:631–642

57 Shy ME, Rowland LP, Latov N, Pesce MA, Sherman W. Characteristics of 40 patients with motor neuron diseases and monoclonal gammopathy. Muscle & Nerve 1986;9:55, 107

58 Freddo L, Yu RK, Latov N, et al. Gangliosides G_{M1} and GD_{1b} are antigens for lgM M protein in a patient with motor neuron disease. Neurology 1986;36:454–458

59 Ilyas A, Dalakas MC, Quarles RH. Unpublished observations 1987

60 Ilyas AA, Li SC, Chou DKH, Li YT, Jungalwala FB, Dalakas MC, Quarles RH. Gangliosides as antigens for monoclonal lgM in two patients with neuropathy. J Biol Chem 1988;263:4369–4373

61 Dalakas MC, Galdi A. Unpublished observations 1987

62 Engel WK, Brook MH. Muscle Biopsy in ALS and Other Motor Neuron Diseases: Research on ALS and Related Disorders. New York, Grune and Stratton, 1964;154–159

63 Carpenter S, Karpati G. Pathology of Skeletal Muscle. New York, Churchill Livingston, 1984

64 Wiechers DO. Reinnervation after acute poliomyelitis. In: Halstead LS, Wiechers DO, eds. Research and Clinical Aspects of the Late Effects of Poliomyelitis. March of Dimes 1987;23:213–221

65 Cashman NR, et al. Late denervation in patients with ancecedent paralytic poliomyelitis. New Eng J Med 1987;317:7–12

66 Buchthal F, Pinelli P. Action potentials in muscular atrophy of neurogenic origin. Neurology (Minneap) 1953;3:591–603

67 Lütschg J, Ludin HP. Electromyographic findings in patients after recovery from peripheral nerve lesions and poliomyelitis. J Neurol 1981;225:25–32

68 Fetell MR, et al. A benign motor neuron disorder: delayed cramps and fasciculation after poliomyelitis or myelitis. Ann Neurol 1982;11:423–427

69 Cruz Martinez A, Ferrer MT, Perez Conde MC. Electrophysiological features in patients with non-progressive and late progressive weakness after paralytic poliomyelitis. Conventional EMG automatic analysis of the electromyogram and single fibre electromyography study. Electromyogr Clin Neurophysiol 1984;24:469–479

70 Cruz Martinez A, Perez Conde MC, Ferrer, MT. Chronic partial denervation is more widespread than is suspected clinically in paralytic poliomyelitis: Electrophysiological study. Eur Neurol 1983;22:314–321

71 McComas AJ, et al. Three novel electrophysiologic tests for patients with muscle weakness. In: Halstead LS, Wiechers DO, eds. Research and Clinical Aspects of the Late Effects of Poliomyelitis. March of Dimes 1987;23:201–212

72 Maselli RA, Cashman N, Salazar E, Spire JP, Roos R. Impairment of neuromuscular transmission in patients with prior history of poliomyelitis. Muscle & Nerve 1987;10:665

73 Borg K, Borg J. Conduction velocity and refractory period of single motor nerve fibres in antecedent poliomyelitis. J Neurol Neurosurg Psychiat 1987;50:443–446

74 Carpenter J. Proximal axonal enlargement in motor neuron disease. Neurology 1968;18:842–851

75 Griffin JW, Price DL. Proximal axonopathies induced by toxic chemicals. In: Spencer PS, Shaunberg HH, eds. Experimental and Clinical Neurotoxicology. Baltimore, Williams and Wilkins, 1980;161–178

76 Hatazawa J, Brooks RA, Dalakas MC, Di Chiro G. Regional cerebral hypometabolism in amyotrophic lateral sclerosis. J Comput Assist Tomography 1988;12:630–636

77 Sharrad WJW. Correlation between changes in the spinal cord and muscle paralysis in poliomyelitis. Proc R Soc Med 1953;40:346

78 Tomlison BE, Irving D. The numbers of limb motor neurons in the human lumbosacral cord throughout life. J Neurol Sci 1977;34:213–219

79 Hicks JE, Cutler NA, Dalakas MC. Assessment of peripheral nervous system involvement in normal aged and Alzheimer's patients. Arch Phys Med Rehab 1985;16:10

80 Rosenheimer JL, Smith DO. Differential changes in the end-plate architecture of functionally diverse muscles during ageing. J Neurophysiol 1985;53:1567

81 Perstronk A, Drachman DB, Griffin JW. Effects of aging on nerve sprouting and regeneration. Exp Neurol 1980;70:65

82 Kawamura Y, Dyck PJ. Permanent axotomy by amputation results in loss of motor neurons in man. J Neuropath Exp Neurol 1981;40:658–666

Recent Developments in PET Scanning Related to Amyotrophic Lateral Sclerosis and Primary Lateral Sclerosis

E. STEPHEN GARNETT, RAMAN CHIRAKAL,
GUNTER FIRNAU, CLAUDE NAHMIAS, AND
ARTHUR J.HUDSON

Positron computerized tomography (PCT), also called positron emission tomography (PET), is a technique by which the metabolic behaviour or blood flow in a prescribed volume of tissue can be investigated simply and atraumatically during life. The technique comprises two components, the tomograph itself and a source of tracer molecules that are labelled with suitable positron-emitting isotopes. In this chapter we will discuss some of the principles that underlie PCT and then describe what we found when PCT was used with [^{18}F]fluoro-2-deoxyglucose (^{18}FDG) to examine cortical glucose consumption in the brains of patients with primary lateral sclerosis and amyotrophic lateral sclerosis.

Positron Computerized Tomography Procedure and Rationale

When the atoms of a radioactive isotope decay they do so by emitting energy. This energy is carried away either as electromagnetic radiation or as the rest mass and kinetic energy of particles or as a combination of both. Some radioactive atoms contain fewer neutrons than their stable counterparts. For example, carbon-11 contains five neutrons whereas its stable counterpart, carbon-12, contains six. Many of these neutron-deficient radioactive atoms, including those of biological interest such as carbon-11, nitrogen-13, oxygen-15, and fluorine-18, decay by emitting a combination of electromagnetic energy and a particle. This particle is a positron, and a radioisotope that decays by emitting it is called a positron emitter. All positrons have the same mass, the mass of an electron or about 1/2000th that of a hydrogen atom. They differ from each other in having different kinetic energies. However, all positrons from one species of radioactive atom have the same kinetic energy when they are emitted. Because of this kinetic energy positrons travel through space. They are brought to rest when they collide with electrons. The distance positrons will travel in brain tissue depends upon their atom of origin but ranges up to 7 mm. Because positrons are not detected by PCT until they have collided with an electron a point source of positrons will always be perceived as a sphere. In practice this means that there is a theoretical limit to the spatial resolution of PET below which even the most advanced instruments cannot go. Contemporary PET devices are approaching this limit; their in-plane and axial resolutions are approximately 5 mm.

When a positron which has lost all or most of its kinetic energy collides with an electron the combined mass of the two oppositely charged particles is transformed into electromagnetic energy in accordance with Einstein's famous equation. $E = mc^2$. This energy is emitted from the site of the collision as a pair of photons travelling in not quite opposite directions. Because the mass of all positrons is the same, the energy of all photons arising from the annihilation of a positron-electron pair will also be the same. This means that PET has no potential for energy resolution and consequently different positron-emitting isotopes, such as carbon-11 and oxygen-15, cannot be distinguished from each other by the tomograph. It is not therefore possible to measure oxygen consumption and glucose utilization simultaneously using oxygen-15 and ^{11}C-labelled glucose as tracers.

The overriding advantage of PCT compared to other imaging modalities is its ability to measure the time course of the concentration of a radioisotope in a defined volume anywhere within an organ or tissue of interest. Then, having defined an operational equation for the system under consideration, the time course of the radioactivity in the tissue and the time course of radioactivity in the blood supplied to the tissue can be used to calculate a local transfer rate, metabolic rate, or binding capacity. These sorts of measurement cannot be made by other techniques: single photon emission computerized tomography (SPECT) is too slow. Proton imaging using magnetic resonance and computerized axial tomography (CAT) are used almost exclusively to define anatomy. Phosphorus-31 MR spectroscopy gives a measure of phosphorus metabolism in volumes of brain close to 30 cm^3. However, it should not be forgotten that it was Kuhl and Edwards's [1] pioneering efforts with single photon tomography and Hounsefield et al's [2] and Cormack's [3] development of x-ray–based axial tomography that provided the technical and mathematical foundations on which contemporary positron tomography is built.

Positron emission tomography, like the other techniques of nuclear medicine, relies on a source of radioisotopes – in this case positron-emitting radioisotopes. The half-lives of the biologically interesting positron emitters are measured in minutes, and consequently the source of these isotopes has to be close to the tomograph. To date, this geographical restriction has greatly reduced the availability of PCT to major centres, often university based, with access to an existing cyclotron or nuclear reactor. However, as PCT gains recognition and its use is extended toward all of the organ systems of the body, small, dedicated medical cyclotrons are being installed in major medical institutions. These cyclotrons generate positron-emitting isotopes of elements. The radioactive element has then to be incorporated into a molecule of biological interest. In the present case the positron emitter fluorine-18, made by bombarding neon atoms with deuterons in a cyclotron, is incorporated into 2-dexoy-D-glucose to give [^{18}F]fluoro-2-deoxy-D-glucose (^{18}FDG). ^{18}FDG, like glucose itself, crosses the blood/brain barrier, equilibrates with the cerebral interstitial fluid, and passes into the neurones, where it is phosphorylated by the enzyme hexokinase. This is the first step in the glycolytic pathway from glucose to pyruvate and thence into Krebs cycle. For ^{18}FDG it is the only step along the pathway. Deoxyglucose and its fluorine-labelled analogue are not substrates for the enzyme phosphoglucose isomerase, the second step. [^{18}F]fluoro-deoxyglucose that has entered a neurone is converted by hexokinase to [^{18}F]fluoro-deoxyglucose-6-phosphate but cannot be metabolized further. Equally important, from the perspective of PCT, the phosphorylated deoxyglucose remains trapped in the neurone. It does not diffuse from the cell; nor is it dephosphorylated, except very slowly. The neurone behaves as a closed sink into which ^{18}FDG enters but from which it cannot escape.

When ^{18}FDG is used as a radiopharmaceutical in positron tomography to measure local cerebral metabolic rates for glucose it is injected intravenously as a bolus. The time course of the ^{18}F radioactivity in the blood is monitored over the next 50 or so minutes and, assuming there has been no fluctuation in the concentration of blood glucose, an average specific activity in units of ^{18}F activity per gram of glucose in the blood can be calculated. At the end of the 50-minute period the patient is positioned in the tomograph and the concentration of ^{18}F in a defined volume of brain is measured. This ^{18}F is trapped in the neurones as described above. The rate at which glucose has been accumulated by the neurones in the defined volume of brain is then given by dividing the value for ^{18}F trapped by the product of the average specific activity and the time between injecting the ^{18}FDG and making the measurement in the tomograph.

Unfortunately this simple quotient does not tell the whole story. It does not allow for ^{18}F in the cerebral interstitial fluid as opposed to the neurones and it does not allow for the fact that the combined transport and enzyme kinetics of natural glucose and [^{18}F]fluoro-2-deoxyglucose differ by a factor of almost 2. In the now famous and much-debated operational equation of Sokoloff et al [4] these complicating factors are taken into account. This operational equation was first described to measure regional cerebral glucose consumption by an autoradiographic technique in rats. With no, or only minor, modification it is now used to measure regional cerebral glucose consumption by the PCT technique in man.

This discussion has avoided the issue of what the neurones do with the energy derived from the combustion of glucose and it has not considered whether the glucose is consumed aerobically or anaerobically. Under normal conditions it is assumed that the glucose is used aerobically and that the energy released when it is consumed is used by the nerve cells to maintain their transmembrane ionic gradients [5] and hence their ability to transfer information through trains of action potentials.

Clinical Studies

Regional brain glucose metabolism was determined by PET using [18]FDG in three patients suffering from *primary lateral sclerosis*, two patients with *amyotrophic lateral sclerosis*, and three age-matched control subjects (Table 1)

Methods

The positron tomograph used in these studies was a single ring device [6] with a spatial resolution in the plane of 8 mm (full width at half-maximum, FWHM) and an axial resolution of 16 mm, FWHM. Sixteen slices of brain were examined sequentially in each patient. The lowest slice included the hippocampal gyri; the highest was at the level of the vertex. The slices were taken in planes parallel to a plane 5° to the orbitomeatal line. Each slice overlapped its predecessor by 5 mm. Approximately a million counts were used to generate an image of one slice. This took 3–5 minutes so that the whole brain was examined in about 1 hour.

[^{18}F]fluoro-deoxyglucose was prepared from glycal [7]. In each patient it was injected iv an hour before tomography. In the interval between the injection of [18]FDG and the tomographic study patients lay quietly on a couch in a normally lit room in which the only sound was that of

TABLE 1
Clinical, electromyographic, and magnetic resonance findings in PLS and ALS

	Diagnosis	Sex	Age (yr)	Duration (yr)	Clinical features	Electromyographic findings	Magnetic resonance images
Patient 1	PLS	F	48	14	-Marked generalized spasticity; almost totally immobile, communicates by grunts -Brisk deep tendon reflexes and bilateral upgoing toes	No evidence of lower motor neurone lesions or of denervation	-Atrophy of temporal lobes, parietal opercula, frontal and parietal lobes superiorly. Corpus callosum thin -Several small areas of increased signal density in subcortical white -Marked iron deposition in globus pallidus
Patient 2	PLS	F	56	6	-Extreme spasticity in all limbs -Cannot walk -No wasting or fasciculation -No sensory loss	-Nothing to suggest lower motor neurone lesions -Normal peripheral and central sensory conduction times	Normal
Patient 3	PLS	M	56	5	-Generalized spasticity with pseudo bulbar palsy -Walks with difficulty -Brisk deep tendon reflexes and bilaterally upgoing toes -No wasting or fasciculation -No sensory loss	-Nothing to suggest lower motor neurone lesions -Normal peripheral and central sensory conduction times	-Mild cortical atrophy -A few areas of increased signal density in subcortical white matter

Patient 4	ALS	F	57	3	-Bulbar and pseudobulbar paresis -Wasted arms and hands with fasciculation -Brisk deep tendon reflexes and bilaterally upgoing toes -No sensory loss	-Denervation potentials -Normal sensory nerve conduction	-Mild widening of cortical sulci, 2–5 mm -Several areas of increased signal density in deep and subcortical white matter -Otherwise normal
Patient 5	ALS	M	64	2	-Bulbar and pseudobulbar paresis -Wasted hands with fasciculation in arms, upper torso, and legs -Brisk deep tendon reflexes and bilateral upgoing toes -No sensory loss	-Denervation potentials	Refused investigation

the air-handling system. During the interval samples of arterialized venous blood were taken from which a value for the mean specific activity was derived.

In each tomographic slice the anatomical distribution of glucose consumption was assigned by comparing the PCT scan with an image obtained by magnetic resonance at an identical level in the brain. The cortical distribution of glucose was also examined by a new projection method [8]. In this method the inner and outer margins of the cortical mantle of each hemisphere of a single tomographic slice are defined electronically. The strip of mantle is then divided into 10° sectors and the ^{18}F content of each sector determined. A colour-coded map of the cortical distribution of regional cerebral glucose consumption is then made by displaying the ^{18}F content of each sector from one slice as coloured rectangles arranged in a sequence along a row starting from the mid-line anteriorly and ending at the mid-line posteriorly. Each tomographic slice is thus represented as a row of blocks of colour. By arranging the rows obtained from adjacent slices one above the other it is possible to make a display of the cortex of each hemisphere. In this display the area of any region of cortex is a 1:1 representation of the cortex examined in each tomographic slice; it has not been diminished by projecting the hemisphere onto a plane. The illustrations of Figures 1 and 2 were made by this method.

Results

Figure 1 is a black-and-white display of the cortical glucose accumulation in patient 1. This individual, a woman, was the most severely affected of the three patients suffering from primary lateral sclerosis. In her, glucose consumption in the whole of the pericentral cortex of both sides was reduced by approximately 50% compared to the rest of the cortex. It was also reduced in the superior parietal cortex on both sides. PCT slices taken at levels above the corpus callosum showed that both zones of reduced glucose consumption extended over the vertex and down the medial aspects of the parietal lobes. Tomographic slices taken at levels below the corpus callosum showed symmetrically reduced glucose consumption in the caudate and putamen and in the thalamus.

Patient 2, another female, was less severely incapacitated than the first, but had a similar distribution of reduced cortical glucose consumption. The pericentral region was most affected but, as in patient 1, glucose accumulation was also reduced in the superior parietal cortex. She also showed the same symmetrical reduction of glucose consumption in the striatum and thalamus. Patient 3 was the least affected of those who had

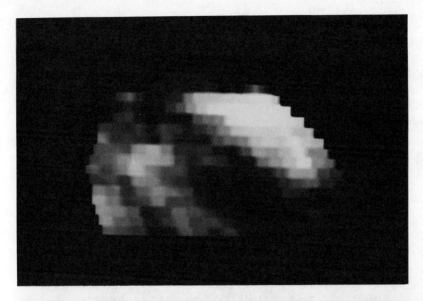

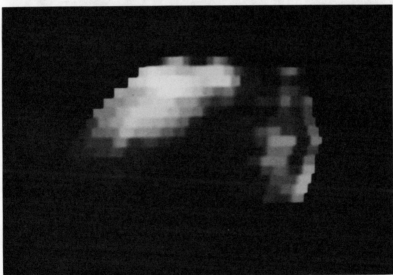

Figure 1. Display of cortical glucose consumption obtained from a 48-year-old female suffering from severe primary lateral sclerosis (patient 1). The shades of grey indicate local glucose consumption relative to that in the whole of the cortical mantle. White represents regions of highest glucose consumption; black, regions of lowest glucose consumption. (In the display of the right hemisphere [upper panel], the patient's nose is on the reader's right. In the display of the left hemisphere [lower panel], the patient's nose is on the reader's left.)

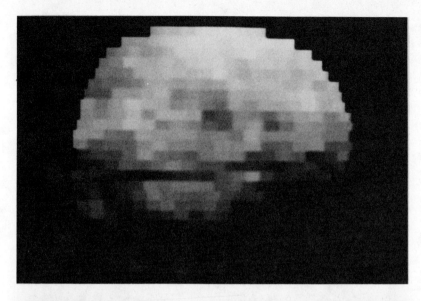

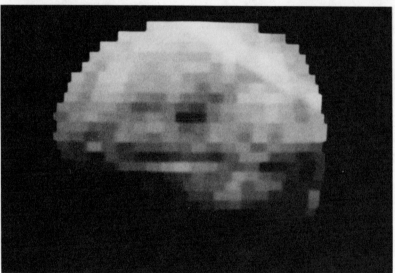

Figure 2. Display of cortical glucose consumption obtained from a 50-year-old, neurologically normal, woman. The grey scale and orientation are the same as those used in Figure 1.

primary lateral sclerosis. He was still able to walk. His distribution of cortical and deep glucose consumption, as seen from the tomographic study, was indistinguishable from normal. The pericentral region accumulated glucose normally and so did the basal ganglia and thalamus. Clinically the two patients who had amyotrophic lateral sclerosis, both of whom had pseudobulbar palsy, were about as incapacitated as patient 3. In both of them the distribution of cortical and deep glucose consumption was indistinguishable from normal (Fig. 2).

Four of the five patients were also examined by MRI. Some degree of cortical atrophy was seen in three (Table 1). It was most severe in patient 1 but involved almost the whole cortex to the same extent. The regions of the central sulci were not particularly atrophic.

Discussion

As far as we know, this is the first time that patients suffering from primary lateral sclerosis have been studied by positron tomography. Primary lateral sclerosis is rare. It is a diagnosis by exclusion in patients with slowly progressing spastic paraparesis [9]. It is distinguished from amyotrophic lateral sclerosis by the absence of muscle wasting and fasciculation and the presence of normal electromyographic patterns from the proximal and distal muscles of both upper and lower extremities. It tends to run a longer course than ALS; our most severely affected patient had manifested the disease for 14 years. The striking tomographic abnormality in our two severely affected patients was the marked reduction of glucose consumption in the pericentral regions of the cortex. The whole length of the central sulcus was equally involved. Because the method of image reconstruction and display used in our studies does not distort the picture it is possible to calculate that the width of the swath of reduced cortical glucose consumption is approximately 4 cm. This is wider than the strip of precentral cortex usually assigned to the primary motor area and probably includes the post-central gyrus as well. If the reduction in glucose consumption that we observed is due to loss of cells that directly subserve a motor function it is perhaps not surprising to find that a broad band around the central sulcus is abnormal. Penfield and Rasmussen [10], using direct cortical stimulation at craniotomy, found that the primary motor area seemed to coincide with Vogts' cytological field 4 and with subordinate motor areas in the post-central gyrus as well as in the remainder of the precentral gyrus (area 6a, beta). Beal and Richardson [11] examined the brain of a 66-year-old woman who died from bronchopnuemonia after having suffered from primary lateral sclerosis for approximately 3 years. They sectioned the pre- and post-central gyri bilaterally. Superiorly there was a minimal loss of neurones but in sections from the arm and face regions of the pre-central gyri there was complete loss of Betz cells in cortical layer 5 and decreased numbers of pyramidal neurons in layers 3 and 5. The loss of neurons was accompanied by marked gliosis. Unfortunately there is no comment on the cells of the post-central gyri or any other cortical regions.

Mata et al [5], using the autoradiographic method for ^{14}C-deoxy-glucose developed by Sokoloff, concluded that local cerebral glucose consumption was largely due to metabolic activity in the dendrites and synapses. In the motor cortex, typified by its agranular appearance, layer 5 contains a variety of pyramidal cells, among them the giant pyramids of Betz. As already mentioned, these cells are, eventually, completely lost in PLS. However, in the precentral cortex they only number a few tens of thousands and, overall, these cells only contribute 3–4% of the fibres in the pyramid [12]. The 50% reduction in cortical glucose consumption therefore cannot be explained merely by the loss of Betz cells. Loss of the other more numerous pyramidal cells and their interconnections is much more likely to account for the fall in glucose consumption in the pericentral regions.

The reduction in glucose consumption in the superior parietal region abutting the central sulcus was unexpected. It occurred in Brodmann areas 5 and 7. Like the pericentral reduction of glucose utilization, it was only seen in the two most severely affected patients suffering from primary lateral sclerosis. Areas 5 and 7 receive association fibres from somatic sensory region SmI, and are concerned in controlling movements in relation to visual targets [13] as well as with the motor functions of the face [14]. Our findings may mean that cells in these association areas are lost in primary lateral sclerosis or that in man there is major projection from the primary sensorimotor cortex to area 7. The MRI finding of cortical atrophy in the superior parietal regions of patient 1 supports the first interpretation.

Reduced glucose consumption in the striatum and thalamus is probably a consequence of loss of afferent input from the cortex. Both central grey structures receive input from the motor cortex; in the case of striatum to putamen and in the case of thalamus to the VL nucleus [15]. Neurons need not be lost from a region to explain its reduced glucose consumption. For example, the accumulation of ^{18}FDG in the visual cortex can be readily reduced by occluding the eyes. However, it should be noted that there was a mild loss of neurons in the posterior part of the putamen of the patient described by Beal and Richardson [11].

Finally, it should be noted that there were no changes in glucose consumption in the pericentral or superior parietal regions of the two patients suffering from amyotrophic lateral sclerosis. Neither of these patients was as motorically incapacitated as those with primary lateral sclerosis although both had major problems due to bulbar and pseudo-bulbar palsies. Patient 5 and patient 1 of the primary lateral sclerosis group, however, did have reduced frontal glucose consumption, compared to age-matched control subjects. This is at variance with an abstract from Dalakas et al [16] that claimed that glucose consumption is reduced by a quarter in all neuronal regions of the cortex in ALS patients with upper motor neuron signs.

In summary three patients suffering from primary lateral sclerosis and two suffering from amyotrophic lateral sclerosis have been examined by positron computerized tomography using [^{18}F]fluoro-2-deoxy-D-glucose. In addition to examining the tomographic sections, individual maps of cortical glucose consumption were generated for each patient by summing the data obtained from all PCT sections.

In the patients suffering from PLS the most striking feature was a 50% reduction in pericentral glucose consumption and a similar loss from the superior parietal regions. These cortical changes were accompanied by a reduction in striatal and thalamic glucose consumption that is probably due to a loss of afferents from the cortex. The reduction in pericentral glucose consumption is probably due to loss of pyramidal neurones and their local connections. The loss of parietal activity, we suggest, is due to loss of association fibres arising in the pericentral region.

References

1 Kuhl DE, Edwards RQ. Image separation radioisotope scanning. Radiology 1963;30:653–661
2 Hounsfield G, Ambrose J, Perry J, et al. Computerized transverse axial scanning. Br J Radiol 1973;46:1016
3 Cormack AM. Reconstruction of densities from their projections, with applications in radiological physics. Phys Med Biol 1973;18:195–207
4 Sokoloff L, Reivich M, Kennedy C, et al. The [^{14}C]deoxyglucose method for the measurement of local cerebral glucose utilization: Theory, procedure and normal values in the conscious and anaesthetized albino rat. J Neurochem 1977;28:897–916
5 Mata M, Fink DJ, Gainer H, et al. Activity dependent energy metabolism in rat posterior pituitary primarily reflects sodium pump activity. J Neurochem 1980;34:213–221

6 Nahmias C, Firnau G, Garnett ES. Performance characteristics of the Mc-Master positron emission tomograph. IEEE Trans 1984;NS-31:637–639

7 Bida GT, Satyamurthy N, Barrio JR. The synthesis of 2-[F-18]fluoro-2-deoxy-D-glucose using glycals: A reexamination. J Nucl Med 1984;25:1327–1334

8 Nahmias C, Loken M, Garnett ES. Display of hemispheric local metabolic rates from human brain. In: Meyer-Ebrecht D, ed. Proc Sixth Aachen Symposium. Heidelberg, Springer Verlag, 1987

9 Sotaniemi KA, Myllayla VV. Primary lateral sclerosis; a debated entity. Acta Neurol Scand 1985;71:334–336

10 Penfield W, Rasmussen T. The Cerebral Cortex of Man. A Clinical Study of Localization of Function. New York, Hafner, 1968;58–59

11 Beal MF, Richardson EP. Primary lateral sclerosis. A case report. Arch Neurol 1981;38:630–633

12 Brodal A. Neurological Anatomy in Relation to Clinical Medicine. Oxford, Oxford University Press, 1981;184

13 Stein J. Effects of parietal lobe cooling on manipulative behaviour in the conscious monkey. In: Gordon G, ed. Active Touch. Oxford, Pergamon Press, 1978;79–90

14 Leinonen L, Nyman G. Functional properties of cells in antero-lateral part of area 7 associative face area of awake monkeys. Exp Brain Res 1979;34:321–333

15 Carpenter MB, Sutin J. Human neuroanatomy. Baltimore, Williams & Wilkins, 1983;519–587

16 Dalakas M, DiChiro G, Hatazawa, Brooks R. Metabolic status of cortical neurons in patients with motor neuron disease (MND): A study with positron emission tomography (PET). Neurology 1986;36:138

Index